Handbook on Neurovascular Ultrasound

Frontiers of Neurology and Neuroscience

Vol. 21

Series Editor

J. Bogousslavsky *Lausanne*

KARGER

Handbook on Neurovascular Ultrasound

Volume Editor

R.W. Baumgartner *Zürich*

74 figures, 42 in color, and 26 tables, 2006

KARGER

Basel · Freiburg · Paris · London · New York ·
Bangalore · Bangkok · Singapore · Tokyo · Sydney

Prof. Dr. Ralf W. Baumgartner
Department of Neurology
University Hospital
Frauenklinikstrasse 26
CH–8091 Zürich (Switzerland)

Library of Congress Cataloging-in-Publication Data

Handbook on neurovascular ultrasound / volume editor, R.W. Baumgartner.
p. ; cm. – (Frontiers of neurology and neuroscience ; v. 21)
Includes bibliographical references and index.
ISBN 3-8055-8022-3 (hard cover : alk. paper)
1. Cerebovascular disease–Ultrasonic imaging.
[DNLM: 1. Cerebrovascular Disorders–ultrasonography. 2.
Ultrasonography, Doppler–methods. WL 355 H2368 2006] I. Baumgartner, R.
W. (Ralf W.) II. Series.
RC388.5.H3455 2006
616.8′047543–dc22

2006004152

Bibliographic Indices. This publication is listed in bibliographic services, including Current Contents® and Index Medicus.

www.karger.com
Printed in Switzerland on acid-free paper by Reinhardt Druck, Basel
ISSN 1660–4431
ISBN 3–8055–8022–3

Contents

Preface

This volume of *Frontiers of Neurology and Neuroscience* is devoted to neurovascular ultrasound, which has shown fascinating developments in the last years. Written by international experts it reviews the present knowledge and presents research topics of diagnostic and therapeutic neurovascular ultrasound.

The first chapter gives an overview about physical and technical principles of ultrasound. Then, arterial wall imaging, endothelial function testing and modern assessment of atherosclerotic obstruction of the carotid and vertebro-basilar systems are described. Subsequently, typical ultrasound findings in cervical artery dissection, dural fistula, glomus tumor and vasculitis are reported. The next chapters describe diagnostic and therapeutic transcranial ultrasound and clinical applications of transcranial Doppler monitoring, and in the last chapter future developments are presented.

I hope that this volume will be useful in the daily work and stimulate sonographers to use this fascinating and essentially non-invasive technique, which allows the real-time assessment of the human cerebral vessels.

Ralf W. Baumgartner

Baumgartner RW (ed): Handbook on Neurovascular Ultrasound.
Front Neurol Neurosci. Basel, Karger, 2006, vol 21, pp 1–18

Physical and Technical Principles

David H. Evans

Department of Cardiovascular Sciences, University of Leicester, Leicester, UK

Abstract

Ultrasound is an important technique for studying neurovascular pathology. As with any measurement or imaging technique, it has strengths and weaknesses, and there are a number of potential pitfalls for those interpreting its results. This chapter describes the basic physics and instrumentation behind both imaging and Doppler ultrasound techniques, with a special emphasis on their application to the cerebral circulation. The nature of ultrasound propagation in tissue is described, and the speed of ultrasound, its attenuation, and its behaviour at boundaries of various types are discussed. A description of pulse–echo B-mode techniques includes a section on transducers and artefacts. Doppler ultrasound is particularly important in the study of blood flow, and embolus detection, and its basic principles and various instrument types are described. The uses of transcranial Doppler for the measurement of velocity, flow changes, cerebrovascular resistance, and embolus detection are described. Finally the safety of ultrasound techniques in the context of cerebral vessels and in particularly transcranial Doppler is discussed.

Medical ultrasound is used to image the body in much the same way as radar is used to detect the range (and often speed) of an aircraft, except that instead of using radio waves, pulses of high-frequency sound (usually in the region of 2–15 MHz or about a thousand times higher than audible sound) are used. A transducer sends a very short pulse of ultrasound (often lasting much less than one-millionth of a second) into the body, and then gathers any reflected sound returning from the body. Once a sufficient time has elapsed for all the reflections to return from the tissue of interest, another pulse is emitted in a slightly different direction and the sequence repeated. The position of any structure producing a reflection can be calculated from the direction in which the pulse has been transmitted, and from the delay between the transmission of the pulse and the reception of the reflection, which is proportional to the distance to the structure. Further information about the characteristics of the structure can be determined from the size of the echo and information about the velocity of the structure relative to the transducer (particularly important for echoes from blood) can be extracted from slight changes in the ultrasound frequency (the so-called Doppler effect). Ultrasound is an ideal technique for imaging soft tissues, but cannot penetrate gas, and is distorted and rapidly attenuated by bone. One of its distinctive properties is its superb temporal resolution – it is possible to acquire many tens of new images every second so that it is possible to record the movement of structures such as the heart or arteries in great detail. Furthermore with Doppler colour flow imaging it is possible to observe blood flow patterns, and their relationship to vascular anatomy.

The Nature of Ultrasound and Propagation in Tissue

Ultrasound is generally taken to mean any sound that has a frequency above the limit of human hearing (about 20 kHz or 20,000 cycles/s). In medical diagnostic applications, however, the frequencies used are approximately 100–1,000 times higher than this, i.e., in the range of 2 MHz (2 million cycles/s) to 20 MHz. The reason for this higher range in frequency is that spatial resolution is limited by the wavelength, which is inversely related to the frequency. Ultrasonic waves in soft tissue, like audible sound waves, are compressional waves produced by the push–pull action of the source on the propagating media. These waves are also known as 'longitudinal' waves, since the oscillatory motion of the particles in the tissue is parallel to the direction of propagation. Other modes of vibration such as 'shear' or 'transverse' waves can occur in bone, but are not usually of great importance.

Speed of Ultrasound in Tissue

The speed of sound in tissue is important for many reasons. It must be known in order to convert the time delay between the transmission of a pulse and the subsequent reception of echoes into physical distances, it determines the maximum rate at which pulses can be transmitted (it is usually necessary to wait until all the relevant echoes from one pulse return to the transducer before transmitting another), it determines the wavelength of the ultrasound (and hence resolution), it determines the amount of refraction that takes place at tissue interfaces, and it is needed to convert Doppler shift frequencies into tissue velocities. The speed of sound in tissue depends on the elastic properties and density of the tissue, and in general, the less compressible the tissue the higher the speed of sound, so that, sound propagates much more quickly through a bone than through a soft tissue. Table 1 gives approximate values for the speed of sound in some relevant tissues. The important thing to be noted from this table is that, with the exception of air

Table 1. Speed of sound and acoustic impedance of some common biological materials

Material	Speed (m/s)	Acoustic impedance (rayls)
Air	330	0.0004×10^6
Aqueous humour	1,500	1.50×10^6
Blood	1,570	1.61×10^6
Bone	3,500	7.80×10^6
Brain	1,540	1.58×10^6
CSF	1,510	–
Fat	1,450	1.38×10^6
Lens of eye	1,620	1.84×10^6
Muscle	1,580	1.70×10^6
Skin	1,600	–
Soft tissue average	1,540	1.63×10^6
Vitreous humour	1,520	1.52×10^6

and bone, all the values are very similar, at around 1,540 ms^{-1}. The value for air is much lower, but since ultrasound does not propagate through air this is of little significance; the value for bone is much higher which is of some relevance when performing transcranial examinations. Taking the value of 1,540 ms^{-1} as representative, it is easy to calculate that it takes pulses of ultrasound approximately 6.5 μs to travel 1 cm, and therefore to convert the delay between the transmission of a pulse and the reception of an echo into a depth (remembering that it will take 13 μs for a round trip of 1 cm). Of course ultrasound scanners do this automatically, but it should be noted that a scanner has no way of determining what tissues the pulse has travelled through, and must use the same conversion factor for all acoustic paths. Because, the speed of sound is much higher in bone than soft tissue the apparent thickness of bone will be less than half its actual thickness. This may not matter when making transcranial measurements on the brain through a relatively small aperture because it may simply mean the entire image is shifted, but where there are significant variations in the thickness of bone underlying the transducer it can obviously introduce undesirable distortions into the image of the brain. Knowing the speed of ultrasound enables us to calculate the wavelength (given by sound speed divided by frequency) which gives us an idea of the best spatial resolution available from the technique, and in soft tissue it will be approximately 0.77 mm at 2 MHz and 0.1 mm at 15 MHz.

Attenuation of Ultrasound by Tissue

As ultrasound propagates through tissue it is attenuated; that is to say the energy in the beam is reduced. This happens through two main mechanisms, i.e.

Table 2. Attenuation coefficients for some biological materials at 1 MHz. The values at a higher frequency may be obtained approximately by multiplying by the frequency in MHz. (Note however that for water the value should be multiplied by the square of frequency.)

Material	Attenuation coefficient (dB cm^{-1})
Blood	0.2
Bone	10
Brain (adult)	0.8
Brain (infant)	0.3
Fat	0.6
Muscle	1.5
Water	0.002
Soft tissue average	0.7

absorption and scattering. Absorption is the conversion of the mechanical energy in the beam into heat (which will cause a temperature rise in the tissue – see section on ultrasound safety), whilst scattering is the process by which energy is redirected out of the beam. In most soft tissues, the most important mechanism that takes place is absorption, but in blood, scattering dominates. Attenuation varies from tissue to tissue, and is strongly frequency dependent. It is usually measured in decibels (dB), and may be written as

$$\text{Attenuation (dB)} = -10 \log_{10} (I_x/I_0) \tag{1}$$

where I_0 is the initial intensity and I_x is the final intensity. Thus if the final intensity is one-tenth of the initial intensity, the attenuation is said to be -10 dB, likewise reductions in intensity to one-hundredth and one-thousandth of the initial intensity would be written as -20 dB and -30 dB, respectively. Typical values of attenuation in some biological materials are given in table 2. Note that with the exception of water, the attenuation coefficients for higher frequencies may be obtained approximately by multiplying the attenuation at 1 MHz by the frequency in MHz. For example, the attenuation in soft tissue at 2 MHz would be 1.4 dB cm^{-1}, and at 10 MHz would be 7 dB cm^{-1}. The strong frequency dependency of attenuation is the factor that limits the highest frequency that can be used in any particular situation (ideally we would always use the highest frequency possible because the shorter the wavelength, the better the spatial resolution). The higher the attenuation coefficient, the higher the frequency, and the deeper the target, then the smaller will be the return echoes. We are able to obtain extremely high-resolution images of arteries like the extra-cranial carotid arteries because they are relatively superficial and the overlying tissue has a relatively low-attenuation coefficient, the same is not true for deep

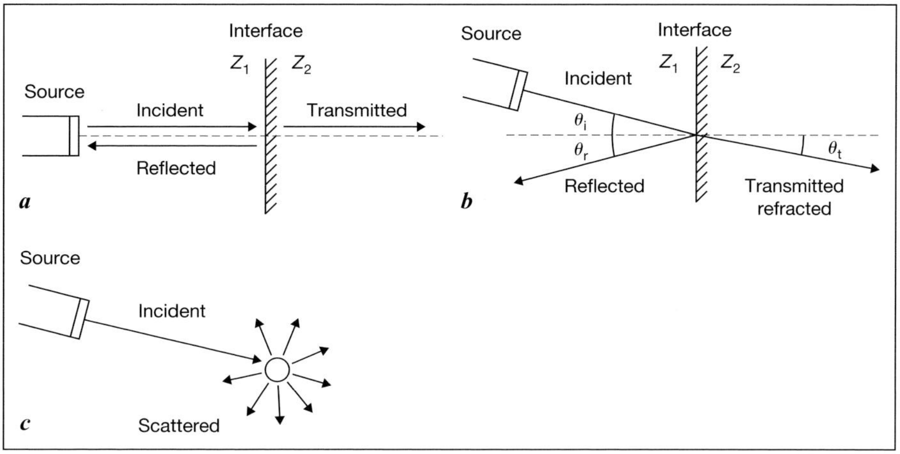

Fig. 1. ***a*** Reflection of ultrasound at a plane boundary (perpendicular incidence). ***b*** Reflection and refraction of ultrasound at a plane boundary (nonperpendicular incidence). ***c*** Scattering of ultrasound by a target with dimensions smaller or comparable to the ultrasound wavelength.

vessels. The rapid attenuation of ultrasound by bone means that if we wish to insonate through the skull then we have to use relatively low-ultrasound frequencies. (Note however, that the poor resolution we obtain when imaging the brain is both a result of using a low frequency and of the distortion of the ultrasound beam by the skull bone, see next section.)

Ultrasound Behaviour at Acoustic Boundaries

Ultrasonic imaging is reliant on variations in the acoustic properties of tissues to generate the echoes that reveal the range and direction a myriad of 'targets'. The behaviour of sound when it encounters a change in acoustic properties depends on the relative dimensions of the ultrasound wavelength and the target in its path. If the target is small compared with the wavelength (such as might be the case with a red blood cell or the inhomogeneities in the parenchyma of an organ) then the wave is said to be scattered. If the target is large (such as might be the case at the interface between two organs) then the wave is said to be reflected or refracted. Both types of behaviour are important in ultrasonic scanning. In the case of scattering the incident energy is re-transmitted in all directions (though not necessarily equally) whilst in the case of reflection and refraction the incident energy remains confined to a well-defined reflected and transmitted beam.

Figure 1a and b illustrate the behaviour of ultrasound at a plain boundary for perpendicular and nonperpendicular incidence, respectively. In the first case, a proportion of the ultrasound is reflected directly back to the source (the angle of incidence and reflection are both equal to zero) and a proportion continues along the original path. In the second case the angle of incidence and reflection are also equal, but not to zero, and therefore the reflected wave does not return to the transducer (that is why it is much more difficult to image large surfaces, which are not perpendicular to the ultrasound beam). In the second case there is also a transmitted wave, but its direction depends both on the angle of incidence and the relative speeds of ultrasound on either side of the boundary. The relationship between the angle of the incident wave θ_i and the transmitted wave θ_t is given by

$$\frac{\sin \theta_i}{\sin \theta_t} = \frac{c_1}{c_2} \tag{2}$$

where c_1 is the speed of sound before the boundary and c_2 is the speed of sound after the boundary. If the speeds of sound on either side of the boundary are similar, the direction of propagation changes very little, but if they are dissimilar then the direction may change significantly (i.e., it is said to be refracted). Refraction effects are particularly important at interfaces between soft tissue and bone (recall the speed of sound in bone is 2–3 times higher than in soft tissue) and can lead to considerable distortion as an ultrasound beam propagates through the skull. The proportion of energy transmitted and reflected at a boundary depends on the difference in the acoustic impedance on the two sides of the boundary and for normal incidence may be written as

$$\alpha_t = \frac{I_t}{I_i} = \frac{4Z_1Z_2}{(Z_1 + Z_2)^2} \tag{3a}$$

and

$$\alpha_r = \frac{I_r}{I_i} = \left(\frac{Z_2 - Z_1}{Z_2 + Z_1}\right)^2 \tag{3b}$$

respectively, where I_i, I_t, and I_r, are the incident, transmitted, and reflected intensities, and Z_1 and Z_2 are the acoustic impedance of the tissue before and after the boundary. If Z_1 and Z_2 are similar then most of the energy is transmitted, and little is reflected, if Z_1 and Z_2 are very dissimilar then the converse is true. Values of acoustic impedance for some relevant tissues are given in table 1. It can be seen that the values for most soft tissues are very similar, but that air has a very low value and bone has a relatively high value. The result of this is that the percentage of energy reflected at soft tissue interfaces is of the order of 1%, but that at soft tissue/bone interfaces, approximately 50% of the energy is reflected. The impedance of air is so low that effectively no transmission takes place at a soft tissue/air interface. The low-acoustic impedance of air is the main reason why it is impossible to image through air and why it is essential to exclude air from the interface between the transducer and the skin surface (the other reason is that the attenuation of ultrasound in the megaHertz region by gas is extremely high).

Figure 1c illustrates the phenomenon of scattering. Scattering is an important phenomenon because it is the process that allows us to image the parenchyma of organs and to image blood flow. The scattering pattern and the amount of scattering that occurs at a target depend on the size of the target, and the distribution of compressibility and density in the target volume. For targets that are very much smaller than the ultrasound wavelength, the wave is scattered more or less uniformly in all directions, whilst for larger targets the scattering pattern is more complex but still takes place over a wide range of angles. For very small targets, such as red blood cells, the scattering phenomenon is called Rayleigh scattering, and is proportional to the fourth power of frequency and the sixth power of the radius of the scatterer; for larger targets the scattered power still increases with frequency but less rapidly so. It should be noted that the power returned to the ultrasound transducer by scattering is much less than that returned by specular reflectors, but is also much less angle dependent. Therefore echoes from the internal structure of organs and from blood are much weaker than those from distinct boundaries, but do not change significantly as the angle of insonation changes.

Pulse-Echo Principles (B-Mode Techniques)

The basic principle behind B-scanning has been described earlier in this chapter. A B-mode display is essentially a cross-sectional image of the tissue in the scan plane, built up using an echo-ranging technique. A transducer transmits a short-ultrasound pulse into the tissue in a predetermined direction, and then switches to receive mode, and gathers echoes due to reflection or scattering in the tissue from that same direction. Since the direction of transmission and reception and the time delay between pulse transmission and echo reception are known, the position of any structure producing an echo can be determined. The size of each of the echoes provides information about the amount of ultrasound that is reflected or back-scattered by the structure (although it is necessary to compensate for the attenuation of the pulse by intervening tissue). Once all the echoes have been received from depths of interest then another pulse is transmitted along a slightly different path and then the whole process is repeated until the required plane, perpendicular to the transducer face, has been interrogated. The rate at which pulses can be transmitted (the pulse repetition frequency or PRF) is limited by the speed of ultrasound in the tissue, and the maximum depth of interest, so, if it is required to image to a depth of 10 cm, it will be necessary to wait 13 μs × 10, i.e., 130 μs, before another pulse is transmitted. This means that in this case it is possible to transmit pulses at a rate of approximately 7.7 kHz without introducing range ambiguity. If then, it is required to update the image at a rate of 25 frames/s, it is possible to interrogate the tissue in approximately 300 different directions. The limitations on image formation due to the finite speed of sound are not likely to be of much significance in neurovascular B-scanning, but as will be seen later may be a limitation in colour flow mapping. Clearly considerable processing by the ultrasound scanner is necessary to produce acceptable images from the simple echo information described above, and the interested reader is referred to the recommended reading list for further information.

Transducers

At one time the method used for scanning the ultrasound beam through tissue involved physical movements within the transducer. Now, all transducers for B-scan imaging are array transducers where the beam is steered electronically. There are two basic types of arrays, i.e. linear arrays and phased arrays, both of which contain a large number of very small piezo-electric elements capable of transmitting and receiving ultrasound.

In linear arrays, each beam is generated using only a limited number of adjacent array elements at any one time. Each successive beam is generated by selecting another group of elements, so if the first beam is generated using elements 1–8 then the second beam might be generated using elements 2–9, and so on. Thus the beam steps along the array. Linear array transducers produce rectangular or parallelogram shaped fields where all the scan lines are parallel to each other and are the transducers of choice for imaging the extra-cranial carotid arteries.

In phased arrays, each beam is generated using most or even all of the elements at the same time. Each successive beam is generated by steering the direction of transmission and reception by appropriate phasing of the signals applied to the transducer elements. Phased arrays produce sector shaped fields where the scan lines are not parallel to each other and are the transducers of choice for intracranial imaging because their small foot-print, which allows them to be used with the limited acoustic windows available in the skull.

Modern ultrasound systems not only move the beam electronically, but dynamically vary their aperture (the number of elements used) and apodization (relative weighting of the contribution of different elements), and also use electronic focussing on both transmit (multiple zone focussing) and receive (dynamic focussing) to achieve excellent lateral resolution in the scan plane.

Some modern transducers also use more than one row of elements to improve the focussing in the elevation plane (i.e., the out of plain dimension or the slice thickness).

Artefacts

It is important that users of ultrasound instruments are aware of the many image artefacts that can arise. Two of the most important one are described briefly in the following sections.

Speed of Sound and Beam Deviation Artefacts

To generate ultrasound images, it is necessary to assume that the beam has followed a straight path through the tissue, and that the speed of sound in the tissue is constant and known. Anything that invalidates these assumptions will lead to misregistration of targets. Beam direction may be changed either by refraction effects (i.e., where the beam meets a boundary between two tissues with different ultrasound velocities at non-normal incidence) or by very strong specular reflectors that are not at right-angles to the beam. Deviations from the assumed velocity of sound will make targets to appear closer or farther away than they should. If the tissue with the higher or lower velocity is a parallel-sided layer then all the structures behind the layer will be moved so as to appear closer or farther from the transducer, which may not matter. On the other hand if the layer is not parallel-sided or is incomplete, then some parts of the structure behind the layer will be moved more than others, so that a straight boundary might appear ragged.

Shadowing and Flaring Artefacts

Attenuation of ultrasound in bodily tissues is very significant so that echoes returning from deep structures are always very much smaller than those returning from similar superficial structures. In order to overcome this, ultrasound instruments employ what is known as time-gain compensation (TGC) to the returning echoes, so that echoes from deeper structures are amplified more than those from superficial structures. In order to do this, the instrument needs to assume an average rate of attenuation in the tissue so that it can calculate the appropriate gain to apply to echoes from each depth. Shadowing and flaring artefacts occur when the attenuation is either underestimated or overestimated, respectively. One common example of shadowing occurs behind an atheromatous plaque in the carotid artery, where the plaque attenuates the ultrasound much more rapidly than soft tissue, and so the TGC does not adequately compensate for the reduction in the size of the echoes returning from behind the plaque. The converse effect can be seen when there is a cyst in the tissue. The fluid in the cyst does not attenuate ultrasound as rapidly as soft tissue, but the TGC continues to increase gain with depth as though there is soft tissue present. The result of this is that the echoes from behind the cyst are amplified more than is appropriate, and the region behind the cyst appears to be very highly reflecting. Although these are artefacts, they do in fact convey diagnostic information, in that they reveal the presence of tissue with an unexpectedly high- or low-attenuation values.

Doppler Principles

If an observer is stationary relative to a source of waves, then the frequency the observer measures is the same as the frequency transmitted. If, however, the observer is moving towards or away from the source of waves, then a greater or lesser number of wave fronts will pass the observer in a given time interval, and so the observer will measure a higher or lower frequency than that which was transmitted. This effect is known as the Doppler effect after the Austrian physicist, Christian Doppler, who first described the phenomenon in 1842. In medical ultrasound the targets do not emit spontaneously, and therefore to make use of this effect it is necessary to transmit ultrasound into the body, and to observe the change of frequency as the wave is reflected or scattered from the target. Under these conditions it can be shown that the 'Doppler frequency', f_d, i.e., the difference between the transmitted frequency f_t and the received frequency f_r, is given by

$$f_d = f_t - f_r = 2 f_t v \cos\theta / c \qquad (4)$$

where v is the velocity of the target, c is the speed of sound in tissue, and θ is the angle between the ultrasound beam and the direction of motion of the target. The speed of sound and the transmitted frequency are known in any situation and therefore the velocity of a target can be found from the following equation:

$$v = K f_d \cos\theta \qquad (5)$$

where K is a known constant ($c/2f_t$). This equation may be used to monitor changes in velocity and if the angle θ can be determined then absolute velocity may be calculated. In practice, where blood flow is concerned, there will be many targets in the Doppler sample volume with a range of velocities, and so the Doppler shift signal will contain a spectrum of frequencies. Figure 2 shows the spectral display (usually called a sonogram) of the Doppler signal recorded from an internal carotid artery. The horizontal axis represents time, the vertical axis represents the Doppler shift frequency, and the grey-level of each pixel represents the power of the Doppler signal at the corresponding frequency and time.

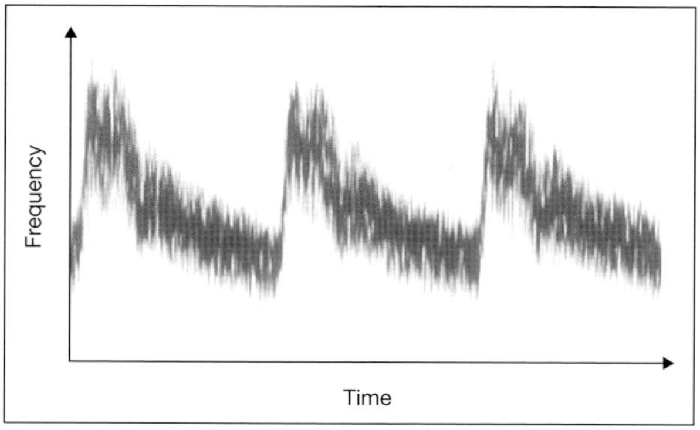

Fig. 2. Sonogram of the Doppler signal from a normal internal carotid artery. The horizontal axis represents time, the vertical axis represents Doppler shift frequency (or velocity), and the grey scale represents the power of the Doppler shift frequency at the corresponding time and frequency. The three complete cardiac cycles are shown.

Under 'ideal' conditions the spectrum of Doppler frequencies at any moment in time would correspond to the distribution of velocities in the sample volume, but there are a number of factors which distort the spectrum and limit the accuracy with which the velocity distribution can be determined. (Note also that the shape of the sample volume itself will mean that the flow within a vessel is unlikely to be sampled uniformly, and therefore the distribution of velocities in the sample volume may not exactly correspond to the distribution of velocities in the vessel as a whole.) The reader is referred to [1] for an in depth discussion of these effects but the effect of 'wall-thump' filters is briefly described here, because of its importance. As already mentioned, the signals reflected by structures such as blood vessel walls are orders of magnitude greater than those scattered by blood, and therefore it is necessary to reject such signals if we wish to study the motion of the blood. This is possible because in general such solid structures move with much lower velocities than those of blood flow, and therefore these signals can be rejected using a high-pass (wall-thump) filter. Whilst this can be quite effective, the filter will also reject the signals from slowly moving blood. This means that blood flow close to a vessel wall cannot be studied, and that the mean blood flow velocity in a vessel tends to be slightly overestimated, but is not usually a major problem as long as the operator is aware of the effect.

Pulsed-Wave Doppler

The earliest Doppler ultrasound devices were continuous wave devices (that is to say they both transmitted and received ultrasound continuously) but such devices had little or no range resolution. Because in general it is important to be able to select signals from a particular depth, nowadays, nearly all ultrasound Doppler instruments use pulsed transmission. Pulses of ultrasound are transmitted at regular intervals, and after a fixed (but controllable) delay a receive gate attached to the transducer opens for a brief period of time and allows signals from a pre-determined range of depths to be collected for Doppler processing. The delay between pulse transmission and the opening of the receive gate determines the depth from which signal samples are collected, and the time for which the receive gate is open in combination with the transmitted pulse length determine the sample volume length. It is common for the transmitted pulse length and the receive gate opening time to be similar (this leads to an optimum signal-to-noise ratio) in which case the sample volume sensitivity has a triangular shape in the axial direction, such that the maximum sensitivity occurs in the middle of the sample volume and falls both towards and away from the transducer.

Pulsed-wave (PW) ultrasound systems actually operate by measuring the rate of change of phase of the returning ultrasound pulses rather than the Doppler shift frequency per se (the reasons for this are beyond the scope of this discussion and make little or no difference to the 'Doppler shift' actually measured) and because of this are subject to the effects of aliasing. Aliasing is the phenomenon that occurs when a moving object is not sampled sufficiently rapidly to be able to reconstruct its true movement. If a Doppler signal is to be correctly interpreted, then the rate at which it is sampled (i.e., the PRF) must be at least twice the maximum frequency component of the Doppler signal (with certain caveats). Failure to respect this limit can lead to artefacts such as rapid forward flow being interpreted as reverse flow. The obvious way to avoid this problem is to increase the PRF, but as we have already seen this is limited by the fact that if we wish to avoid range ambiguity we must collect all the returning echoes of interest before transmitting a further pulse. It can be shown that there is a maximum range-velocity product limit given by

$$z_{\text{max}} v_{\text{max}} = c^2/8 f_{\text{t}} \cos\theta \tag{6}$$

where z_{max} is the maximum range a PW system can gather echoes from unambiguously and v_{max} is the maximum velocity that can be unambiguously measured. Therefore, it is possible to measure high velocities in superficial structures correctly and low velocities in deep structures correctly, but not high velocities in deep structures. This limit is particularly troublesome in cardiac work where there may be very high velocities through stenosed heart valves, but it is possible to encounter aliasing in more superficial structures such as stenosed carotid arteries. Equation (6) reveals that one of the ways to avoid aliasing is to use a lower transmitted ultrasound frequency, and this is one of the reasons why Doppler studies are often performed at slightly lower frequencies than imaging studies.

Duplex Scanning

Duplex scanners are scanners that combine B-mode imaging with PW Doppler measurements. The B-scan image is used to guide the Doppler beam and to place a Doppler sample volume in a region of interest. Since blood vessels may be imaged, the Doppler angle, θ, can also be measured (by assuming that the blood flow is parallel to the vessel wall) and therefore the Doppler shift frequency can be calibrated in terms of blood flow velocity. Also where the blood vessels are relatively large, their diameters can be measured, and converted to a cross-sectional area, thus allowing blood flow velocity to be converted into volumetric blood flow. It is important to realise, however, that there are many potential errors in this process, and the reader is referred to [1] for an in depth discussion of volumetric blood flow measurements using Doppler ultrasound.

Colour Flow Imaging

Colour flow imaging (CFI) systems are similar to pulse–echo B-mode systems, except that both the amplitude and the 'Doppler shift' on the returning echoes are measured. Where no Doppler shift is detected the usual grey-scale information is written to the display device, but where a Doppler shift is detected, it is colour-coded to show the measured relative velocity between the transducer and the detected target. Usually the flow towards the transducer will be coded in one colour (often red), and the flow away from the transducer in another colour (usually blue).

CFI is an extremely good technique for imaging anatomy and related blood flow, but it has a number of limitations that the operator must bear in mind. First and foremost it must be remembered that equation (4) is equally applicable to CFI as to ordinary PW Doppler; in other words the Doppler angle, θ, will dramatically affect the measured Doppler shift, and therefore flow with the same speed in different parts of the image may be represented by different shades of colour, or even completely different colours, depending on the component of their velocity relative to the transducer. Also CFI, just as ordinary PW Doppler, is susceptible to aliasing, and it is important to differentiate between regions of reverse flow in a vessel and regions of aliasing, both of which lead to a change in the displayed flow direction (it is usually possible to make this distinction by examining the boundary between the colours representing different flow directions). Frame rates in CFI are significantly lower than in standard B-mode imaging because in order to detect and quantify a Doppler shift it is necessary to interrogate a sample volume several times (typically between 8 and 16) and this is the reason why the so-called 'colour box' (where colour information is displayed) is often significantly smaller than the total area of the scan. Finally, colour flow estimates of velocity, are based on a relatively small number of samples when compared with PW Doppler, and so their velocity resolution is much lower. CFI is an excellent way to gain an impression of the overall haemodynamics in a region of the body, but if quantitative measurements are to be made, CFI should be used to identify a region of interest, and PW Doppler used to make the measurements.

Power Doppler Imaging

An alternative to coding and displaying the Doppler shift frequency measured from each sample volume is to measure and display the total Doppler power, which is determined mainly by the volume of moving blood rather than its velocity. Thus changes in angle and even aliasing do not alter the colour coding – indeed because of a mechanism known as intrinsic spectral broadening it is even possible to image flow perpendicular to the transducer face, which is not possible with ordinary CFI. The result is that images of tortuous vessel can often be more complete and easier to understand. Power Doppler imaging (PDI) can also be more sensitive to flow in networks of small vessels. PDI also has disadvantages in that it is particularly susceptible to movement artefacts, and it must not be forgotten that its apparent advantages are gained at the expense of suppressing all information about velocity, which clearly can contain diagnostic information.

Transcranial Doppler Ultrasound

Transcranial Doppler ultrasound (TCD) is simply the application of Doppler ultrasound techniques through the intact skull. Where imaging techniques are involved, such techniques are usually called transcranial colour coded sonography (TCCS). In general the skull bone is too thick to penetrate with ultrasound, but there are a number of 'acoustic windows' where there is a natural foramina, or the bone is sufficiently thin for a significant percentage of ultrasound energy to penetrate. The most commonly used window is the temporal bone window, which allows insonation of the middle, anterior, and posterior cerebral arteries. The foramen magnum window (or sub-occipital approach) allows insonation of the basilar and vertebral arteries, and the orbital approach allows insonation of the ophthalmic arteries and the internal carotid siphon. TCD techniques not only have many similarities to ordinary pulsed Doppler techniques but also differ in a number of ways. In order to penetrate the skull it is necessary to use very low-transmitted frequencies (recall that attenuation increases with frequency) and most simple TCD examinations are performed with 2 MHz ultrasound or thereabouts, and in some applications even lower frequencies are used. Low frequencies generate much lower levels of scattering from blood (an advantage when monitoring for emboli since small signals from small emboli are less likely to be masked by the blood flow signal, but a disadvantage if it is the blood flow itself that is to be studied). Low frequencies also give poor spatial resolution, but the major contribution to poor spatial resolution in transcranial studies is the distortion of the ultrasound beam by the skull.

TCD – Velocity Measurement

The method used to estimate blood flow velocity in TCD applications is different from that used elsewhere in the body. The standard method is to average the instantaneous intensity weighted mean velocity over the cardiac cycle, but in TCD it is the instantaneous maximum velocity that is usually averaged. The reason for this is that it is easier to extract a good maximum frequency envelope than a good mean envelope when the signal-to-noise ratio is poor. Fortunately, because of the type of flow found in cerebral vessels, the mean of the maximum over the cardiac cycle is more or less proportional to the true mean, and the constant of proportionality is approximately two. In other words the true mean velocity is half the figure usually quoted as 'mean velocity'. It is vital when reporting TCD velocity measurements that investigators explain exactly which velocity they have calculated. Another particular issue with TCD velocity measurements is that they are usually made blind, and the Doppler angle, θ, assumed. Although this may be valid for some patients, in others it can introduce significant errors which must be recognised if absolute velocity values are of interest.

TCD – Flow Changes

In most arteries in the body it is reasonable to assume that, in the short term at least, changes in blood flow velocity are proportional to changes in flow. This is not necessarily a valid assumption in TCD as there is evidence that even the major arteries exhibit considerable vasoactivity. Certainly arterial spasm leads to dramatic increases in blood flow velocity that are not representative of changes in flow, and other stimuli are thought to affect cerebral arterial diameter. It is vital that this fact is borne in mind when interpreting velocity changes in TCD. Unfortunately cerebral vessels are too small to have their diameters accurately measured by ultrasound, but attempts have been made to monitor changes in diameter by measuring changes in the total amount of power backscattered by the moving blood within the sample volume. This technique can only be partially successful because it relies on uniform insonation of the blood vessel, which cannot be achieved due to the distortion of the ultrasound beam by the skull bone.

TCD – Cerebrovascular Resistance

Cerebrovascular resistance (CVR) can be calculated by dividing mean blood pressure by mean blood flow. TCD, however, measures velocity (i.e., flow divided by vessel cross-section). Therefore dividing mean blood pressure by mean blood flow velocity leads to a value of CVR multiplied by vessel cross-section (at the point of ultrasound insonation). This quantity has been called 'resistance–area product' or RAP both to distinguish it from true CVR, and to emphasise that it is also dependent on any changes in the cross-section of the vessel where the measurement is being made.

TCD – Embolus Detection

Embolus detection has become a major application of TCD. The basis of embolus detection is very simple. As an embolus passes through the Doppler sample volume, if its scattering cross-section is sufficiently large, it will give rise to an additional Doppler component that can be heard or seen on the Doppler display. Whether or not an embolus can be detected depends on its size and composition, the ultrasound frequency, the size of the sample volume, the embolus trajectory, and its interaction with the ultrasound beam. In general even relatively small gas bubbles will be detected, but some larger solid emboli may not. Several techniques have been proposed for distinguishing between different types of emboli, and whilst some progress has been made towards this goal, there are still significant challenges. Microembolic signals are discussed in a later chapter of this book, and for an in depth discussion of the physics of embolus detection the reader is referred to [2].

Transcranial Colour Coded Sonography

Transcranial Colour Coded Sonography is simply CFI or PDI performed through the cranial bones. As for simple TCD it can only be done through the 'bone windows', must be done at relatively low frequencies to achieve adequate penetration, and is subject to the effects of beam distortion (and therefore image distortion) by the skull.

Ultrasound Safety

No chapter on the physical and technical principles of neurovascular ultrasound would be complete without a mention of ultrasound safety. Diagnostic ultrasound is generally assumed to be perfectly safe, and that even if there are potential hazards, that these are greatly outweighed by the benefits to the patient. It is, however, important to remember that it is impossible to show that any technique is completely safe, and that there are known mechanisms whereby ultrasound can damage tissue (it is after all capable of smashing kidney-stones and 'cooking' liver tumours albeit using very different peak pressures and intensities from those used in diagnosis). There are two broad classes of mechanism by which ultrasound is capable of damaging tissue, the 'thermal effects', and the 'nonthermal effects' which may be further broken down into cavitation, streaming, and other direct effects.

Thermal effects, i.e., heating of the tissue, are related to the conversion of ultrasound energy into heat energy, and hence to the temporal average intensity of the ultrasound beam, and the rate at which it is absorbed by the tissue. Nonthermal effects are related to the peak negative pressure of the ultrasound wave as it propagates through the tissue. It should be noted that these may be independent of each other, as the relationship between average intensity and peak negative pressure depends completely on the pulsing regime selected.

One potential area for caution in neurovascular ultrasound is TCD. There are three reasons for this. Firstly, in order to overcome the rapid attenuation of ultrasound by the skull it is necessary to use relatively high ultrasound intensities, secondly, bone is a rapid absorber of ultrasound, and thirdly, TCD monitoring may last for considerable periods of time (well in excess of an hour) where the same region of tissue is being insonated continuously. All these effects can lead to significant heating of the skull bone, and potentially to secondary heating of brain tissue by conduction from the bone.

There are two indices that are of value in evaluating the potential hazard of ultrasonic examinations, the thermal index (TI) and the mechanical index (MI). The TI is an estimate of the rise in tissue temperature in °C under worse case conditions. The MI is an attempt to indicate the probability of mechanical damage by nonthermal processes. When these indices have a value of 1 or more, the possibility of hazard should be considered. There are in fact three different thermal indices, the soft tissue index (TIS), and bone index (TIB), and most relevant to TCD, the cranial index (TIC), which is the TI that should be used when there is bone at the surface (this is because in this situation the greatest temperature rise occurs in the bone and adjacent tissue). The TIC can be calculated as

$$\mathrm{TIC} = 0.025 W_0 \sqrt{\pi/4A} \qquad (7)$$

where W_0 is the time averaged power at the source (in mW), and A is the active aperture area (in cm^2). Operators of TCD instruments should strive to maintain as low a value of TIC as is compatible with obtaining a good signal, and have clear justification for using unusually high values.

One final area of caution with TCD is in relation to the use of contrast agents, as they significantly lower the threshold for cavitational activity. Clearly it is important with respect to any potential for hazard related to ultrasound, that the operator must do all they can to reduce unnecessary exposure, and to ensure that the benefits to the patient outweigh potential hazards. It is also important that ultrasound practitioners keep up-to-date with the current literature on safety. The European Federation of Societies for Ultrasound in Medicine and Biology (EFSUMB) issue safety statements regularly, and can be found on their web site at www.efsumb.org. Much more in depth discussions of ultrasound safety can be found in [3].

Recent Advances

Improvements in ultrasound images continue unabated as a result of both technological advances and of the introduction of new modalities. There have been important developments in many areas including transducer technology, pulse encoding, harmonic imaging, contrast agents, and 3-D imaging, but this list is certainly not exhaustive.

Conclusion

Ultrasound is a powerful diagnostic technique, which continues to develop at a tremendous pace. It is important that any user of the technique is familiar with the physical and technical principles behind the method, as these provide an insight into its strengths and weaknesses, and sources of possible artefacts.

Further Reading

It is not possible in a single chapter to do more than provide a superficial overview of the physical and technical principles behind the use of ultrasound as a diagnostic technique. The reader is referred to the following references for more in depth information on these aspects of diagnostic ultrasound techniques.

1 Evans DH, McDicken WN: Doppler Ultrasound: Physics, Instrumentation and Signal Processing, ed 2. Chichester, John Wiley & Sons, 2000.

2 Evans DH: Ultrasonic detection of cerebral emboli; in Yuhas DE, Schneider SC (eds): Proceedings of IEEE Ultrasonics Symposium. Piscataway, IEEE, 2003, pp 316–326.

3 ter Haar G, Duck FA (eds): The Safe Use of Ultrasound in Medical Diagnosis. London, British Institute of Radiology, 2000.

4 Hedrick WR, Hykes DL, Starchman DE: Ultrasound Physics and Instrumentation, ed 3. St Louis, Mosby, 1995.

5 Hoskins PR, Thrush A, Martin K, Whittingham TA (eds): Diagnostic Ultrasound: Physics and Equipment. London, GMM, 2003.

6 Zagzebski JA: Essentials of Ultrasound Physics. St Louis, Mosby, 1996.

David H. Evans
Department of Medical Physics
Leicester Royal Infirmary
Leicester LE1 5WW (UK)
Tel. +44 116 2585610, Fax +44 116 2586070, E-Mail dhe@le.ac.uk

Baumgartner RW (ed): Handbook on Neurovascular Ultrasound.
Front Neurol Neurosci. Basel, Karger, 2006, vol 21, pp 19–26

Arterial Wall Imaging

Gérald Devuyst[a], *Bartłomiej Piechowski-Jóźwiak*[a,b], *Julien Bogousslavsky*[a]

[a]Department of Neurology, Centre Hospitalier Universitaire Vaudois, Lausanne, Switzerland; [b]Department of Neurology, The Medical University of Warsaw, Warsaw, Poland

Abstract

Not so long ago atherosclerotic plaque formation was considered to be the consequence of a slow, ongoing process leading to artery stenosis or occlusion. Now it is well recognized that arterial narrowing and occlusion develop rapidly after the rupture of an atherosclerotic plaque. Thus, the assessment of the vulnerability of atheromatous plaques is an important issue in ultrasound of the carotid arteries, and will be discussed in this chapter.

Atherosclerosis is a serious medical and health care problem, as it is one of the major causes of death worldwide. In 2002, there were 16.7 million deaths from cardiovascular disease, including 5.5 million deaths due to stroke, and 7.2 million deaths due to coronary heart disease [1]. Strokes from 80% to 90% are due to ischemia, and 20% to 25% of them are due to large artery disease [2]. Echotomography and spectrum analysis of the Doppler signal was the first method allowing for an in vivo demonstration of carotid wall structures [3]. B-mode sonography is a high resolution, noninvasive, readily available, and easily applicable imaging technique. It allows for visualization of arterial wall structures including the intima-media thickness (IMT), plaque morphology, plaque surface, fibrous cap, and plaque motion. Moreover, color duplex flow imaging (CDFI) and power duplex imaging (PDI) allow to detect carotid stenosis. However, conventional angiography remains the 'gold standard' for diagnosis of carotid stenosis or occlusion. A recent systematic review showed that when referring to digital subtraction angiography (DSA), magnetic resonance angiography (MRA) has a higher specificity and sensitivity than ultrasound (US) in diagnosing carotid stenosis >70%, and both methods are

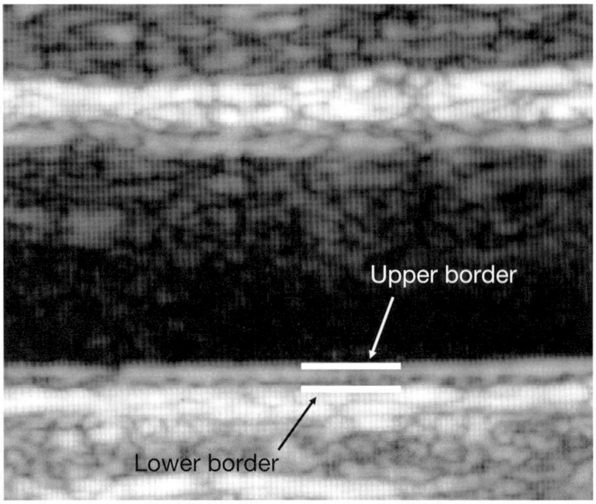

Fig. 1. Intima-media complex.

comparable in detecting carotid occlusion. The sensitivity for detecting severe carotid stenosis was 86% (95% CI, 84–89%), and the specificity was 87% (84–90%) [4]. Using US contrast agents the accuracy of detecting the carotid stenosis may improve in selected cases [5]. Although bearing some disadvantages, carotid US is a useful diagnostic tool in primary and secondary stroke prevention. In this review, we will concentrate on the imaging of carotid wall morphology and pathology.

Intima-Media Thickness

The arterial wall is composed of three layers, the intima, the media, and the adventitia. As seen with B-mode sonography, a transition from the hypoechogenic lumen into the hyperechogenic intima (lumen-intima boundary) represents the internal border of intima-media complex. A transition from the hypoechogenic media into the hyperechogenic adventitia (media-adventitia boundary) represents the external border of the complex. Thus, B-mode sonography depicts the intima-media complex as a double-line structure (fig. 1). Due to the properties of US the far wall can be better visualized than the near wall as with B-mode sonography. The ultrasonographic appearance of IMT was confirmed by histological and in vitro studies [6, 7]. Moreover, B-mode assessment of IMT was shown to yield highly reproducible measures [8]. The thickness of intima-media complex has been used in atherosclerosis prevention trials, such as for statins, as a surrogate marker of efficacy of tested interventions and the surrogate of a control of cardiovascular risk factors. The increased common carotid artery (CCA) IMT assessed with B-mode sonography has shown to be correlated with fluctuations of blood pressure, and hyperglycemia in hypertensive subjects [9, 10]. Hypercholesterolemia, smoking, advanced age, the history of coronary artery disease, peripheral arterial disease, and cerebrovascular disease were also shown to increase the CCA IMT [11, 12]. Furthermore, CCA IMT measured with B-mode sonography was shown to be a risk factor for first-ever stroke and myocardial infarction. The risk increased for each quintile of combined CCA and internal carotid IMT, from the 2nd quintile (RR 1.54; 95% CI, 1.04–2.28), to the 5th (3.15; 2.19–4.52) [13]. The GENIC study has shown that IMT was predictive of stroke, in particularly for lacunar stroke [14].

The criteria for IMT measurements, and the distinction of thickened intima-media from an early plaque are still the matter of debate [5], and were recently summarized in an international consensus. According to the consensus, a plaque can be differentiated from a thickened intima-media complex by its focal invasion into the arterial lumen of at least 0.5 mm, or >50% of the surrounding IMT. A focal thickness of at least 1.5 mm, as measured from the media-adventitia to the intima-lumen border, is another criterion of a plaque. The IMT should be measured in a longitudinal view in a plaque-free area in the common carotid, proximal internal carotid or carotid bulb far wall [15].

Carotid Plaque

The search for surrogate markers of stroke risk is ongoing. With the use of high resolution B-mode imaging that is a noninvasive, easily available and vastly utilized technique for morphological assessment of carotid artery, the echogenicity, texture, surface contour, motion, total area and volume of a plaque can be detected. Several studies demonstrated that hypoechoic or anechoic carotid plaques, either independently or together with stenosis, carry an increased risk of cardiovascular events, such as stroke, transient ischemic attack, myocardial infarction and even to death [16–20]. The hypoechoic appearance of carotid plaques may be related to the presence of elastin fibers [21], hemorrhage [22], lipids and neointimal hyperplasia [23]. There were several studies on visual classification of plaque morphology that yielded the interobserver and intraobserver reliability with very low kappa values ranging from 0.47 to 0.73 depending on the assessed parameters [24, 25]. However, the unaided visual assessment of plaque morphology was recently shown to give the low-interrater agreement with kappa values of 0.05 (95% CI, 0.07–0.16) for plaque surface structure, 0.15 (0.02–0.28) for plaque heterogeneity, 0.18 (0.09–0.29) for plaque echogenicity, and 0.29 (0.19–0.39) for plaque calcification [26]. Moreover, the B-mode plaque categorization did not show any significant correlation with the actual volume of fibrosis and lipids [27]. Recently, computerized methods of echogenicity categorization were introduced, and some promising results were showed [28, 29].

The characterization of plaque surface with B-mode US is a great challenge, as an irregular, ulcerated surface may suggest an emboligenic potential and an increased risk of stroke [30]. The early reports were promising and showed a potential to differentiate between regular and ulcerated plaque surface in post-mortem carotid specimens [31]. However, the irregular plaque surface was demonstrated with B-mode imaging only in 27% of irregular endarterectomy specimens [32]. As reported by other authors, the B-mode sensitivity in detecting ulcerations when compared to histological assessment of endarterectomy specimens was 77% in plaques causing stenosis less than 50%, and it was 41% in plaques causing more than 50% stenosis [32, 33].

Except for static determination of plaque morphology, recently a novel technique of plaque motion based on temporal three dimensional ultrasound imaging was introduced. It is believed that the arterial wall distensibility may be related to the properties of the atheromatous plaque, and features such as asymmetrical plaque movements may prognosticate plaque rupture [5]. A study demonstrated that asymptomatic carotid plaques had similar motion properties as internal carotid artery, while symptomatic ones showed inherent plaque movements [34].

Total plaque area is considered to be an another surrogate marker of cardiovascular risk. The plaque area detected with B-mode US has shown to be linked to smoking and serum cholesterol levels [35]. Total plaque area was also demonstrated to be a better predictor of stroke, myocardial infarction and vascular death than carotid stenosis [36]. Another parameter allowing for monitoring the progression of atherosclerosis is the total plaque volume. The accuracy and reliability of its measurement was shown to be as high as 95% [37]. Recently, the total plaque volume was linked with the presence of diabetes mellitus [35].

All of these potential surrogate markers are interesting, but further studies are needed to determine their utility in determining the risk of stroke and the efficacy of preventive treatment.

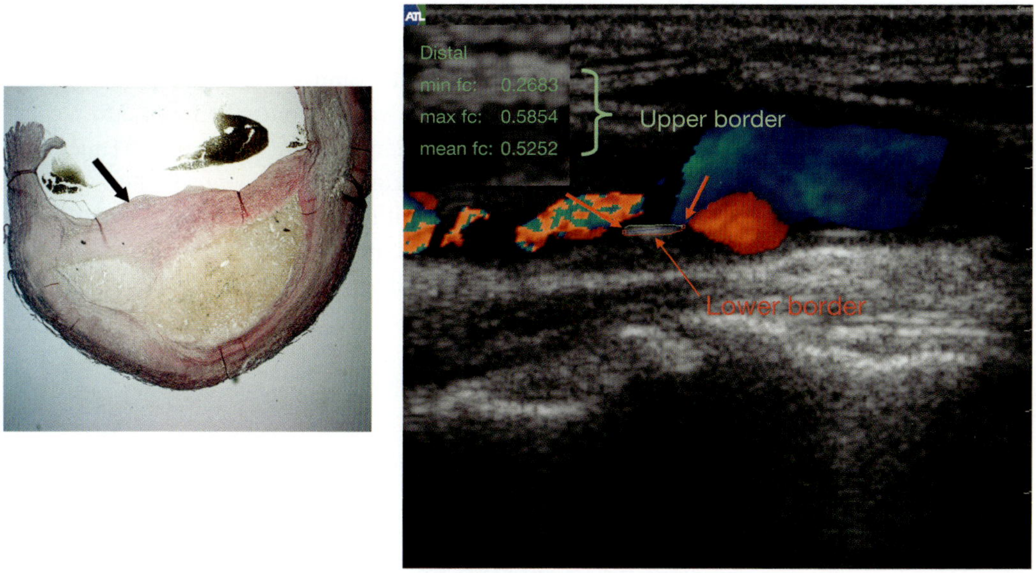

Fig. 2. Measurement of fibrous cap thickness in a carotid atheromatous plaque by a new semi-automatic system. Fibrous cap is defined as the hyperechoic structure existing between two anechoic surroundings (blood and lipid core).

'Unstable' Carotid Plaque

A border-zone infarct due to cerebral hypoperfusion is relatively rare, while the majority of strokes results from brain embolism originating from an atheromatous stenosis or occlusion of the carotid artery with a thrombus. The different behavior of the atheromatous plaque in symptomatic and asymptomatic carotids suggests that other factors than aging play a role. Some authors compared the histology findings of symptomatic and asymptomatic carotid plaques. They observed that symptomatic unstable plaques were characterized by surface ulceration, plaque rupture, thinning of the fibrous cap, and infiltration of the cap by greater load of macrophages and T cells [38]. Others also reported in an another review about the features of US and unstable carotid plaques. Their conclusion was that ultrasound is able to predict lipid-rich and rupture-prone plaques [39]. To make a diagnosis of an unstable carotid plaque in vivo, in contrast with cardiologists who perform intravascular ultrasound (IVUS) to investigate coronary plaques, noninvasive methods such as MR imaging (MRI), CT or US must be used. Recently, MRI and CT begin the exploration of the carotid arterial wall, and have a lower resolution in comparison to US (B-mode imaging). Lammie et al. presented a paper comparing histology and US on endarterectomy about the following features: ulceration, inflammation, size of necrotic core, and thickness of fibrous cap, hemorrhage and luminal thrombosis [40]. The thickness of fibrous cap and any necrosis or hemorrhage were identified with some reliability, kappa values being 0.53 and 0.5, respectively. With a new Doppler instrument (large band with multifrequencies, 5–12 MHz) and a semi-automatic system (fig. 2), we have separated symptomatic carotid plaques from asymptomatic with a sensitivity of 82% and a specificity of 83% for the best threshold, 650 microns [41]. But, this diagnostic tool must be validated by future prospective studies.

Acknowledgements

B.P-J. is supported by research grants from the International Stroke Society and World Federation of Neurology.

References

1 The Atlas of heart Disease and Stroke. Geneva, The World Health Organization, 2004.

2 Bogousslavsky J, Van MG, Regli F: The Lausanne stroke registry: Analysis of 1,000 consecutive patients with first stroke. Stroke 1988;19:1083–1092.

3 Arbeille P, Berson M, Fleury G, Besse D, Pourcelot L: Demonstration of atheromatous structures at the carotid level by echotomography and spectrum analysis of the Doppler signal. J Neuroradiol 1983;10:188–191.

4 Nederkoorn PJ, van der Graaf Y, Hunink MGM: Duplex ultrasound and magnetic resonance angiography compared with digital subtraction angiography in carotid artery stenosis: A systematic review. Stroke 2003;34:1324–1331.

5 Hennerici M, Baezner H, Daffertshofer M: Ultrasound and arterial wall disease. Cerebrovasc Dis 2004;17(suppl 1):19–33.

6 Pignoli P, Tremoli E, Poli A, Oreste P, Paoletti R: Intimal plus medial thickness of the arterial wall: A direct measurement with ultrasound imaging. Circulation 1986;74:1399–1406.

7 Wong M, Edelstein J, Wollman J, Bond MG: Ultrasonic-pathological comparison of the human arterial wall. Verification of intima-media thickness. Arterioscler Thromb 1993;13:482–486.

8 Riley WA, Barnes RW, Applegate WB, et al: Reproducibility of noninvasive ultrasonic measurement of carotid atherosclerosis. The asymptomatic carotid artery plaque study. Stroke 1992;23: 1062–1068.

9 Zakopoulos NA, Tsivgoulis G, Barlas G, et al: Time rate of blood pressure variation is associated with increased common carotid artery intima-media thickness. Hypertension 2005;01.

10 Tropeano AI, Boutouyrie P, Katsahian S, Laloux B, Laurent S: Glucose level is a major determinant of carotid intima-media thickness in patients with hypertension and hyperglycemia. J Hypertens 2004;22:2153–2160.

11 Poli A, Tremoli E, Colombo A, Sirtori M, Pignoli P, Paoletti R: Ultrasonographic measurement of the common carotid artery wall thickness in hypercholesterolemic patients. A new model for the quantitation and follow-up of preclinical atherosclerosis in living human subjects. Atherosclerosis 1988;70:253–261.

12 O'Leary DH, Polak JF, Kronmal RA, et al: Thickening of the carotid wall: A marker for atherosclerosis in the elderly? Stroke 1996;27:224–231.

13 O'Leary DH, Polak JF, Kronmal RA, et al: Carotid-artery intima and media thickness as a risk factor for myocardial infarction and stroke in older adults. N Engl J Med 1999;340:14–22.
14 Touboul PJ, Elbaz A, Koller C, et al: Common carotid artery intima-media thickness and brain infarction: The Etude du Profil Genetique de l'Infarctus Cerebral (GENIC) case-control study. The GENIC investigators. Circulation 2000;102:313–318.
15 Touboul PJ, Hennerici MG, Meairs S, et al: Mannheim intima-media thickness consensus. Cerebrovasc Dis 2004;18:346–349.
16 Schmidt C, Fagerberg B, Wikstrand J, Hulthe J: Multiple risk factor intervention reduces cardiovascular risk in hypertensive patients with echolucent plaques in the carotid artery. J Int Med 2003;253:430–438.
17 Biasi GM, Froio A, Diethrich EB, et al: Carotid plaque echolucency increases the risk of stroke in carotid stenting: The imaging in carotid angioplasty and risk of stroke (ICAROS) study. Circulation 2004;110:756–762.
18 Mathiesen EB, Bonaa KH, Joakimsen O: Echolucent plaques are associated with high risk of ischemic cerebrovascular events in carotid stenosis: The tromso study. Circulation 2001;103: 2171–2175.
19 Gronholdt ML, Nordestgaard BG, Schroeder TV, Vorstrup S, Sillesen H: Ultrasonic echolucent carotid plaques predict future strokes. Circulation 2001;104:68–73.
20 Tegos TJ, Kalomiris KJ, Sabetai MM, Kalodiki E, Nicolaides AN: Significance of sonographic tissue and surface characteristics of carotid plaques. AJNR Am J Neuroradiol 2001;22: 1605–1612.
21 Goncalves I, Lindholm MW, Pedro LM, et al: Elastin and calcium rather than collagen or lipid content are associated with echogenicity of human carotid plaques. Stroke 2004;35:2795–2800.
22 Tegos TJ, Sohail M, Sabetai MM, et al: Echomorphologic and histopathologic characteristics of unstable carotid plaques. AJNR Am J Neuroradiol 2000;21:1937–1944.
23 Gronholdt ML, Wiebe BM, Laursen H, Nielsen TG, Schroeder TV, Sillesen H: Lipid-rich carotid artery plaques appear echolucent on ultrasound B-mode images and may be associated with intraplaque haemorrhage. Eur J Vasc Endovasc Surg 1997;14:439–445.
24 de Bray JM, Baud JM, Delanoy P, et al: Reproducibility in ultrasonic characterization of carotid plaques. Cerebrovasc Dis 1998;8:273–277.
25 Joakimsen O, Bonaa KH, Stensland-Bugge E: Reproducibility of ultrasound assessment of carotid plaque occurrence, thickness, and morphology: The tromso study. Stroke 1997;28:2201–2207.
26 Hartmann A, Mohr JP, Thompson JL, Ramos O, Mast H: Interrater reliability of plaque morphology classification in patients with severe carotid artery stenosis. Acta Neurol Scand 1999;99: 61–64.
27 Montauban van Swijndregt AD, Elbers HRJ, Moll FL, de Letter J, Ackerstaff RGA: Ultrasonographic characterization of carotid plaques. Ultrasound Med & Biol 1998;24: 489–493.
28 Elatrozy T, Nicolaides A, Tegos T, Griffin M: The objective characterisation of ultrasonic carotid plaque features. Eur J Vasc Endovasc Surg 1998;16:223–230.
29 Gronholdt ML, Nordestgaard BG, Wiebe BM, Wilhjelm JE, Sillesen H: Echo-lucency of computerized ultrasound images of carotid atherosclerotic plaques are associated with increased levels of triglyceride-rich lipoproteins as well as increased plaque lipid content. Circulation 1998;97: 34–40.
30 Eliasziw M, Streifler JY, Fox AJ, Hachinski VC, Ferguson GG, Barnett HJ: Significance of plaque ulceration in symptomatic patients with high-grade carotid stenosis. North American symptomatic carotid endarterectomy trial. Stroke 1994;25:304–308.
31 Hennerici M, Reifschneider G, Trockel U, Aulich A: Detection of early atherosclerotic lesions by duplex scanning of the carotid artery. J Clin Ultrasound 1984;12:455–463.
32 Widder B, Paulat K, Hackspacher J, et al: Morphological characterization of carotid artery stenoses by ultrasound duplex scanning. Ultrasound Med Biol 1990;16:349–354.
33 Comerota AJ, Katz ML, White JV, Grosh JD: The preoperative diagnosis of the ulcerated carotid atheroma. J Vasc Surg 1990;11:505–510.
34 Meairs S, Hennerici M: Four-dimensional ultrasonographic characterization of plaque surface motion in patients with symptomatic and asymptomatic carotid artery stenosis. Stroke 1999;30: 1807–1813.

35 Al-Shali K, House AA, Hanley AJG, et al: Differences between carotid wall morphological phenotypes measured by ultrasound in one, two and three dimensions. Atherosclerosis 2005;178: 319–325.
36 Iemolo F, Martiniuk A, Steinman DA, Spence JD: Sex differences in carotid plaque and stenosis. Stroke 2004;35:477–481.
37 Spence JD, Blake C, Landry A, Fenster A: Measurement of carotid plaque and effect of vitamin therapy for total homocysteine. Clin Chem Lab Med 2003;41:1498–1504.
38 Golledge J, Greenhalgh RM, Davies AH: The symptomatic carotid plaque. Stroke 2000;31: 774–781.
39 Gronholdt ML: Ultrasound and lipoproteins as predictors of lipid-rich, rupture-prone plaques in the carotid artery. Arterioscler Thromb Vasc Biol 1999;19:2–13.
40 Lammie GA, Wardlaw J, Allan P, Ruckley CV, Peek R, Signorini DF: What pathological components indicate carotid atheroma activity and can these be identified reliably using ultrasound? Eur J Ultrasound 2000;11:77–86.
41 Devuyst G, Karapanayiotides T, Pusztaszeri M, Lobrinus J-A, Jonasson L, Cuisinaire O, Kalangos A, Despland P-A, Thiran J-P, Ruchat P, Bogousslavsky J: Ultrasound measurement of the fibrous cap in symptomatic and asymptomatic atheromatous carotid plaques. Circulation 2005;76: 797–803.

PD Dr. Gérald Devuyst
Department of Neurology
CHUV
CH–1011 Lausanne (Switzerland)
Tel. +41 21 314 1111, Fax +41 21 314 1231, E-Mail gerald.devuyst@chuv.ch

Baumgartner RW (ed): Handbook on Neurovascular Ultrasound.
Front Neurol Neurosci. Basel, Karger, 2006, vol 21, pp 27–35

Endothelial Function Testing

László Csiba

Department of Neurology, University of Debrecen, Health Science Center, Debrecen, Hungary

Abstract

It has been shown that the presence of well-preserved brachial artery vasoreactivity predicts the absence of coronary artery disease. The recent findings that coronary endothelial dysfunction is associated with an increased risk of stroke or transient ischemic attack in middle-aged patients without coronary artery disease support the concept that endothelial dysfunction is a systemic and prognostically relevant disorder and assessment of endothelial function may play a role as an additional strategy to identify patients who would benefit from aggressive preventive measures. It remains unknown whether an improvement in endothelial function directly translates into improved outcome.

The endothelial cells play an important role in the regulation of vascular tone by the release of vasoactive substances such as nitrous oxide (NO) [1]. Besides its vascular effects, NO also influences the atherogenesis, platelet aggregation, leukocyte adhesion, and inflammatory mechanisms. In addition to NO, the principal endothelium-derived vasodilators are prostacyclin, endothelium-derived hyperpolarizing factor, and adenosine. In general, the healthy endothelium maintains a vasodilator, antithrombotic, and anti-inflammatory state. Endothelial function is impaired in the early phase of atherogenic process, and diminishes the normal vasodilator response.

Impaired endothelium-dependent vasorelaxation can be diagnosed by measuring the response to different stressors before the development of atherosclerosis in the coronary or peripheral vasculature.

Endothelium-independent vasodilation can also be evaluated in the coronary or peripheral circulation after administration of agents that directly relax smooth muscle (e.g., nitroglycerin or sodium nitroprusside). This technique assesses the ability of the artery to maximally dilate. Because vascular smooth muscle cell is the final common pathway mediating vasorelaxation, it is important to realize that individuals with decreased endothelium-independent vasodilation responses, by definition, will have decreased endothelium-dependent vasodilation [2, 3].

Well-known vascular risk factors, including age, gender, hypertension, hyperlipidemia, diabetes mellitus, and smoking, as well as novel risk factors, such as inflammation and hyperhomocysteinemia, have been associated with abnormal vasorelaxation. Because atherosclerosis is a diffuse disease process, endothelial function can be assessed in either the coronary or peripheral circulation [4]. Recently, invasive and noninvasive techniques have been developed to evaluate endothelial function [5].

Endothelial Function Assessed by Invasive Techniques

Vasoactive Agents: Intracoronary Infusion

Acetylcholine produces a dose-dependent vasodilation in patients with angiographically smooth coronary arteries. Previous studies have shown that acetylcholine results in vasoconstriction in patients with risk factors (smoking, hypertension, hypercholesterolemia, diabetes), even when the coronary arteries are normal by angiography or intracoronary ultrasonography [5]. Intracoronary agonist infusion is the direct method for quantification of endothelial function in the coronary arteries, since it allows both the evaluation of endothelial agonists and antagonists as well as assessing the endothelial function. If endothelial dysfunction is present, acetylcholine leads to vasoconstriction (instead of vasodilatation) of smooth muscle cells. The abnormal reaction could be detected by Doppler probe. The protocol of Vita [6], is summarized below:

- Clinically stable patients undergoing diagnostic catheterization or percutaneous revascularization
- Hold vasodilators for 24 h (nitrates, calcium channel blockers, ACE inhibitors, β-blockers)
- Select vessel for study: one with no significant stenosis, subtends normal myocardium that is less than 1/3 of functional myocardium, and does not supply AV nodal artery
- Administer heparin 10,000 units. Instrument coronary using Judkins guide and 3-F infusion catheter and Doppler flow wire
- Serial drug infusions, including acetylcholine, nitroglycerin, nitroprusside, substance P, phenylephrine, *L*-arginine, bicycle exercise, pacing, or cold pressor testing etc
- Quantitative angiography using nonionic contrast to assess changes in epicardial coronary diameter
- Resistance vessel function assessed as changes in coronary blood flow

Serial drug infusions are made via the catheter for 2–3 min. After steady state is achieved, coronary angiography is performed with nonionic contrast and changes in vessel diameter measured using quantitative angiography. Changes in coronary blood flow could be estimated from the coronary flow velocity and the simultaneously determined cross-sectional area of the vessel lumen at the site of the Doppler [6]. Acetylcholine is infused at increasing rates (1–10 μg/min) with normal saline as vehicle. The presence or absence of endothelial dysfunction is diagnosed by analyzing the dose-response curves. If the endothelium is intact, a dose-dependent dilatation could be observed, while in the presence of endothelial dysfunction, acetylcholine results in a decreased vasodilatory response or even vasoconstriction of the coronary artery. Unfortunately, the method needs experienced investigators and could be associated with complications like dissection, embolization, myocardial infarction, arrhythmia, etc. The intracoronary studies are considered to be the gold standard for early detection of endothelial dysfunction, but they are invasive and cannot be used as a screening test.

Intrabrachial Infusion of Vasoactive Agents

If the endothelial function in the coronary arteries reflects that of peripheral arteries (as assumed), then the intracoronary infusions of vasoactive agents can also be applied in the brachial artery, which is better accessible, and its investigation is easier. Although the brachial artery circulation is most commonly investigated to determine changes in blood vessel diameter during reactive hyperemia, other peripheral arteries may also be evaluated, including the carotid, femoral, and radial arteries [7]. These studies involve insertion of an arterial catheter into the brachial or femoral artery for intra-arterial drug infusions and use of venous occlusion plethysmography to measure changes in limb blood flow, which reflect the vasomotor responses of limb microvessels. The protocol of Vita [6] is presented here:

- Clinically stable patients
- Hold vasodilators for 24 h (nitrates, calcium channel blockers, ACE inhibitors, β-blockers)
- Insert 20-gauge or smaller catheter into nondominant brachial artery using sterile technique and local anesthesia
- Continuously monitor arterial pressure
- Cuffs and strain gauge for venous occlusion plethysmography
- Serial drug infusions, including acetylcholine, methacholine (some investigators use this drug, because of the rapid metabolism of acetylcholine), nitroglycerin, nitroprusside, substance P, bradykinin, isoproterenol, phenylephrine, *L*-arginine, etc
- Assess resistance vessel vasomotor function as changes in forearm blood flow (FBF)

- FBF is measured by gauge-strain plethysmography
- During each FBF determination, the circulation of the hand is excluded for one minute before and during the measurements, by inflation of a cuff around the wrist at suprasystolic blood pressure

After saline infusion, and estimation of baseline FBF, acetylcholine is infused into the brachial artery with an increasing infusion rate by the normal saline displacement method, where the total pump infusion rate remains constant with a simultaneous decrease of the normal saline infusion rate. Each infusion rate of acetylcholine remains constant for 5 min (3 min before and during the 2 min of each FBF determination). FBF under acetylcholine infusion is measured as the average of at least three consecutive steady state measurements at the end of each infusion period [8].

Each dosing is followed by a 30-min resting period (with normal saline infusion at a constant rate), before the next dosing effect is evaluated, to allow the vascular endothelium to return to rest levels. The same protocol is usually repeated with nitroprusside infusion instead of acetylcholine, for evaluation of endothelium independent dilatation. The endothelium-dependent and endothelium-independent dilation could be calculated from the changes in FBF during acetylcholine or nitroprusside infusions [9]. This method has a high reproducibility but still remains invasive; therefore, noninvasive methods are needed for screening and follow-up [10].

Endothelial Function Assessed by Noninvasive Techniques

Assessment of Endothelium-Dependent Flow-Mediated Vasodilation

Many blood vessels respond to an increase in shear stress, by dilating. This phenomenon is designated flow-mediated dilation (FMD). A principal mediator of FMD is endothelium-derived NO. Endothelium-dependent FMD of the brachial artery was first reported by Laurent et al. [11], and later developed by others [12].

The recommendations of International Brachial Artery Reactivity Task Force Factors are summarized here [13].

- The patients should fast for at least 8 h before the study
- All vasoactive medications should be withdrawn. In addition, subjects should not exercise, consume caffeine, vitamin C, or smoke for at least 6 h before the study
- At rest the diameter of the brachial artery should be determined with high resolution B-mode ultrasound from multiple places (averaging), and blood flow must be calculated using the pulsed Doppler velocity signal. Ultrasound systems must be equipped with an internal electrocardiogram monitor and a high-frequency vascular transducer

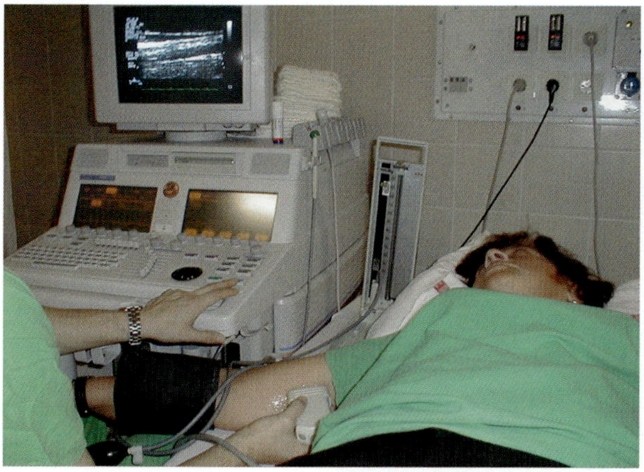

Fig. 1. Investigational set-up for ultrasound measurement (courtesy Dr. Soltesz).

- The subject is positioned supine with the arm in a comfortable position for imaging the brachial artery
- The brachial artery is imaged above the antecubital fossa in the longitudinal plane (fig. 1). In addition to two-dimensional grayscale imaging, both M-mode and A-mode (wall tracking) can be used to continuously measure the diameter (fig. 2)

After baseline diameter determination and blood flow estimation (by time-averaging the pulsed Doppler velocity signal obtained from a midartery sample volume), ischemia is caused by inflating a cuff placed at the distal forearm, at a pressure 50 mm Hg greater than the systolic blood pressure (5-min occlusion is typically used). Subsequent cuff deflation induces a brief high-flow state through the brachial artery (reactive hyperemia) to accommodate the dilated resistance vessels. The resulting increase in shear stress causes the brachial artery to dilate. The longitudinal image of the artery is recorded continuously from 30 s before to 2 min after cuff deflation (fig. 3). The diameter of the brachial artery should be measured from longitudinal images. A midartery pulsed Doppler signal is obtained upon immediate cuff release and no later than 15 s after cuff deflation to assess hyperemic velocity [13].

Studies have variably used either upper arm or forearm cuff occlusion, and there is no consensus as to which technique provides more accurate or precise information [14]. The maximum blood flow velocity is detected immediately or up to 15 s after cuff release, while the maximum diameter of the brachial artery is determined approximately 60 s after release. About 70% of the dilation observed 1 min after cuff release is attributable to NO synthesis [15]. The increase in diameter at this time could be prevented by *L*-arginine (NO synthase

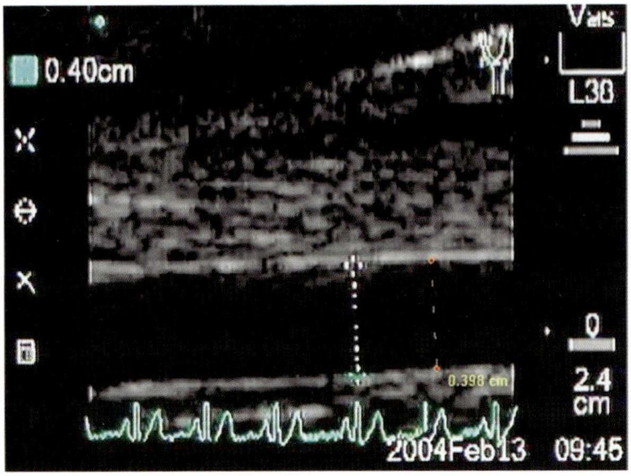

Fig. 2. B-mode picture and diameter of brachial artery (courtesy Dr. Soltesz).

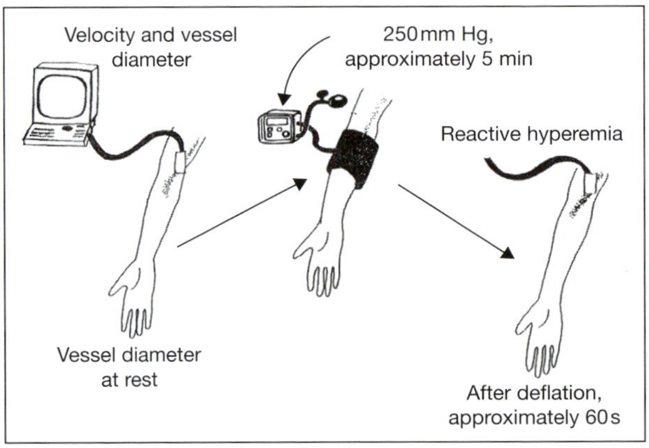

Fig. 3. Measurement of flow-mediated dilatation of brachial artery (modified figure of Hashimoto et al. [22]).

inhibitor), indicating that it is an endothelium-dependent process mediated by NO. Simultaneous electrocardiographic recordings are essential to achieve the most reliable results. Most laboratories define FMD as the percentage change of the brachial artery diameter from rest to the diameter 60 s after ischemia cuff release. The magnitude of systolic expansion is affected by the vessel compliance, and it may be reduced by factors such as aging and hypertension (possibly by reduced bioavailability of NO) [14]. The present technology makes it possible to examine the entire time course of brachial dilation in response to reactive hyperemia, the true peak response, the time to peak, and the overall duration of FMD. The investigation is operator dependent, requires patient cooperation, and has a relatively poor resolution [16].

Endothelium-Independent Vasodilation with Nitroglycerin

After FMD measurement 10 min of waiting time is necessary. Thereafter the endothelium-independent vasodilation could be tested by nitroglycerin (0.4 mg sublingual) to determine the maximum vasodilator response reflecting vascular smooth muscle function [17]. Maximal vasodilation occurs 3–4 min after nitroglycerin administration; images should be continuously recorded during this time. Determining the vasodilator responses to increasing doses of nitroglycerin, rather than a single dose, may further elucidate changes in smooth muscle function. Although most studies have detected little effect of disease states on this response, there is evidence that cardiovascular risk factors might impair the vasodilator response to nitroglycerin especially when a dose-response curve is measured [18].

Gauge-Strain Plethysmography (Evaluation of Reactive Hyperemia)

Another index currently used for the noninvasive evaluation of endothelial function in the brachial artery is evaluation of the changes in FBF during reactive hyperemia. The technique estimates the percentage change of flow from baseline to the maximum flow during reactive hyperemia following a short time of ischemia of the forearm. The endogenous NO has a minor role in vasodilation during reactive hyperemia, and the reactive hyperemia is caused by adenosine, prostaglandins, and endothelium-derived factor.

FBF is measured using a strain-gauge plethysmograph. The strain-gauge is attached to the upper forearm, at the position with the maximum diameter; it is supported above the level of the right atrium and it is connected to a plethysmographic device. The upper-arm-congesting cuff is inflated to 40 mm Hg for 7 s in each 15-sec cycle to occlude venous outflow from the arm by using a rapid cuff inflator. The final FBF is calculated by the mean of ten subsequent measurements, and always by two independent observers. A second wrist cuff is placed distal to the gauge-strain, and inflated at 50 mm Hg over the systolic blood pressure for 5 min, to produce ischemia. The FBF is measured every 15 s after the release of the ischemia cuff, and the time-flow curve is plotted. The percentage flow change from rest to the maximum hyperemic flow [19] and the dilatory capacity of resistance arteries [19, 20] could be measured.

Cold Pressor Stress

The technique investigates the endothelium-dependent vasodilation by releasing catecholamines [13, 21]. Cold pressor stress is provoked by immersing one hand in cold water (ice water) for 2 min, and determination of coronary blood flow (invasive technique), FBF by gauge-strain plethysmography, or the diameter of the brachial artery by high-resolution ultrasound occur by the end of the test. The percentage change of coronary blood flow or FBF from baseline to the maximum flow after cold pressor stress, as well as the percentage change of the diameter of the brachial artery from baseline to the diameter after the test, are also indexes of endothelial function.

Carotid Artery Reactivity to Isometric Handgrip Exercise

The static isometric handgrip exercise could induce changes in the carotid artery diameter.

The protocol [7] includes 10 min of rest at baseline and 10–15 min between interventions. High-resolution B-mode ultrasound scans should be performed. Isometric peak handgrip strength is tested on the nondominant hand with a handgrip dynamometer 30 min prior to the study. Then subjects are asked to sustain a handgrip at 33% of peak effort for 120 s in the left hand, and can visually see the assigned target force. The hemodynamic response is recorded at baseline and each minute following isometric handgrip for 10 min. Care should be taken not to inflate the blood pressure cuff for 45 s after release to allow washout of all metabolites. The carotid diameter is measured at baseline and in every 30-sec interval sample during isometric handgrip, immediately following, and every 30 s for 10 min.

References

1 Pepine C: Clinical implications of endothelial dysfunction. Clin Cardiol 1998;1:795–799.
2 Kuvin JT, Karas RH: Clinical utility of endothelial function testing. Ready for prime time? Circulation 2003;107:3243–3247.
3 Gocke N, Keaney J, Vita J: Endotheliopathies: Clinical manifestations of endothelial dysfunction; in Loscalzo J, Shafer AI (eds): Thrombosis and Hemorrhage. Baltimore, MD, Williams and Wilkins, 1998, pp 901–924.
4 Neunteufl T, Katzenschlager R, Hassan A, Klaar U, Schwarzacher S, Glogar D, Bauer P, Weidinger F: Systemic endothelial dysfunction is related to the extent and severity of coronary artery disease. Atherosclerosis 1997;129:111–118.
5 Tousoulis D, Antoniades C, Stefanadis C: Evaluating endothelial function in humans: A guide to invasive and non-invasive techniques. Heart 2005;91:553–558.
6 Vita JA: Clinical assessment of endothelial function; in Lanzer P, Topol EJ (eds): Panvascular Medicine. Berlin, Springer 2002, pp 691–700.
7 Rubenfire M, Cao N, Smith DE, Mosca L: Carotid artery reactivity to isometric hand grip exercise identifies persons at risk and with coronary disease. Atherosclerosis 2002;160:241–248.
8 Schlaich MP, John S, Langenfeld RW, Lackner KJ, Schmitz G, Schmieder RE: Does lipoprotein(a) impair endothelial function? J Am Coll Cardiol 1998;31:359–365.
9 Virdis A, Ghiadoni L, Cardinal H, Favilla S, Duranti P, Birindelli R, Magagna A, Bernini G, Salvetti G, Taddei S, Salvetti A: Mechanisms responsible for endothelial dysfunction induced by fasting hyperhomocystinemia in normotensive subjects and patients with essential hypertension. J Am Coll Cardiol 2001;38:1106–1115.

10 Lind L, Hall J, Johansson K: Evaluation of four different methods to measure endothelium-dependent vasodilation in the human peripheral circulation. Clin Sci 2002;102:561–567.

11 Laurent S, Brunel P, Lacolley P, Billaud E, Pannier B, Safar M: Flow-dependent vasodilation of the brachial artery in essential hypertension: Preliminary report. J Hypertens Suppl 1988;6: S182–S184.

12 Celermajer DS, Sorensen KE, Gooch VM: Non-invasive detection of endothelial dysfunction in children and adults at risk of atherosclerosis. Lancet 1992;340:1111–1115.

13 Corretti MC, Anderson TJ, Benjamin EJ, Celermajer D, Charbonneau F, Creager MA, Deanfield J, Drexler H, Gerhard-Herman M, Herrington D, Vallance P, Vita J, Vogel R: International Brachial Artery Reactivity Task Force. Guidelines for the ultrasound assessment of endothelial-dependent flow-mediated vasodilation of the brachial artery. J Am Coll Cardiol 2002;39: 257–265.

14 Corretti MC, Plotnick GD, Vogel RA: Technical aspects of evaluating brachial artery vasodilatation using high-frequency ultrasound. Am J Physiol 1995;268:H1397–H1404.

15 Lieberman EH, Gerhard MD, Uehata A, Selwyn AP, Ganz P, Yeung AC, Creager MA: Flow-induced vasodilation of the human brachial artery is impaired in patients 40 years of age with coronary artery disease. Am J Cardiol 1996;78:1210–1214.

16 Kuvin J, Patel A, Karas R: Need for standardization of non-invasive assessment of vascular endothelial function. Am Heart J 2001;141:327–328.

17 Ducharme A, Dupuis J, McNicoll S, Harel F, Tardif JC: Comparison of nitroglycerin lingual spray and sublingual tablet on time of onset and duration of brachial artery vasodilation in normal subjects. Am J Cardiol 1999;84:952–954.

18 Adams MR, Robinson J, McCredie R, Seale JP, Sorensen KE, Deanfield JE, Celermajer DS: Smooth muscle dysfunction occurs independently of impaired endothelium-dependent dilation in adults at risk of atherosclerosis. J Am Coll Cardiol 1998;32:123–127.

19 Kornerup K, Nordestgaard BG, Feldt-Rasmussen B, Borch-Johnsen K, Jensen KS: Antioxidant vitamins C and E administration in smokers: Effects on endothelial function and adhesion molecules. Atherosclerosis 2003;170:263–269.

20 Higashi Y, Sasaki S, Nakagawa K, Matsuura H, Kajiyama G, Oshima T: Effect of angiotensin-converting enzyme inhibitor imidapril on reactive hyperemia in patients with essential hypertension: Relationship between treatment periods and resistance artery endothelial function. J Am Coll Cardiol 2001;37:863–870.

21 Nabel EG, Ganz P, Gordon JB, Alexander RW, Selwyn AP: Dilation of normal and constriction of atherosclerotic coronary arteries caused by the cold pressor test. Circulation 1988;77:43–52.

22 Hashimoto M, Miyamoto Y, Matsuda Y, Akita H: New methods to evaluate endothelial function. Non-invasive method of evaluating endothelial function in humans. J Pharmacol Sci 2003;93: 405–408.

Dr. László Csiba
Department of Neurology, University of Debrecen, Health Science Center
Nagyerdei krt. 98
HR–4012 Debrecen (Hungary)
Tel. +36 52 415 176, Fax +36 52 453 590, E-Mail csiba@jaguar.dote.hu

Baumgartner RW (ed): Handbook on Neurovascular Ultrasound.
Front Neurol Neurosci. Basel, Karger, 2006, vol 21, pp 36–56

Atherosclerotic Carotid Stenosis and Occlusion

Matthias Sitzer

Department of Neurology, Centre for Neurology and Neurosurgery, Johann Wolfgang Goethe-University, Frankfurt am Main, Germany

Abstract

Ultrasonic techniques can determine both the presence and degree of atherosclerotic lesions around the internal carotid artery bifurcation with a high degree of accuracy. Carried out by experienced sonographers, who are aware of the relevant limitations and the most common pitfalls, noninvasive ultrasound can serve as a screening tool, supply the vascular surgeon or interventionalist with sufficient information for determining treatment, and is an optimal tool for follow-up examinations. In this context, it will be of importance that ultrasound also facilitates the delineation of blood flow in a stented internal carotid artery. This will open up the possibility of using ultrasound to detect restenosis after endovascular treatment.

Atherosclerotic stenoses of the proximal part of the internal carotid artery (ICA) are a major cause of stroke. Approximately 10–15% of all ischemic strokes and transitory ischemic attacks occur in the territory of a severely stenosed ICA [1, 2]. Carotid endarterectomy is a very successful preventive therapy, not only in previously symptomatic, but also in a subset of asymptomatic patients [3–6]. Endovascular stent placement may be of comparable benefit to these patients, but final data are still lacking. Noninvasive cervical ultrasound can be used to delineate the carotid system from the middle part of the common carotid artery (CCA) up to the submandibular part of the ICA. In almost all cases, this facilitates the detection and quantification of stenotic lesions in the proximal part of the ICA, the predilection site for atherosclerotic lesions in the extracranial carotid system. Cervical ultrasound is therefore the diagnostic procedure most frequently used to detect and quantify atherosclerotic lesions in the ICA. It is not only important for determining stroke etiology in acute management but also for determining the individual stroke risk in asymptomatic patients. In the future, the stented ICA could be closely monitored using ultrasound technology.

Frequency of Carotid Stenosis and the Associated Stroke Risk

Approximately 5–10% of all individuals aged 65 years or over harbor an asymptomatic ICA stenosis of 50% luminal narrowing or more [1]. The annual risk of a major stroke varies from 1 to 3.2% in cases of luminal narrowing ranging from 50 to 99% [4, 6–8]. This risk remains almost stable over a long period of time [6]. An increasing degree of luminal narrowing is associated with an increasing risk of stroke in asymptomatic ICA stenosis. For every 10% increase in luminal narrowing, the stroke risk increases by nearly 31%, or 0.6% (in absolute terms) per year [8]. Stenoses with more than 95% luminal narrowing may be associated with a reduced stroke risk in comparison with stenosis of between 80 and 95% [8]. After an ischemic event in the territory of the stenosed ICA (i.e., transitory ischemic attacks or nondisabling stroke), the annual major stroke risk increases to between 8 and 13% [3, 5]. This risk is substantially higher within the first 6 months after the index event than thereafter [9]. In symptomatic patients too, the degree of stenosis modulates the risk of stroke; for every 10% increase in ICA luminal narrowing, the stroke risk increases by approximately 10% (absolute risk increase of approximately 0.4% per year) [8]. Similarly, the risk decreases in cases of more than 90% luminal narrowing [8].

The prevalence of unilateral carotid occlusion is around 0.5% in older patients (Carotid Atherosclerosis Progression Study, own unpubl. data). The annual risk of major ipsilateral stroke associated with ICA occlusion is approximately between 1.9 and 3.8% per year [8, 10].

Carotid Stenosis

Definition and Detection of Atherosclerotic Carotid Plaque

Stenotic atherosclerotic lesions grow continuously from the focal intimal-medial wall thickening at atherosclerosis-prone sites [11]. From a pathoanatomical point of view, an atherosclerotic plaque (i.e., type (III-) IV/V lesion) is present if two criteria are fulfilled: (1) the arterial wall is focally and eccentrically thickened and the tissue is protruding into the vessel lumen to an increasing degree and (2) the plaque tissue is characterized by lipid-laden macrophages, extracellular lipid accumulation forming the necrotic core, and the fibrous cap [12–15]. Since the precise tissue composition cannot be reliably determined by standard ultrasound, the latter criterion cannot be

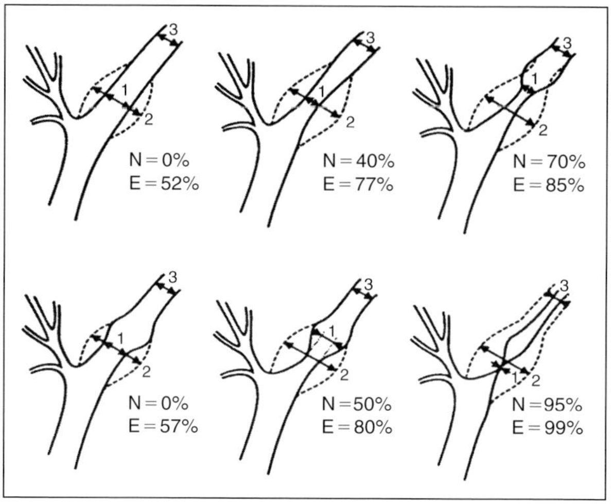

Fig. 1. Schematic examples of intra-arterial angiographic measurements for the degree of stenosis for different configurations of ICA lesions. N = 'NASCET method'; E = 'ECST method'. See text for details. Modified from [19].

established by routine examination. Ultrasonographic diagnosis of atheroma was therefore solely based on the focal appearance and thickness of an intraluminal obscuration. Thus, in the extracranial carotid system, any tissue protruding into the vessel lumen with a distance of more than 1.7 mm between the luminal interface and the medial-adventitial interface should be termed 'atherosclerotic plaque' (fig. 2a) [16–18]. Notwithstanding the arbitrariness of this cutoff point, this definition enables the reliable detection of atherosclerotic plaque using B-mode ultrasound in routine clinical as well as in scientific examinations. More diffuse wall changes or thinner lesions should be termed 'intima-media thickening'.

The benchmark for determining the degree of ICA stenosis is digital subtraction intra-arterial catheter angiography (IA) of the carotid system. Based on the IA images, the degree of luminal narrowing can be determined using two different methods: (1) the distal method, which calculates the ratio of the minimal residual diameter of the stenosed segment ('1' in fig. 1) to the diameter of a distal, clearly nondiseased segment of the ICA ('3' in fig. 1; 'North American Symptomatic Carotid Endarterectomy Trial (NASCET) method') [19]; (2) the local method, which calculates the ratio of the minimal residual diameter of the stenosed segment ('1' in fig. 1) to the presumed former diameter of the same segment ('2' in fig. 1; 'European Carotid Surgery Trial (ECST) method') [20]. Both methods rely on the IA projection showing the minimal residual lumen

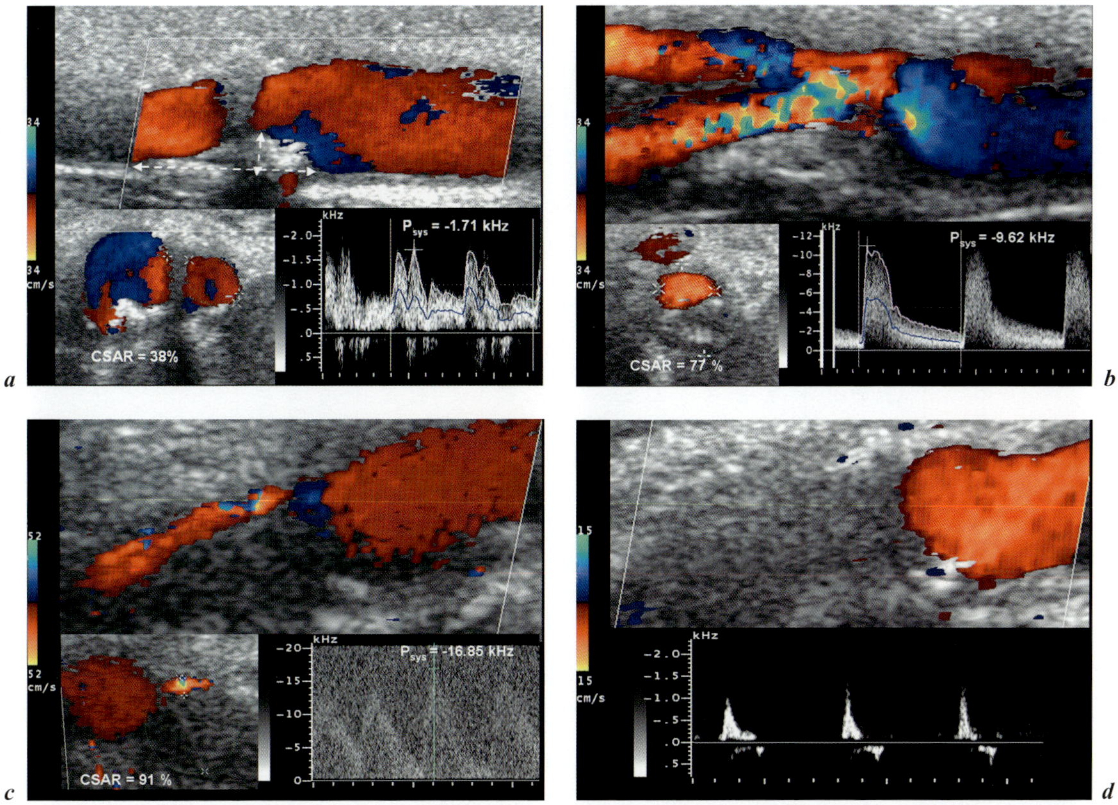

Fig. 2. Multimodality imaging of internal carotid artery (ICA) atherosclerotic lesions. ***a*** Nonstenotic ICA plaque without hemodynamic changes, plaque length is about 15 mm, plaque thickness 3.9 mm; ***b*** approximately 60–70% ICA stenosis; ***c*** approximately 90% ICA stenosis; and ***d*** proximal ICA occlusion. ***a–d*** The upper panel shows longitudinal color Doppler-assisted duplex imaging where right is proximal, the bottom left panel shows the transverse view of the narrowest part of the stenosis and cross-sectional luminal area reduction measurement (velocity coding is the same for both longitudinal and transverse views, see far left color panel). The bottom right panel displays the Doppler shift recording and spectrum analysis, the maximum peak systolic shift is given in kilo Hertz (kHz).

[20]. It is important to note that the NASCET method describes predominantly the hemodynamic significance of ICA stenosis (relation of the inflow to outflow diameter), whereas the ESCT method reflects more the amount of atherosclerotic tissue at the stenosed segment. As shown in figure 1, the degree of luminal narrowing determined can vary significantly between the two different methods. In most cases, the ECST method results in a 10–30% higher degree of ICA stenosis, especially in the middle range (i.e., 50–80%) [20]. The validity of

Table 1. Diagnostic criteria for different hemodynamic parameters for determining the degree of luminal narrowing in ICA stenosis by means of cervical ultrasound

Degree of luminal narrowing	PSV m/s	ΔF kHz	FFT spectrum		STA	CCA spectrum	ICA/CCA PSV ratio	ICA/ICA MV ratio
			intrastenotic	poststenotic				
<40%	<1.2	<4	laminar	laminar	orthograde	normal	<1.5	<2
40–50%	~1.2	~4	laminar	laminar	orthograde	normal	<1.5	<2
51–70%	~2.0	4–7	laminar • spectrum broadening	turbulences • PSV ↓	orthograde	normal	1.5–2.0	2–3 sometimes >3
71–90%	~3.0	>7	nonlaminar • inverse velocity parts • spectrum broadening ↑ • sys/dias amplitude ↓	turbulences • PSV ↓↓ • EDV ↑	reduced orthograde or retrograde	PSV ↓ PI ↑	2–4 sometimes >4	5–10
>90%	variable	variable	nonlaminar • inverse velocity parts • spectrum broadening ↑ • sys/dias amplitude ↓↓	turbulences • PSV ↓↓↓ • EDV ↑	mostly retrograde	PSV ↓↓ PI ↑	>4	>10 often not reliable
Occlusion	0	0	stump flow signal at the proximal part of the ICA	not detectable	mostly retrograde	PSV ↓↓ PI ↑↑	0	0

ΔF = Doppler shift frequency; CCA = common carotid artery; EDV = end-diastolic velocity; FFT = fast Fourier transformed; ICA/CCA = internal/common carotid artery velocity ratio; ICA/ICA = intra/poststenotic internal carotid artery velocity ratio; MV = mean velocity; PI = pulsatility index; PSV = peak systolic velocity, insonation angle corrected; STA = supratrochlear artery; sys/dias = systolic/diastolic.

the various ultrasonographic measurements should be determined against the IA standard, either according to the NASCET or ECST method [20–24].

Degree of Stenosis

Indirect Signs

Indirect signs of an ICA stenosis stem predominantly from hemodynamic alterations in the carotid system. It is therefore plausible that these indirect signs may only be detectable in cases of high-grade ICA stenosis, with significant flow reduction (>80% luminal narrowing) on the affected side. Under normal conditions, the blood flow in the periorbital arteries, mainly in the supratrochlear artery, is intracranial to extracranial. Owing to the higher perfusion pressure in the ophthalmic artery, originating from the intracranial portion of the ICA, than in the facial artery, as a branch of the external carotid artery, the blood flow in this anastomosis is directed towards the ultrasonic probe. A significant reduction of blood flow compared with the nonaffected side, an oscillating flow pattern, no flow, or most frequently, an inverse flow direction, all indicate increasing hemodynamic compromise in the case of ICA stenosis or occlusion (table 1) [25–27]. Nevertheless, owing to the considerable variation in the flow pattern in the supratrochlear artery in the case of ICA disease, the accuracy of supraorbital Doppler, on its own, is only moderate, with wide confidence intervals: sensitivities for the detection of a 50%, 70% ICA stenosis, or ICA occlusion were 0.81 (0.57–0.95), 0.88 (0.74–0.95), and 0.87 (0.53–0.99), respectively [28]. The corresponding specificities were higher: 0.97 (0.89–1.0), 0.97 (0.92–0.99), and 0.90 (0.74–0.98), respectively [28].

In cases of significant ICA stenosis, the Doppler flow pattern derived from the ipsilateral CCA changes showed an increase in the pulsatility index (decrease in diastolic velocity) and a reduction in the blood flow [29]. Comparing the CCA peak systolic (PSV) or mean velocity (MV) or pulsatility index of the affected with those of the nonaffected side can help to identify high-grade ICA stenosis.

In conclusion, the comparison of indirect parameters, such as supraorbital Doppler findings and CCA Doppler spectrum parameters, with the nonaffected side serves as a confirmatory test to affirm the direct findings in cases of high-grade ICA stenosis or occlusion (see below). The diagnosis and grading of carotid lesions should not be determined using this test alone.

Peak Systolic Velocity and Doppler Spectrum Analysis

The most important hemodynamic parameter derived directly from the stenotic lesion is the peak systolic Doppler shift (measured in kHz) or the peak

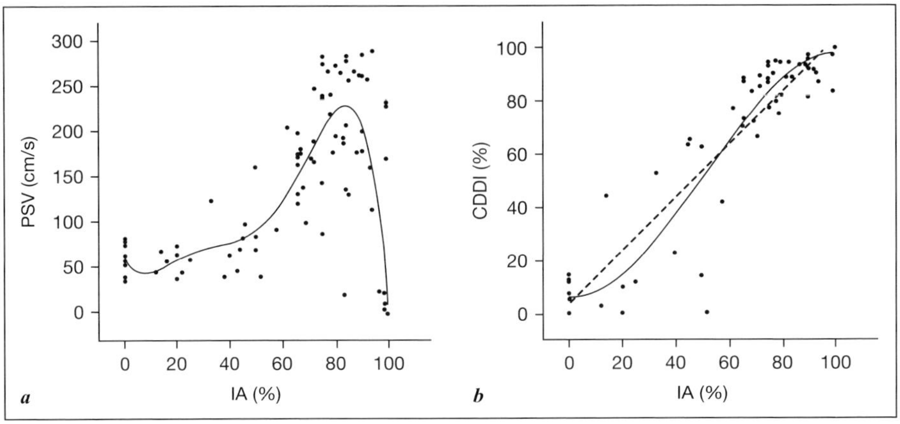

Fig. 3. Correlation analyses between peak systolic velocity (PSV; ***a***)- and color Doppler-assisted duplex imaging (CDDI; ***b***)- derived cross-sectional luminal area reduction measurements and intra-arterial digital subtraction angiography (IA) in determining the degree of internal carotid artery stenosis (modified from [17]). The dotted line in (***b***) indicates first-order regression and the solid lines indicate the best-fitting higher-order regression (***a***, ***b***). The correlation coefficients were $R_5 = 0.85$ in (***a***), and $R_1 = 0.94$, $R_3 = 0.96$ in (***b***).

systolic velocity PSV corrected for the insonation angle in meters per sec (m/s) (table 1) [17, 30–34]. The relationship between an increasing degree of luminal narrowing and the corresponding PSV is nonlinear, as shown in figure 3a. As the degree of luminal narrowing increases up to 80%, the PSV also increases, reaching maximum velocities of up to 3.0 m/s. In luminal narrowing >80%, the PSV decreases due to a significant reduction in blood flow volume through the stenosed segment. In 95–99% stenosis, it may be difficult to detect any residual flow through the stenosed segment, suggesting ICA occlusion (this is known as 'pseudo-occlusion'; see below) [35]. As summarized in table 2, systematic meta-analyses of 70 published articles revealed an approximate 90% sensitivity and specificity for the detection of both medium- and high-grade ICA stenosis [28]. Nevertheless, the grading of ICA stenosis using PSV alone poses some potential pitfalls: (1) As mentioned above, PSV decreases above 80–90% stenosis. A 50–60% stenosis can therefore reveal similar PSV values to a 95% stenosis. (2) PSV depends not only on the degree of luminal narrowing, but also on the length of the stenosis. PSV also decreases if a further, more distally located second stenosis is present ('tandem lesion'). (3) Contralateral lesions can increase the recorded PSV by 25–35%, potentially leading to an overestimation of the ipsilateral lesion [36–38]. (4) Extensive tortuosity of the extracranial vessel can influence the Doppler shift, as it causes a change in the insonation angle [39]. In conclusion, these limitations are responsible for the high but not

Table 2. Diagnostic accuracy of different ultrasonic modalities in detecting 50–69% and 70–99% internal carotid artery (ICA) stenosis, respectively. Accuracy measurements (confidence interval) were derived from a systematic meta-analysis [28]

	Number of arteries	50–69% ICA stenosis		70–99% ICA stenosis	
		sensitivity	specificity	sensitivity	specificity
B-mode sonography	1,698	0.80 (0.55–0.95)	0.82 (0.43–0.99)	0.59 (0.22–0.89)	0.85 (0.51–1.0)
PSV or ΔF measurements	1,888	0.90 (0.86–0.94)	0.91 (0.87–0.94)	0.85 (0.79–0.89)	0.93 (0.90–0.96)
CDDI	2,646	0.91 (0.87–0.94)	0.91 (0.87–0.93)	0.87 (0.80–0.93)	0.92 (0.88–0.95)

ΔF = Doppler shift frequency; CDDI = color Doppler-assisted duplex imaging; PSV = peak systolic velocity, insonation angle corrected.

perfect diagnostic accuracy of PSV measurements for assessing the degree of ICA stenosis [40].

Furthermore, there are some features of Doppler spectrum analyses that may be observed in cases of high-grade stenosis: (1) Spectrum broadening indicates an increase in the frequency bandwidth, which means that the range between the lowest and highest measurable frequency component increases in cases of stenosis [41, 42]. This is mainly because slow flow components and turbulences appear in the poststenotic region. (2) In the jet stream of the stenosis, inverse velocity components can occur as a result of vortices in the outer part of the jet stream (fig. 4). In 70–80% stenosis, these appear only during early systole, but in 80–90% stenosis they appear continuously during systole and diastole. In conclusion, the assessment of such phenomena is predominantly observer-dependent and can only support findings derived from more reliable parameters.

ICA/CCA Velocity Ratios

The combination of direct and indirect signs has resulted in the definition and evaluation of various velocity indices, the most important ones being the ICA/CCA PSV ratio and the ICA/ICA MV ratio (table 1):

ICA/CCA PSV Ratio. This ratio is obtained by dividing the ICA intrastenotic PSV by the PSV derived from the ipsilateral CCA 3 cm proximal to the bifurcation. As shown in table 1, the ICA/CCA PSV ratio varies between 1.5 and 2 in cases of 50–70% stenosis, between 2 and 4 in cases of 70–90%

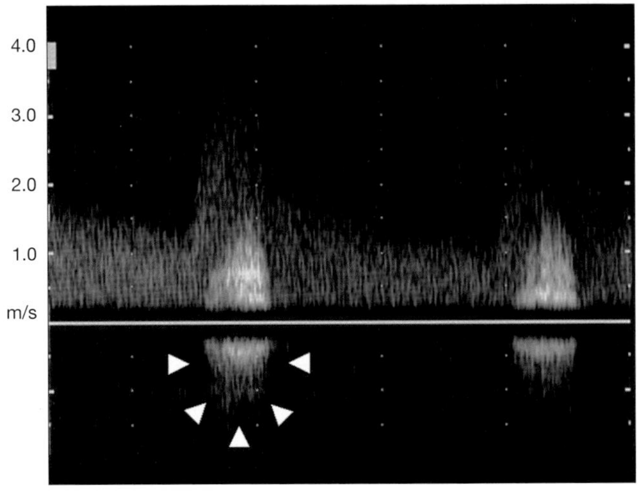

Fig. 4. Doppler spectrum analyses from the jet stream of an 80% internal carotid artery stenosis. Inverse velocity components are present predominantly during the systole (white arrows).

stenosis, and is above 4 in cases of >90% stenosis [32, 40, 43, 44]. The predictive value of this index is moderate. Moneta et al. [45] found for an ICA/CCA PSV ratio of >4 a sensitivity of 0.91 and a specificity of 0.87 for a >70% stenosis according to the NASCET method. Grant et al. [44] found in their series that only 80% of all stenoses were correctly classified as >70% by an ICA/CCA PSV ratio >4.

ICA/ICA MV Ratio. Poststenotically, up to 80% luminal narrowing, flow velocity is normal at around 0.7–0.8 m/s. In narrowing >80%, flow velocity decreases. The ICA/ICA MV ratio is the ratio of the intrastenotic MV to the poststenotic MV of the stenosed ICA. There is a nonlinear relationship between the angiographically determined degree of luminal narrowing, with a regression coefficient of $r^2 = 0.93$ [46]. As summarized in table 1, an ICA/ICA MV ratio >5 indicates >70% stenosis according to angiographic criteria. This threshold confers a sensitivity of 0.97 and a specificity of 0.98 [46].

The ICA/ICA MV ratio, in particular, has some advantages over PSV determination: (1) the prediction of >90% stenosis is more reliable; (2) the MV is more sound than the angle-corrected PSV; (3) the velocity ratio is less susceptible to absolute values and technical differences between ultrasound scanners [46]. The major disadvantages are that (1) the poststenotic velocity cannot be measured in cases of a distal, tandem, or very long ICA stenosis, and (2) this ratio is also influenced by contralateral ICA disease.

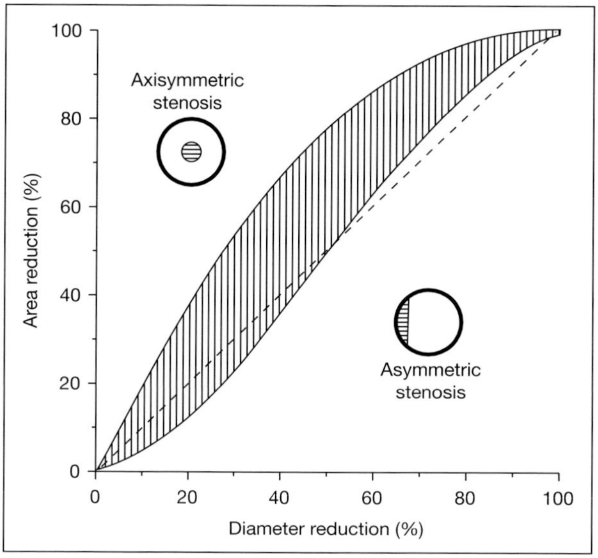

Fig. 5. Graph shows the expected relationship between the diameter and area reduction measurements of increasing luminal narrowing (modified from [47]). The upper and lower solid lines indicate two extreme types of stenosis (axi- and asymmetric); the shaded area represents the variations to be expected within the natural distribution of stenosis. Note that almost all atherosclerotic internal carotid artery stenoses are of asymmetric geometry (compare with fig. 3b).

Cross-Sectional Area Reduction

Based on transverse views of the stenosed segments generated by color Doppler-assisted duplex imaging (CDDI) or power flow imaging (PFI), the local degree of luminal narrowing can be estimated by measuring the former ICA lumen area (A_N) as well as the minimal residual flow lumen (A_S). Using transverse views of the narrowest part of the stenosis (fig. 2a–c), the degree of luminal reduction can be determined as the percentage of cross-sectional area reduction (CSAR; $1-[A_S/A_N]*100\%$) [17]. In a prospective series of 60 consecutive patients with angiographically proven high-grade ICA stenosis, we found a linear correlation coefficient of $r = 0.94$ and a third-order correlation coefficient of $r = 0.96$ for the relationship between the degree of ICA luminal narrowing determined by CSAR measurement and by the NASCET angiographic method (fig. 3b) [17]. It is also worth noting that the correlation between these methods is rather bad in stenosis <50% and better in the higher range, but in such cases the ultrasound measurements tend to overestimate the angiographic findings. Nevertheless, sensitivity to predict >70% stenosis was 0.97 and specificity 0.87 [17]. It is long been known that when comparing diameter- and area-based measurements of stenosis incongruities have to be expected on physical grounds. As shown in figure 5, the shaded area indicates the range of the degree of luminal narrowing based on area measurements (Y-axis) compared with the degree of stenosis based on diameter measurements (X-axis). The tendency for overestimation is most prominent in axisymmetric, but is also seen in asymmetric stenoses [47].

Reliability of Ultrasound Measurements

In our own investigation, we determined interobserver reliabilities from three independent and 'blinded' observers for, among other parameters, CSAR measurements, and the NASCET method from angiograms of high-grade carotid stenosis. For CSAR, we found the correlation coefficient ranged from $r = 0.76$ up to $r = 0.90$ between the observers; for IA, the corresponding values ranged from 0.71 to 0.89 [17]. This was substantiated by other investigators who also reported correlation coefficients of around 0.90 [48]. Furthermore, it has been reported that there is a high degree of interobserver concordance as regards the determination of PSV; Thomson et al. [49] found an intraclass correlation coefficient of 0.91 for the absolute values but only a κ-value of 0.53 ± 0.027 for PSV values above or below the cutoff point, indicating >70% stenosis.

It is important to note that the variation in repeated ultrasonic measurements depends not only on differences between the sonographers but also on technical differences between ultrasound scanners. The PSV of a stenotic lesion can vary by 20–30% between different scanners [46, 50]. Such technical differences can be overcome through the use of velocity ratios (see above) [46].

Pitfalls and Limitations

Calcifications and Shadowing

Extensive calcifications with shadowing can hamper the delineation of the residual lumen, thereby inhibiting the precise determination of the degree of stenosis, either by PSV or CSAR. Consequently, previous authors have noted that imaging conditions are unsatisfactory in 8–13% of images generated by CDDI [17, 48, 51, 52]. The use of a transpulmonary stable intravenous contrast medium can significantly enhance the echogenicity of flowing blood [53]. An earlier study revealed an almost 20-dB increase in the reflected ultrasonic energy for a duration of around 3–5 min after intravenous bolus injection (fig. 6) [53]. In high-grade ICA stenoses, use of a contrast medium can reduce the occurrence of 'insufficient image quality' from around 21 to 6% and improve the delineation of the entire residual lumen from 52 to 83% [53].

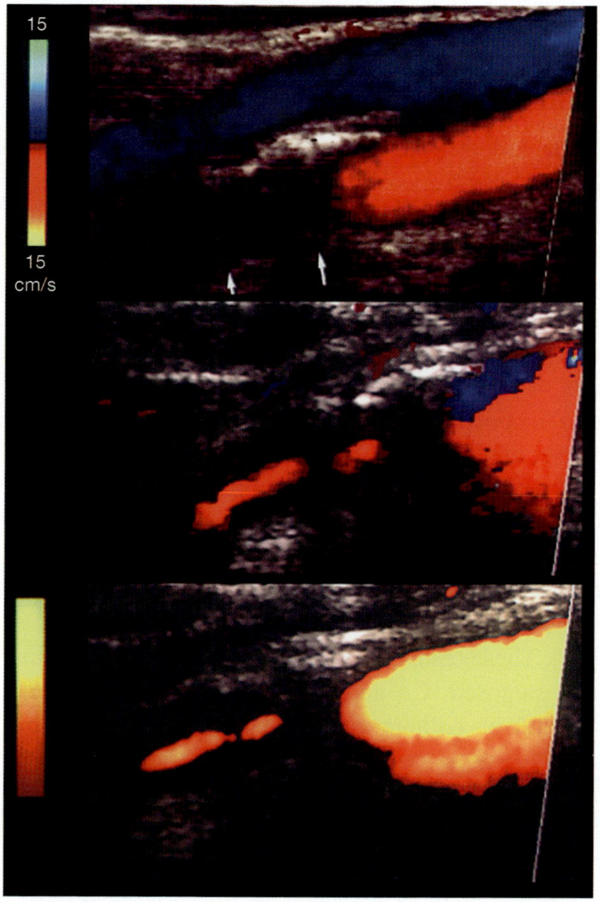

Fig. 6. Multimodality imaging of internal carotid artery (ICA), so-called 'pseudo-occlusion'. ***a*** Nonenhanced color Doppler-assisted duplex imaging (CDDI) failed to detect residual flow through the nearly occluded ICA; ***b*** echo-enhanced CDDI and nonenhanced power flow imaging (***c***) revealed residual flow pattern (modified from [35]).

Overestimation of the Degree of Stenosis in the Middle Range

As previously mentioned, all ultrasound methods tend to overestimate the degree of stenosis in comparison with IA, especially in the 60–80% range. This is an important observation to note because the clinically most important threshold of 70% ICA stenosis lies within this range. The reasons for this are primarily physical, as the ultrasonic criteria rely predominantly on changes in blood flow volume and local area reduction, whereas the angiographic measurements rely on diameter measurements (fig. 5). It is therefore not surprising that, in some studies, the correlation of the degree of stenosis based on ultrasonic measurements and derived from pathoanatomical specimen is better than the correlation with IA [54–56].

Detection of the 'Nearly Occluded' ICA

Clinically, the most common pitfall in neurosonography has always been the diagnosis of ICA occlusion when there is minimal residual blood flow, with percentages of false-positives ranging between 5 and 62% in reported series [17, 57–60]. Compared with Doppler sonography and conventional B-mode imaging, CDDI has already improved the sensitivity for detecting minimal residual blood flow in preocclusive conditions [17, 52, 61]. Enhanced CDDI or PFI go one step further in that they are capable of detecting flow even in the narrowest parts of high-grade ICA stenoses and in the poststenotic flow segment, where flow signal intensities may be below the detection thresholds of nonenhanced CDDI (fig. 6) [35, 53, 62]. In a series of 20 patients with an angiographically proven 'ICA pseudo-occlusion', nonenhanced CDDI revealed a sensitivity of 0.7 and a specificity of 0.92. Under enhanced conditions, these values increased to 0.83 and 0.92, respectively [35]. For PFI, the corresponding accuracy measurements were 0.95 and 0.92 under nonenhanced conditions and 0.94 and 1.0 after the use of a contrast agent, respectively [35]. These results, therefore, clearly show that minimal residual flow in a severely stenosed ICA can be reliably detected by echo-enhanced CDDI and by PFI with or without echo enhancement, but not by nonenhanced CDDI.

Plaque Surface Characteristics

Irregularities and Ulceration

Plaque surface disruption in the ICA, leading to plaque ulceration and intraluminal thrombus formation, is a key stage in the transformation of asymptomatic into symptomatic ICA lesions [63, 64]. Detection of such pathoanatomical features may, therefore, be of clinical relevance. In a pathoanatomical validation study, we compared the ultrasonographic findings of plaque surface ulceration (i.e., plaque niche filled with reversed flow from both a longitudinal and transverse view without aliasing) with the corresponding pathoanatomical findings [65]. Unfortunately, the sonographic diagnosis of ICA plaque ulceration was neither reliable nor valid. Interobserver agreement was only moderate, revealing a κ-value of 0.57, and χ^2-statistics showed no significant link between the ultrasonographic and pathoanatomical findings [65]. In conclusion, plaque surface characteristics cannot be diagnosed from ultrasound examinations with a sufficient degree of accuracy.

Table 3. Diagnostic accuracy of different ultrasonic modalities in detecting internal carotid artery (ICA) occlusion. Accuracy measurements (confidence interval) were derived from a systematic meta-analysis [28]

	Number of arteries	ICA occlusion	
		sensitivity	specificity
B-mode sonography	1,795	0.43 (0.32–0.51)	0.97 (0.96–0.98)
PSV or ΔF measurements	3,574	0.87 (0.78–0.92)	0.97 (0.95–0.98)
CDDI	4,484	0.81 (0.77–0.85)	0.97 (0.86–0.98)

ΔF = Doppler shift frequency; CDDI = color Doppler-assisted duplex imaging; PSV = peak systolic velocity, insonation angle corrected.

Intraluminal Thrombus Formation

Intraluminal thrombus formation is a major precursor of distal arterio-arterial embolization [64]. In some cases, a mobile structure, mostly hypoechoic, can be found at the distal part of an atherosclerotic lesion. This is most probably caused by the tail of an intraluminal thrombus formation, originating from a ruptured plaque surface [66, 67]. Nevertheless, the prevalence of this in symptomatic and asymptomatic patients with high-grade ICA stenosis has not yet been reported. Furthermore, there is some speculation that hypoechoic atherosclerotic plaque is partially composed of thrombotic material, thereby constituting an unstable lesion [68]. At present, the diagnostic accuracy of ultrasound in predicting intraluminal thrombus formation compared with a pathoanatomical standard of reference is still unclear.

Carotid Occlusion

Ultrasonic Criteria

The complete atherosclerotic occlusion of the ICA is ultrasonographically characterized by (1) the absence of detectable flow within the former ICA lumen, (2) the presence of inhomogeneous, calcified material within the former vessel structure, (3) indirect signs of ICA lesions from hemodynamic alterations (see above), and (4) the detection, in almost all cases, of a so-called stump signal directly in front of the occluded segment (fig. 2d) [69]. Using these criteria, ICA occlusion can be diagnosed with a sufficient degree

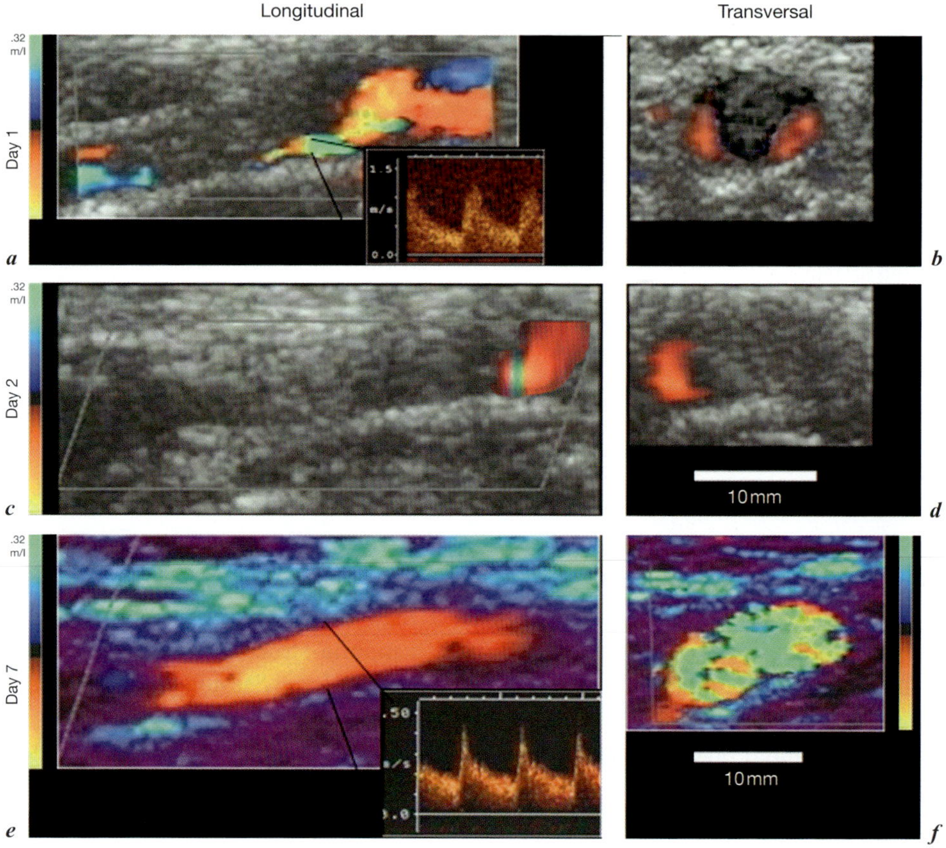

Fig. 7. Color Doppler-assisted duplex imaging of the left extracranial carotid bifurcation in thromboembolic occlusion of the internal carotid artery (ICA) on consecutive days. ***a*** Initial examination on the day of admission revealed hypoechoic material (thromboembolus) within the left carotid bifurcation and the proximal part of the ICA in the longitudinal view (inset of ***a*** shows accelerated Doppler velocities with a peak systolic value of 1.35 m/s, indicating moderate luminal narrowing). ***b*** In the transverse view, color duplex showed only minimal residual flow in both lateral parts of the common carotid artery bifurcation. ***c, d*** Upon a second examination (day 2 after admission), color duplex showed complete thrombotic occlusion of the extracranial portion of the ICA (scale of ***d*** applies to ***a–d***). ***e, f*** A third examination (day 7 after admission) showed complete recanalization of the carotid bifurcation and the proximal part of the ICA (inset of ***e*** shows normalized Doppler velocity spectrum within the recanalized ICA; scale of ***f*** applies to ***e*** and ***f***); blood flow away from the transducer is coded in red to yellow, towards the transducer in blue, and aliasing phenomena in green; numbers at the upper end of the color scales indicate the corresponding blood flow velocity.

of accuracy (table 3). The only moderate sensitivity is mainly attributable to the percentage of false-positive findings that arises because a very low flow in highly stenosed lesions is not always detected (see above). This drawback can be partially overcome through the use of Doppler amplitude-based techniques (PFI) or the use of an ultrasonic contrast agent [35]. On the other hand, false-negative findings (minimal residual flow detected by ultrasound, suggesting high-grade stenosis in cases of angiographically proven ICA occlusion) are mainly caused by the appearance of a vas vasorum arising from the stump [70].

Reliability of Ultrasound Measurements

Interobserver agreement for the diagnosis of ICA occlusion was high using both CDDI and PFI: κ-values were 0.90 for nonenhanced CDDI and 0.93 for nonenhanced PFI respectively [35].

Pitfalls and Limitations

Aplastic Carotid Artery

Aplastic ICA is rarely found in routine clinical examinations and its true prevalence is unknown [71]. It may be difficult to differentiate between carotid occlusion and aplastic ICA. The main criterion for differentiation is that, in ICA occlusion, it is possible to delineate the arterial wall, even behind the perfused segment (fig. 2d), which is not the case in aplastic ICA [71].

Carotid Occlusion Due to Nonatherosclerotic Etiology

ICA occlusion can also be caused by thromboemboli originating from the heart or, as paradoxical emboli, from the venous system (fig. 7) [72, 73]. These lesions can resemble atherosclerotic occlusion, but there are some characteristic differences: (1) the thrombotic mass occluding the ICA is predominantly homogenous and hypoechoic, there is no shadowing resulting from calcifications and (2) the morphology of the lesion changes significantly over time [68, 72, 73]. The case shown in figure 7 suffered from a paradoxical thromboembolism in the proximal ICA, which initially led to a high-grade stenosis, followed by occlusion the day after and complete disappearance one week after symptom onset.

Conclusions

As presented above, ultrasonic techniques can determine both the presence and the degree of atherosclerotic lesions around the ICA bifurcation with a high degree of accuracy. Carried out by experienced sonographers aware of the relevant

a

b

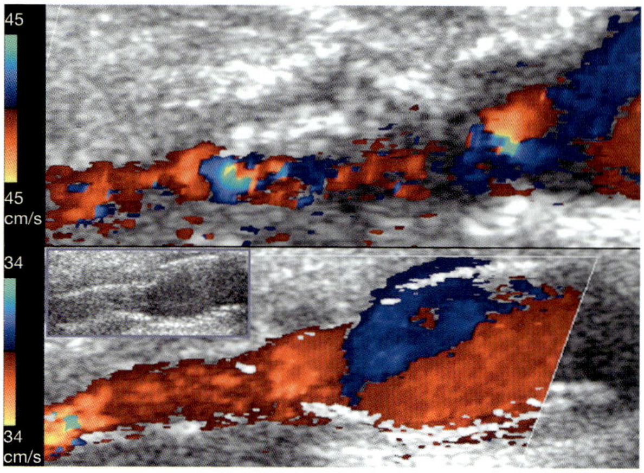

Fig. 8. Color Doppler-assisted duplex imaging of an approximate 80–90% proximal ICA stenosis before (***a***) and after (***b***) percutaneous transluminal angioplasty and stent delivery. Note the ultrasound reflections of the mesh graft at the luminal/intima interface in the inset of ***b*** (B-mode).

limitations and most common pitfalls, noninvasive ultrasound can serve as a screening tool, supply the vascular surgeon or interventionalist with sufficient information for determining treatment, and can be an optimal tool for follow-up examinations. In this context, it will be of importance that ultrasound also facilitates the delineation of blood flow in a stented ICA as shown in figure 8. This will open up the possibility of using cervical ultrasound to detect restenosis after endovascular treatment.

References

1 Fine-Edelstein JS, Wolf PA, O'Leary DH, Poehlman H, Belanger AJ, Kase CS, D'Agostino RB: Precursors of extracranial carotid atherosclerosis in the Framingham Study. Neurology 1994;44: 1046–1050.

2 Sacco R: Ischemic Stroke; in Gorelick P, Alter M (eds): Handbook of Neuroepidemiology. New York/Basel/Hong Kong, Marcel Decker, 1994, pp 77–119.

3 Beneficial effect of carotid endarterectomy in symptomatic patients with high-grade carotid stenosis. North American Symptomatic Carotid Endarterectomy Trial Collaborators. N Engl J Med 1991;325:445–453.

4 Endarterectomy for asymptomatic carotid artery stenosis: Executive Committee for the Asymptomatic Carotid Atherosclerosis Study. JAMA 1995;273:1421–1428.

5 Randomised trial of endarterectomy for recently symptomatic carotid stenosis: Final results of the MRC European Carotid Surgery Trial (ECST). Lancet 1998;351:1379–1387.

6 Halliday A, Mansfield A, Marro J, Peto C, Peto R, Potter J, Thomas D: Prevention of disabling and fatal strokes by successful carotid endarterectomy in patients without recent neurological symptoms: Randomised controlled trial. Lancet 2004;363:1491–1502.

7 Hennerici M, Hulsbomer HB, Hefter H, Lammerts D, Rautenberg W: Natural history of asymptomatic extracranial arterial disease: Results of a long-term prospective study. Brain 1987;110(Pt 3): 777–791.
8 Inzitari D, Eliasziw M, Gates P, Sharpe BL, Chan RK, Meldrum HE, Barnett HJ: The causes and risk of stroke in patients with asymptomatic internal-carotid-artery stenosis: North American Symptomatic Carotid Endarterectomy Trial Collaborators. N Engl J Med 2000;342:1693–1700.
9 Rothwell PM, Eliasziw M, Gutnikov SA, Warlow CP, Barnett HJ: Endarterectomy for symptomatic carotid stenosis in relation to clinical subgroups and timing of surgery. Lancet 2004;363:915–924.
10 Hennerici M, Hulsbomer HB, Rautenberg W, Hefter H: Spontaneous history of asymptomatic internal carotid occlusion. Stroke 1986;17:718–722.
11 Stary HC, Blankenhorn DH, Chandler AB, Glagov S, Insull W Jr, Richardson M, Rosenfeld ME, Schaffer SA, Schwartz CJ, Wagner WD, et al: A definition of the intima of human arteries and of its atherosclerosis-prone regions: A report from the Committee on Vascular Lesions of the Council on Arteriosclerosis, American Heart Association. Circulation 1992;85:391–405.
12 Ross R, Glomset JA: The pathogenesis of atherosclerosis. Part 1. N Engl J Med 1976;295:369–377.
13 Ross R, Glomset JA: The pathogenesis of atherosclerosis. Part 2. N Engl J Med 1976;295:420–425.
14 Stary HC, Chandler AB, Glagov S, Guyton JR, Insull W Jr, Rosenfeld ME, Schaffer SA, Schwartz CJ, Wagner WD, Wissler RW: A definition of initial, fatty streak, and intermediate lesions of atherosclerosis: A report from the Committee on Vascular Lesions of the Council on Arteriosclerosis, American Heart Association. Circulation 1994;89:2462–2478.
15 Trostdorf F, Buchkremer M, Harmjanz A, Kablau M, Jander S, Geiger K, Schmitz-Rixen T, Steinmetz H, Sitzer M: Fibrous cap thickness and smooth muscle cell apoptosis in high-grade carotid artery stenosis. Eur J Vasc Endovasc Surg 2005;29:528–535.
16 Bonithon-Kopp C, Scarabin PY, Taquet A, Touboul PJ, Malmejac A, Guize L: Risk factors for early carotid atherosclerosis in middle-aged French women. Arterioscler Thromb 1991;11:966–972.
17 Sitzer M, Furst G, Fischer H, Siebler M, Fehlings T, Kleinschmidt A, Kahn T, Steinmetz H: Between-method correlation in quantifying internal carotid stenosis. Stroke 1993;24: 1513–1518.
18 Markus HS, Sitzer M, Carrington D, Mendall MA, Steinmetz H: Chlamydia pneumoniae infection and early asymptomatic carotid atherosclerosis. Circulation 1999;100:832–837.
19 North American Symptomatic Carotid Endarterectomy Trial: Methods, patient characteristics, and progress. Stroke 1991;22:711–720.
20 Rothwell PM, Gibson RJ, Slattery J, Sellar RJ, Warlow CP: Equivalence of measurements of carotid stenosis: A comparison of three methods on 1,001 angiograms: European Carotid Surgery Trialists' Collaborative Group. Stroke 1994;25:2435–2439.
21 Toole JF, Castaldo JE: Accurate measurement of carotid stenosis: Chaos in methodology. J Neuroimaging 1994;4:222–230.
22 Wardlaw JM, Lewis S: Carotid stenosis measurement on colour Doppler ultrasound: Agreement of ECST, NASCET and CCA methods applied to ultrasound with intra-arterial angiographic stenosis measurement. Eur J Radiol 2005.
23 Alexandrov AV, Bladin CF, Maggisano R, Norris JW: Measuring carotid stenosis: Time for a reappraisal. Stroke 1993;24:1292–1296.
24 Eliasziw M, Smith RF, Singh N, Holdsworth DW, Fox AJ, Barnett HJ: Further comments on the measurement of carotid stenosis from angiograms: North American Symptomatic Carotid Endarterectomy Trial (NASCET) Group. Stroke 1994;25:2445–2449.
25 Muller HR: The diagnosis of internal carotid artery occlusion by directional Doppler sonography of the ophthalamic artery. Neurology 1972;22:816–823.
26 Barnes RW, Russell HE, Bone GE, Slaymaker EE: Doppler cerebrovascular examination: Improved results with refinements in technique. Stroke 1977;8:468–471.
27 Wise G, Parker J, Burkholder J: Supraorbital Doppler studies, carotid bruits, and arteriography in unilateral ocular or cerebral ischemic disorders. Neurology 1979;29:34–37.
28 Blakeley DD, Oddone EZ, Hasselblad V, Simel DL, Matchar DB: Noninvasive carotid artery testing: A meta-analytic review. Ann Intern Med 1995;122:360–367.
29 Withers CE, Gosink BB, Keightley AM, Casola G, Lee AA, van Sonnenberg E, Rothrock JF, Lyden PD: Duplex carotid sonography. Peak systolic velocity in quantifying internal carotid artery stenosis. J Ultrasound Med 1990;9:345–349.

30 Neale ML, Chambers JL, Kelly AT, Connard S, Lawton MA, Roche J, Appleberg M: Reappraisal of duplex criteria to assess significant carotid stenosis with special reference to reports from the North American Symptomatic Carotid Endarterectomy Trial and the European Carotid Surgery Trial. J Vasc Surg 1994;20:642–649.
31 Browman MW, Cooperberg PL, Harrison PB, Marsh JI, Mallek N: Duplex ultrasonography criteria for internal carotid stenosis of more than 70% diameter: Angiographic correlation and receiver operating characteristic curve analysis. Can Assoc Radiol J 1995;46:291–295.
32 Chen JC, Salvian AJ, Taylor DC, Teal PA, Marotta TR, Hsiang YN: Predictive ability of duplex ultrasonography for internal carotid artery stenosis of 70–99%: A comparative study. Ann Vasc Surg 1998;12:244–247.
33 Jogestrand T, Lindqvist M, Nowak J: Diagnostic performance of duplex ultrasonography in the detection of high grade internal carotid artery stenosis. Eur J Vasc Endovasc Surg 2002;23: 510–518.
34 Grant EG, Benson CB, Moneta GL, Alexandrov AV, Baker JD, Bluth EI, Carroll BA, Eliasziw M, Gocke J, Hertzberg BS, Katanick S, Needleman L, Pellerito J, Polak JF, Rholl KS, Wooster DL, Zierler RE: Carotid artery stenosis: Gray-scale and Doppler US diagnosis – Society of Radiologists in Ultrasound Consensus Conference. Radiology 2003;229:340–346.
35 Furst G, Saleh A, Wenserski F, Malms J, Cohnen M, Aulich A, Neumann-Haefelin T, Schroeter M, Steinmetz H, Sitzer M: Reliability and validity of noninvasive imaging of internal carotid artery pseudo-occlusion. Stroke 1999;30:1444–1449.
36 Busuttil SJ, Franklin DP, Youkey JR, Elmore JR: Carotid duplex overestimation of stenosis due to severe contralateral disease. Am J Surg 1996;172:144–147; discussion 147–148.
37 Henderson RD, Steinman DA, Eliasziw M, Barnett HJ: Effect of contralateral carotid artery stenosis on carotid ultrasound velocity measurements. Stroke 2000;31:2636–2640.
38 Belsky M, Gaitini D, Goldsher D, Hoffman A, Daitzchman M: Color-coded duplex ultrasound compared to CT angiography for detection and quantification of carotid artery stenosis. Eur J Ultrasound 2000;12:49–60.
39 Del Corso L, Moruzzo D, Conte B, Agelli M, Romanelli AM, Pastine F, Protti M, Pentimone F, Baggiani G: Tortuosity, kinking, and coiling of the carotid artery: Expression of atherosclerosis or aging? Angiology 1998;49:361–371.
40 Eliasziw M, Rankin RN, Fox AJ, Haynes RB, Barnett HJ: Accuracy and prognostic consequences of ultrasonography in identifying severe carotid artery stenosis: North American Symptomatic Carotid Endarterectomy Trial (NASCET) Group. Stroke 1995;26:1747–1752.
41 Kassam MS, Cobbold RS, Johnston KW, Graham CM: Method for estimating the Doppler mean velocity waveform. Ultrasound Med Biol 1982;8:537–544.
42 Krause H, Segard M, Carey P, Bernstein EF, Fronek A: Doppler power frequency spectrum analysis in the diagnosis of carotid artery disease. Stroke 1984;15:351–358.
43 Blackshear WM, Phillips DJ, Chikos PM, Harley JD, Thiele BL, Strandness DE Jr: Carotid artery velocity patterns in normal and stenotic vessels. Stroke 1980;11:67–71.
44 Grant EG, Duerinckx AJ, El Saden SM, Melany ML, Hathout GM, Zimmerman PT, Marumoto AK, Cohen SN, Baker JD: Ability to use duplex US to quantify internal carotid arterial stenoses: Fact or fiction? Radiology 2000;214:247–252.
45 Moneta GL, Edwards JM, Chitwood RW, Taylor LM Jr, Lee RW, Cummings CA, Porter JM: Correlation of North American Symptomatic Carotid Endarterectomy Trial (NASCET) angiographic definition of 70% to 99% internal carotid artery stenosis with duplex scanning. J Vasc Surg 1993;17:152–157; discussion 157–159.
46 Ranke C, Creutzig A, Becker H, Trappe HJ: Standardization of carotid ultrasound: A hemodynamic method to normalize for interindividual and interequipment variability. Stroke 1999;30: 402–406.
47 Spencer MP, Reid JM: Quantitation of carotid stenosis with continuous-wave (C-W) Doppler ultrasound. Stroke 1979;10:326–330.
48 Polak JF, Dobkin GR, O'Leary DH, Wang AM, Cutler SS: Internal carotid artery stenosis: Accuracy and reproducibility of color-Doppler-assisted duplex imaging. Radiology 1989;173: 793–798.
49 Thomson H, Woods AE, Iannos J, Sage M: The inter-sonographer reliability of carotid duplex ultrasound. Australas Radiol 2001;45:19–24.

50 Fillinger MF, Baker RJ Jr, Zwolak RM, Musson A, Lenz JE, Mott J, Bech FR, Walsh DB, Cronenwett JL: Carotid duplex criteria for a 60% or greater angiographic stenosis: Variation according to equipment. J Vasc Surg 1996;24:856–864.

51 Erickson SJ, Mewissen MW, Foley WD, Lawson TL, Middleton WD, Quiroz FA, Macrander SJ, Lipchik EO: Stenosis of the internal carotid artery: Assessment using color Doppler imaging compared with angiography. AJR Am J Roentgenol 1989;152:1299–1305.

52 Steinke W, Hennerici M, Rautenberg W, Mohr JP: Symptomatic and asymptomatic high-grade carotid stenoses in Doppler color-flow imaging. Neurology 1992;42:131–138.

53 Sitzer M, Furst G, Siebler M, Steinmetz H: Usefulness of an intravenous contrast medium in the characterization of high-grade internal carotid stenosis with color Doppler-assisted duplex imaging. Stroke 1994;25:385–389.

54 Bladin CF, Alexandrov AV, Murphy J, Maggisano R, Norris JW: Carotid stenosis index: A new method of measuring internal carotid artery Stenosis. Stroke 1995;26:230–234.

55 Eckstein HH, Winter R, Eichbaum M, Klemm K, Schumacher H, Dorfler A, Schulte K, Neuwirth A, Gross W, Schnabel P, Allenberg JR: Grading of internal carotid artery stenosis: Validation of Doppler/duplex ultrasound criteria and angiography against endarterectomy specimen. Eur J Vasc Endovasc Surg 2001;21:301–310.

56 Grant EG, Benson CB, Moneta GL, Alexandrov AV, Baker JD, Bluth EI, Carroll BA, Eliasziw M, Gocke J, Hertzberg BS, Katarick S, Needleman L, Pellerito J, Polak JF, Rholl KS, Wooster DL, Zierler E: Carotid artery stenosis: Grayscale and Doppler ultrasound diagnosis – Society of Radiologists in Ultrasound consensus conference. Ultrasound Q 2003;19:190–198.

57 Trockel U, Hennerici M, Aulich A, Sandmann W: The superiority of combined continuous wave Doppler examination over periorbital Doppler for the detection of extracranial carotid disease. J Neurol Neurosurg Psychiatry 1984;47:43–50.

58 Comerota AJ, Cranley JJ, Cook SE: Real-time B-mode carotid imaging in diagnosis of cerebrovascular disease. Surgery 1981;89:718–729.

59 Ackroyd N, Lane R, Dart L, Appleberg M: Colour-coded carotid Doppler imaging: An angiographic comparison of 324 bifurcations. Aust NZ J Surg 1984;54:509–517.

60 Ricotta JJ, Bryan FA, Bond MG, Kurtz A, O'Leary DH, Raines JK, Berson AS, Clouse ME, Calderon-Ortiz M, Toole JF, et al: Multicenter validation study of real-time (B-mode) ultrasound, arteriography, and pathologic examination. J Vasc Surg 1987;6:512–520.

61 Kessler C, von Maravic C, von Maravic M, Kompf D: Colour Doppler flow imaging of the carotid arteries. Neuroradiology 1991;33:114–117.

62 Berman SS, Devine JJ, Erdoes LS, Hunter GC: Distinguishing carotid artery pseudo-occlusion with color-flow Doppler. Stroke 1995;26:434–438.

63 Ogata J, Masuda J, Yutani C, Yamaguchi T: Rupture of atheromatous plaque as a cause of thrombotic occlusion of stenotic internal carotid artery. Stroke 1990;21:1740–1745.

64 Sitzer M, Muller W, Siebler M, Hort W, Kniemeyer HW, Jancke L, Steinmetz H: Plaque ulceration and lumen thrombus are the main sources of cerebral microemboli in high-grade internal carotid artery stenosis. Stroke 1995;26:1231–1233.

65 Sitzer M, Muller W, Rademacher J, Siebler M, Hort W, Kniemeyer HW, Steinmetz H: Color-flow Doppler-assisted duplex imaging fails to detect ulceration in high-grade internal carotid artery stenosis. J Vasc Surg 1996;23:461–465.

66 Tonizzo M, Fisicaro M, Bussani R, Bollini M, Da Col PG, Fonda M, Cattin L: Carotid atherosclerosis: Echographic patterns versus histological findings. Int Angiol 1994;13:208–214.

67 Stewart J, Gover J, Tridgell D, Frawley J: A mobile lesion in the carotid artery. Aust NZ J Surg 1996;66:639–641.

68 Biasi GM, Sampaolo A, Mingazzini P, De Amicis P, El-Barghouty N, Nicolaides AN: Computer analysis of ultrasonic plaque echolucency in identifying high risk carotid bifurcation lesions. Eur J Vasc Endovasc Surg 1999;17:476–479.

69 AbuRahma AF, Pollack JA, Robinson PA, Mullins D: The reliability of color duplex ultrasound in diagnosing total carotid artery occlusion. Am J Surg 1997;174:185–187.

70 Kemeny V, Droste DW, Nabavi DG, Schulte-Altedorneburg G, Schuierer G, Ringelstein EB: Collateralization of an occluded internal carotid artery via a vas vasorum. Stroke 1998;29: 521–523.

71 Grand CM, Louryan S, Bank WO, Baleriaux D, Brotchi J, Raybaud C: Agenesis of the internal carotid artery and cavernous sinus hypoplasia with contralateral cavernous sinus meningioma. Neuroradiology 1993;35:588–590.
72 Yonemura K, Kimura K, Yonemitsu M, Hashimoto Y, Uchino M: The intravascular mobile structure detected by duplex carotid ultrasonography in cardioembolic internal carotid artery occlusion. Rinsho Shinkeigaku 1996;36:1125–1128.
73 Kimura K, Yasaka M, Minematsu K, Wada K, Uchino M, Yonemura K, Ogata J, Yamaguchi T: Oscillating thromboemboli within the extracranial internal carotid artery demonstrated by ultrasonography in patients with acute cardioembolic stroke. Ultrasound Med Biol 1998;24: 1121–1124.

Matthias Sitzer, MD
Department of Neurology
Centre for Neurology and Neurosurgery
Johann Wolfgang Goethe-University
Schleusenweg 2–16
DE–60528 Frankfurt am Main (Germany)
Tel. +49 69 6301 5942, Fax +49 69 6301 6842, E-Mail sitzer@em.uni-frankfurt.de

Baumgartner RW (ed): Handbook on Neurovascular Ultrasound.
Front Neurol Neurosci. Basel, Karger, 2006, vol 21, pp 57–69

Ultrasound Diagnostics of the Vertebrobasilar System

Hans-Christian von Büdingen[a], *Thomas Staudacher*[b], *Hans Joachim von Büdingen*[b]

[a]Universitätsspital Zürich, Neurologische Klinik und Poliklinik, Zürich, Switzerland; [b]Krankenhaus St. Elisabeth der Oberschwabenklinik GmbH, Abteilung für Neurologie und klinische Neurophysiologie mit regionalem Schlaganfall-Schwerpunkt, Ravensburg, Germany

Abstract

Despite the fact that ischemic stroke in the vertebrobasilar system (VBS) is significantly less frequent than in the carotid system, abnormalities found in Doppler and duplex examinations are about as prevalent in the VBS as in the carotid system. Because of the potentially severe clinical deficits associated with stroke of the VBS and the increased risk for stroke under conditions, such as underlying symptomatic vertebrobasilar stenosis and general anesthesia, it is highly desirable to have reliable methods available to identify pathological changes of the VBS. Furthermore, because the VBS via the circle of Willis can play a significant role as collateral blood supply system when vessels of the anterior circulation have been compromised, the knowledge of the VBS is necessary to estimate the overall integrity of the remaining blood flow to the brain.

In the hands of a well-trained and experienced sonographer, the diagnosis of alterations in the vertebral (VA) and basilar arteries (BA) by ultrasound can help determine noninvasively the etiology of symptomatic VA or BA disease. However, not all parts of the posterior cerebral circulation are easily accessible by ultrasound, which is why both direct and indirect signs of stenosis or occlusion must be interpreted correctly to obtain relevant findings. Nowadays duplex sonography has evolved to a point where, by integrating Doppler examination and information, it is superior to Doppler sonography itself. Nevertheless, in situations where only Doppler equipment is available or applicable, knowing the technique and its limitations, it is reliably possible to evaluate the integrity of the

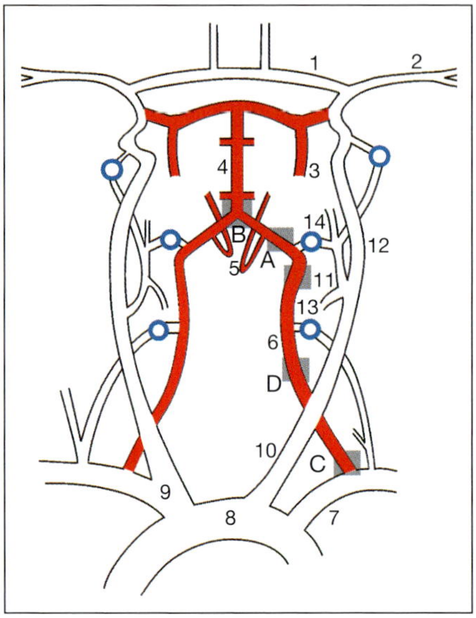

Fig. 1. Schematic of the main vessels of the cerebral circulation. Vessels of the posterior circulation are filled in red. Collaterals to the vertebro-basilar system are shown as blue circles. Gray squares (A–D) refer to arterial segments shown in figures 2, 3, 5. 1 = Anterior cerebral artery, ACA; 2 = middle cerebral artery, MCA; 3 = posterior cerebral artery, PCA; 4 = basilar artery, BA; 5 = posterior inferior cerebellar artery, PICA; 6 = vertebral artery, VA; 7 = subclavian artery, SA; 8 = aortic arch; 9 = brachiocephalic trunk; 10 = common carotid artery, CCA; 11 = external carotid artery (ECA) and branches; 12 = internal carotid artery, ICA; 13 = anastomoses between the cervical arteries and the VA; 14 = anastomosis between occipital arteries and the VA (modified from [1]).

blood flow in the posterior cerebral circulation. This chapter is intended to provide the necessary anatomical basis of the VBS along with ultrasound techniques and findings in healthy and common pathological conditions. Figure 1 is a diagram of the main vessels of the anterior and posterior circulation and provides an overview of the insonation points depicted in the following examples and figures.

Anatomy of the VBS

The clinical relevance of the posterior cerebral circulation is based on its role as the sole blood supply to the brainstem and cerebellum as well as major blood supply to the thalamus and occipital cortex. A number of well-defined clinical syndromes stem from disruption of arterial blood flow in sections of the VBS. The posterior cerebral circulation includes the proximal subclavian arteries (SA), VA, BA, and the posterior cerebral arteries (PCA) as well as the smaller blood vessels that originate from these.

Vertebral Artery

The VA are the first branches off the SA (fig. 1, No. 7), though in approximately 4% of people the left VA has its origin (V0) from the arch of aorta, which is even much less frequent for the right VA. The prevertebral section of the VA (V1) is defined as reaching from the SA to where it enters the spine through the costotransversal foramina of the 6th (90%) or 5th (5%) vertebrae. The pars transversaria of the VA (V2) is the section from the end of the V1 to the exit from the foramen of the transverse process of the second cervical vertebra. From there, the V3 segment, also referred to as the 'atlas-loop', initially winds posteriorly for about 1 cm past the lateral mass of the atlas in sagittal direction, then medially in the VA sulcus of the atlas. Muscular branches going off from this portion of the VA form anastomoses (fig. 1, No. 14) with the occipital artery from the external carotid artery. Posteromedial to the atlanto-occipital joint, the intracranial section of the VA (V4) pierces through the posterior atlanto-occipital membrane, the dura mater and the arachnoid. After entering the subarachnoid space, the VA continues between the brainstem and the clivus to unite with the opposite VA, usually at the caudal border of the pons. The inner diameter of the VA is on average 3.5 mm (1.5–5 mm). In most individuals the diameters of the VA are different, with the left VA usually being of greater diameter. Hypoplasia (diameter <2 mm) of one VA is found in less than 10%. Hypoplastic VA have lower flow velocities and a higher pulsatility than normoplastic VA. It may be difficult to differentiate a hypoplastic VA with slow diastolic velocities and a missed V4 segment from an intracranial V4 occlusion after the origin of the posterior inferior cerebellar artery (PICA), which often causes in the preocclusion VA slow flow velocities with increased pulsatility and a shrinking of the vessel lumen. Furthermore, transforaminal insonation, especially when performed in the sitting position, may show an undulating flow in the hypoplastic VA.

The first brain-supplying branch off the VA is the inferior posterior cerebellar artery (fig. 1, No. 5), which in its course and prominence is highly variable. The PICA sends off branches to the brainstem and cerebellum. A hypoplastic VA may end as PICA, leaving the opposite VA as the only one, sometimes without any connection to the contralateral VA.

Basilar Artery

From the union of both VA, the BA usually runs straight between the clivus and brainstem, and terminates by dividing into the PCA. Its average length is 30 mm (21–41 mm), its average inner diameter is 3 mm (2.5–3.5 mm). Branches off the BA include the anterior inferior cerebellar artery and the superior cerebellar artery. The superior cerebellar artery leaves the BA near its termination.

In less than 1% the BA arises from the primitive trigeminal artery, which originates from the internal carotid artery (ICA). In these cases often both VA are 'hypoplastic'.

Posterior Cerebral Artery

Anatomically and functionally the PCA (fig. 1, No. 3) defines the boundary between the carotid and vertebral arterial systems. Phylo- and ontogenetically the posterior communicating artery (PCoA) and the postcommunicating (P2) PCA and its branches are derived from the carotid artery, whereas its connection with the BA, the precommunicating (P1) PCA, establishes later during development. In about 10–30% of adults the PCA persists to arise directly from the ICA. In such cases ICA stenoses can be responsible for ischemia in the PCA territory. P1 PCA [average diameter 2.1 mm (0.7–3.0 mm)] runs anterolaterally for 5–10 mm to the PCoA, whereas the subsequent P2 PCA [average diameter 2.3 mm (1.3–3.0 mm)] winds laterally and posteriorly around the cerebral peduncle.

Posterior Communicating Artery

The PCoA runs anteriorly and slightly laterally to connect the PCA with the ICA. It shows significant variations in its development. In 22% of cases it is hypoplastic, and may even be aplastic on one side (1%). Rare cases may even present with bilateral aplasia of the PCoA. Its caliber is inversely proportional to that of the P1 segment of the ipsilateral PCA. The average length of the PCoA is 14 mm (8–18 mm) and the average diameter is 1.2 mm (0.5–3.25 mm).

Circle of Willis

The circle of Willis is the most important intracranial collateral system as it connects both carotid systems with each other and the VBS.

Doppler- and Duplex Sonography of the Extracranial Segments of the VBS

Vertebral Artery

To obtain relevant information on the integrity of the VA, it must be examined both at its origin (V0) and at the atlas loop (V3). Insonation of the *V0 segment*, where stenoses are frequently located, is performed in the supraclavicular fossa with the ultrasound probe pointing in caudal and slightly ventral direction. Since other arteries besides the VA (common carotid artery (CCA), inferior thyroid artery, and proximal SA) may be in the probe's focus at this position, the VA must be identified by oscillating compression (fig. 4, 5) of the ipsilateral atlas loop. Placing the index or middle finger between the tip of the mastoid and the transverse processus of the atlas while having the probe positioned in the supraclavicular fossa, an increasing and oscillating pressure can be applied to the atlas loop. This compression leads to an unmistakable signal modulation, which especially in diastole can reach or typically go beyond the baseline of the Doppler spectrum. However, one always has to keep in mind, that this compression may have an, although much less pronounced, effect on the flow in the CCA. Thus a comparison between CCA and VA during compression of the V3 segment is warranted.

Once the VA has been identified, it should be followed in a caudal direction until signals of the SA and CCA are found. A clear separation of which signal is VA and which is SA or CCA can be obtained by compression of the atlas loop and brachial artery, respectively.

Insonation of the *V1 segment* can be achieved by cranial orientation of the probe. However, stenoses are rare in this segment, which is why analysis of the V0 segment is preferred.

The *V2 segment* – in contrast to duplex sonography – is almost inaccessible to Doppler sonography. But especially in younger individuals it is important to follow the entire course of the VA because of dissections which may be located in the V2 segment.

The *V3 segment* of the VA (fig. 2) is accessible to ultrasound by placing the probe near the tip of the mastoid with slight anterior and rostral orientation pointing between the contralateral ear and eye. In this orientation physiological flow in the VA is directed away from the probe; however, it is possible to mistake the signal of a dorsally running ICA with the VA. Thus, to be sure of the VA insonation, the probe can be tilted slightly downwards to obtain a flow direction towards the probe in the near-horizontal section of the VA, just after its exit from the foramen of the transverse process of the axis. To successfully achieve this maneuver, the probe may also have to be slid slightly caudally and may have to be turned into a caudal medial or even slightly caudal dorsal orientation.

In contrast to Doppler sonography, duplex sonography can be applied to visualize the intervertebral portions of the V2 segment (fig. 1, D). Thus, duplex examination of the VA is usually started by insonation of the V2 segment. Here the inner diameter of the VA can be reliably measured. The origin (V0 segment) of the VA can be found either by sliding the duplex probe down from the V2 segment along the V1 segment or by looking at a longitudinal trans-section of

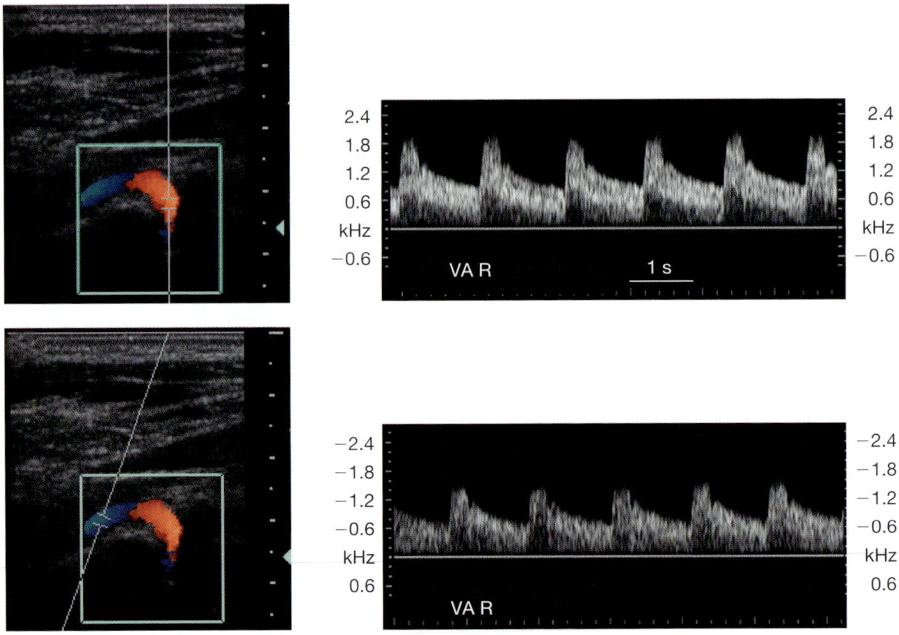

Fig. 2. Color-coded duplex sonography of a normal right V3 segment (atlas loop). In the upper panel the Doppler sample volume is placed in the proximal part of the atlas loop (also see position A in fig. 1) with flow directed towards the probe. In the lower panel the flow is directed away from the probe with the sample volume is located in the more distal part of the atlas loop.

the SA. If, for example, the VA originates from the medial face of the bend of the SA or from the apex of the SA, its origin will be visible in the trans-secting plane. Measures of flow velocity in the VA are, due to a near-ideal angle of insonation, best performed in the atlas loop of the VA.

Subclavian Artery

Insonation of the SA is performed with the tip of the probe located in the supraclavicular fossa pointing in a caudal lateral direction. Flow away from the probe and marked reduction of systolic flow velocity under compression of the ipsilateral brachial artery are characteristics that will permit unequivocal identification of the SA. With the probe pointing in caudal medial direction, flow towards the probe will be detectable in the proximal portion of the SA.

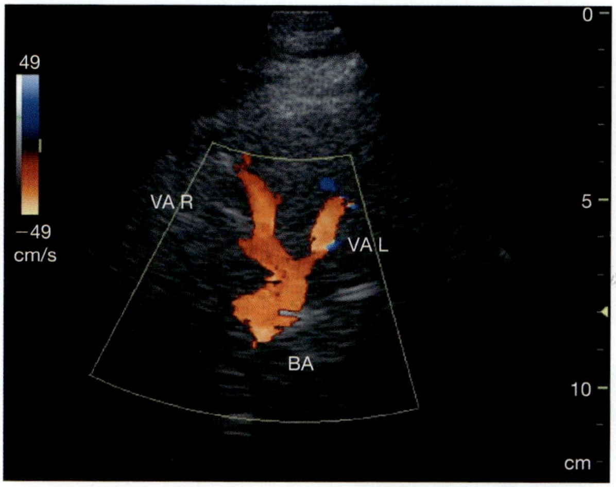

Fig. 3. Color-coded duplex sonography of the intracranial (V4) segment of both vertebral arteries and the proximal part of the basilar artery using transnuchal (transforaminal) insonation. The scale on the right picture border gives the insonation depth in centimeters (also see position B in fig. 1).

Doppler- and Duplex Sonography of the Intracranial Segments of the VBS

The *V4 segment* of the VA (fig. 1, 3) and the proximal segment of the BA can be examined by transnuchal insonation through the foramen magnum by placing the probe in the midline between the occipital bone and the atlas on a person with inclined head position. In ‘blind-mode’ Doppler sonography, the VA can be followed starting from a depth of 50–60 mm. Under normal circumstances it is difficult to differentiate the VA from the BA. Normally, in an examination depth of 70–110 mm, no significant change in flow velocity can be noted, and a slight increase in flow velocity may be due to an increasingly ideal favorable angle of insonation [2]. However, one pathological circumstance allows for a clear discrimination between the two VA: High-grade stenosis or occlusion of the proximal SA with vertebrovertebral steal effect leads to antegrade flow in one VA and retrograde flow in the other VA (fig. 4). The identification of the BA in this situation follows the rule that it must have a flow pattern that differs from that of either VA, which will also permit the identification of the BA origin. In most cases anterograde flow in the BA will be preserved, even when a vertebrovertebral steal is encountered. However, it has to be taken into consideration that with subclavian steal from the VA, flow in the BA manifests as incomplete (systolic deceleration of flow velocity as shown in figure 4, or

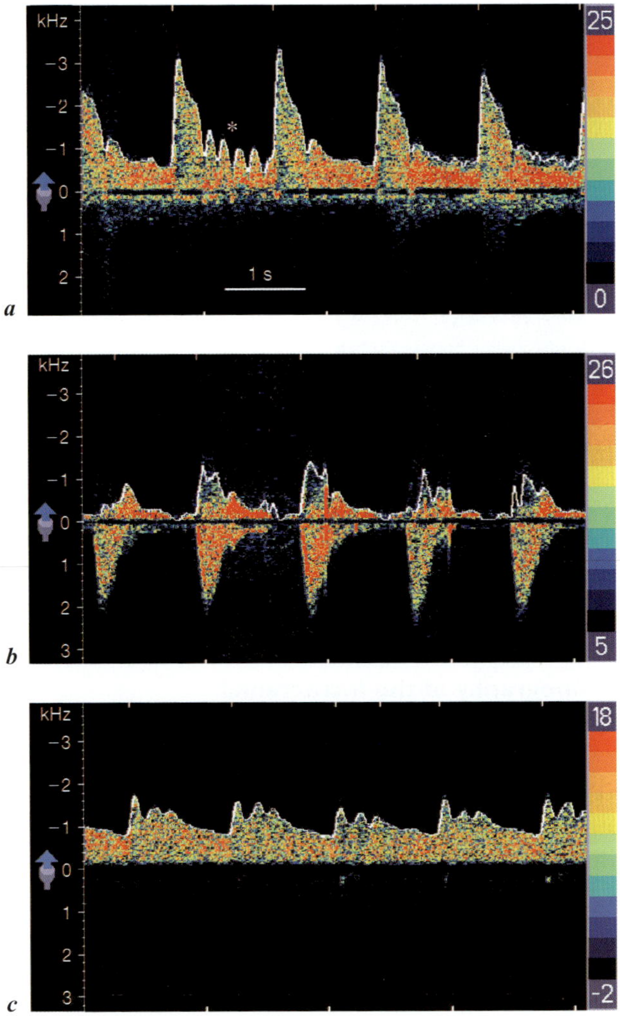

Fig. 4. Doppler spectra of the vertebral and basilar arteries in occlusion of the left proximal subclavian with complete subclavian steal effect. Retrograde flow in the left vertebral artery (***b***), systolic deceleration of flow velocity in the basilar artery (***c***). The antegrade flow velocities in the feeding right vertebral artery (***a***) are determined by the flow resistances of the brain and the left arm. Note flow disturbances (*) due to oscillating compression of the left atlas loop for identification of the ipsilateral vertebral artery.

alternating flow direction) or complete steal effect in ~50% of cases [1]. Very rarely retrograde flow can be observed in the BA [3]. Based on experience and published reports [4–7], by pulsed-wave Doppler sonography the origin of the BA can be expected at a depth of 70–110 mm.

In contrast to transcranial Doppler sonography, transcranial color-coded duplex sonography allows for a clear discrimination between the two VA (fig. 3). For duplex sonography of the distal V3 and V4 segments of the VA as well as the BA, the initial B-picture depth can be set at 100 mm, with the probe producing a transverse to coronal trans-section. The V4 segments can be identified in the foramen magnum, with flow direction away from the probe. In a depth of approximately 70 mm, the VA unite to form the BA which can often be followed up to a depth of about 100 mm, its middle third. The V3 segments of the VA can be visualized by tilting the probe slightly in caudal orientation and will present with flow towards, and then away, from the probe.

Ultrasonographic Findings in Disease of the VBS

A prototypic arterial vessel disease most frequently leading to abnormal ultrasound findings in the posterior circulation is a severe stenosis or occlusion of the proximal SA, leading to the so-called 'subclavian steal effect' or 'subclavian steal phenomenon' [8]. It may cause symptoms and signs of hemodynamic vertebrobasilar ischemia (subclavian steal syndrome) in a few percent of patients [9], and is most frequently due to atherosclerotic disease. Distinct alterations in posterior circulation blood flow permit diagnosis of a subclavian steal effect by ultrasound techniques [10]. If no other arterial occlusions are present, the following features characterize the subclavian steal:

- Depending on the degree of SA stenosis, initially the flow velocity in the ipsilateral VA is reduced with a systolic deceleration of the flow velocity in the Doppler spectrum. When the stenosis progresses, an alternating blood flow can be observed in the ipsilateral VA until, finally at occlusion of the proximal SA, the VA blood flow is completely reversed (fig. 4b).
- Reduced retrograde flow (or retrograde flow components, respectively) in the ipsilateral VA during compression of the ipsilateral brachial artery at the upper arm.
- Accelerated flow velocity in the contralateral VA, due to the greater blood volume required for brain *and* arm supply.
- Monophasic Doppler spectrum in the distal SA in the presence of severe stenosis or occlusion of the SA.

Clinically relevant pathological alterations of the VBS must be differentiated from normal variants such as hypoplasia of the VA. A difference in VA

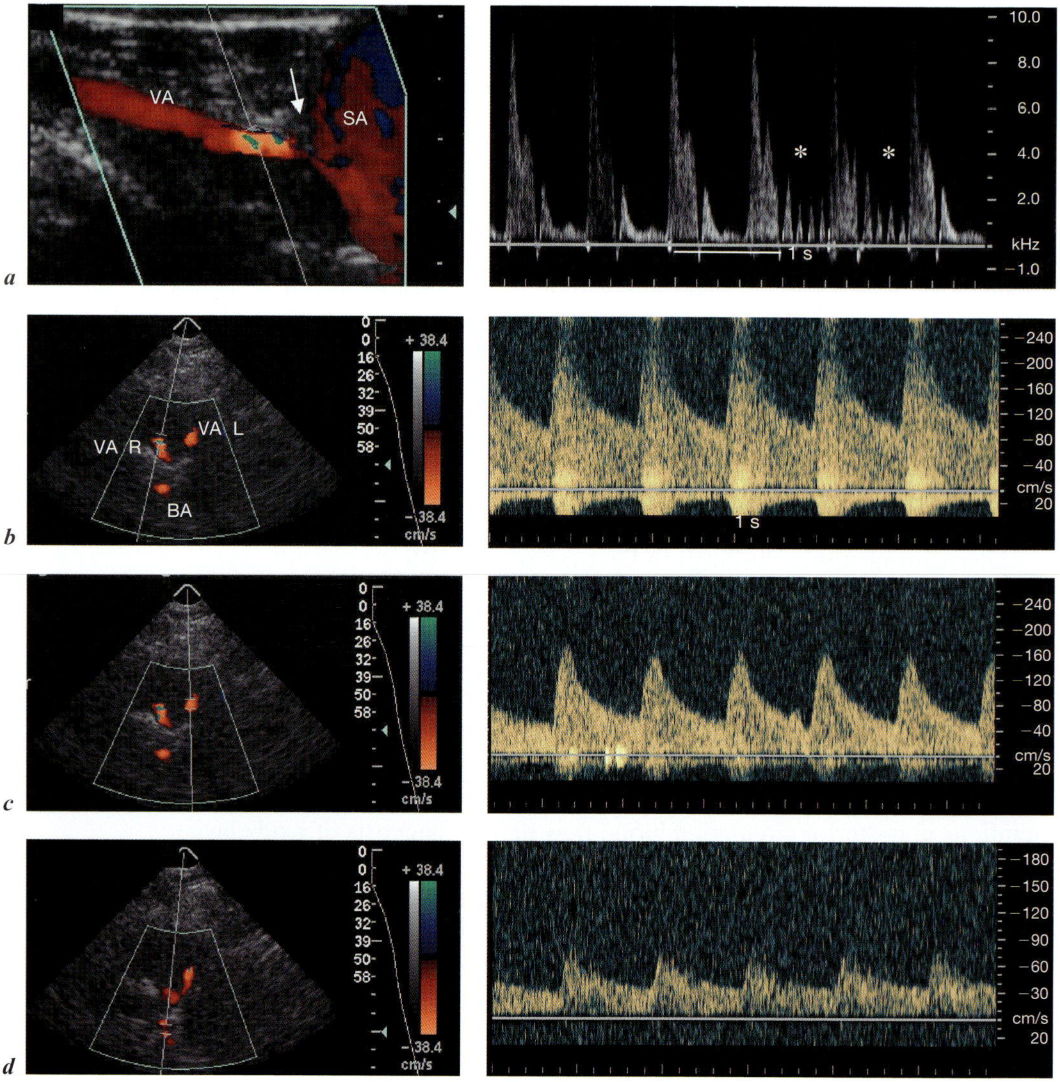

Fig. 5. Color-coded duplex sonography of vertebral artery stenoses. ***a*** Stenosis (white arrow) of the origin of the left VA (V0 segment). In the Doppler spectra note flow disturbances (*) due to oscillating compression of the left atlas loop for identification of the ipsilateral vertebral artery (also see position C in fig. 1). ***b–d*** Transnuchal investigation of a stenosis of the right vertebral artery (V4 segment). Slightly increased flow velocity in the contralateral (left) vertebral artery and 'normal' flow in the basilar artery, (also see position B in fig. 1).

Table 1. Common ultrasound findings in disease of the vertebrobasilar system

Condition	Localization	Ultrasound findings in the VA	
		ipsilateral	contralateral
Hypoplasia	V0–V4	reduced (diastolic) flow velocity, reduced diameter < 2.0 mm), can be difficult to identify	increased diameter (except A. trigemina primitiva), flow velocity in the normal range
Stenosis	extracranial, V0	increased flow velocity in stenosis, poststenotic flow alterations, poststenotic reduced flow velocity and pulsatility, evidence of cervical collaterals	increased flow velocity (severe stenosis)
	intracranial	direct detection via Doppler or Duplex sonography, reduced extracranial diastolic flow velocity	increased flow velocity (severe stenosis)
Occlusion	extracranial, mostly V0–V2	missing flow signal in the VA, postocclusive reduced flow velocity and pulsatility, possible alternating flow, collaterals in V2 and V3 detectable	increased flow velocity
	intracranial proximal to PICA	reduced flow velocity and missing diastolic flow in V0–V3, retrograde blood flow distal to occlusion to supply the PICA	increased flow velocity
	intracranial distal to PICA	reduced flow velocity with preserved diastolic flow	increased flow velocity

PICA = Posterior inferior cerebellar artery; VA = vertebral artery.

caliber can frequently be found, with the left VA usually being of greater diameter [11, 12]. Certain criteria, such as flow volume <30–40 ml/min or diameter <2 mm, may be used to determine whether or not a hypoplastic VA is present [11–13]; however, there is no current consensus on the definition of VA hypoplasia. It has to be kept in mind that differences in the flow signal between both VA are not a safe criteria for a stenosis of the VA, neither extra- nor intracranially.

Stenoses and occlusions of the VA are mostly found at the origin (V0 segment, fig. 5a) or the intracranial (V4) segment [14] (fig. 5b), loops are frequently detectable along the course of the VA, dissections appear in declining frequency in V3, V2, V1 segments, the extracranial parts of the VA are rarely affected in giant cell arteritis and may show typical B-mode findings (see the chapter by Schmidt, pp. 96–104). Patients with occlusion, and rarely severe stenosis of proximal (V0 or V1) VA, develop cervical collaterals, which enter V2 or V3 and lead to undulating or antegrade flow in V4. Cervical collaterals connect the VA with the costocervical and thyrocervical trunks as well as the occipital artery. The aforementioned collaterals show an increased vessel diameter, which allows their detection by ultrasonography.

Table 1 is intended to provide a quick overview on pathological conditions of the VA (hypoplasia, stenosis, occlusion) along with the ultrasonographic findings that are to be expected. Additionally, recent work by Saito et al. [15] provide helpful diagnostic criteria for detecting VA occlusions.

Criteria for assessing VA dissection are discussed in the chapter by Benninger and Baumgartner, pp. 70–84, and those for diagnosing stenoses and occlusions of the intracranial VA, BA, and PCA are discussed in the chapter by Baumgartner, pp. 117–126.

References

1 von Büdingen HJ, Staudacher T: Evaluation of vertebrobasilar disease; in Newell DW, Aaslid R (eds): Transcranial Doppler. New York, Raven Press, 1992, pp 167–195.

2 von Reutern GM, von Büdingen HJ: Ultrasound Diagnosis of Cerebrovascular Disease: Doppler Sonography of the Extra- and Intracranial Arteries, Duplex Scanning. Stuttgart, New York, Thieme, 1993.

3 Klingelhofer J, Conrad B, Benecke R, Frank B: Transcranial Doppler ultrasonography of carotid-basilar collateral circulation in subclavian steal. Stroke 1988;19:1036–1042.

4 Budingen HJ, Staudacher T: Identification of the basilar artery with transcranial Doppler sonography. Ultraschall Med 1987;8:95–101.

5 Budingen HJ, Staudacher T, Stoeter P: Subclavian steal: Transcranial Doppler sonography of the basilar artery. Ultraschall Med 1987;8:218–225.

6 Lindegaard KF, Bakke SJ, Aaslid R, Nornes H: Doppler diagnosis of intracranial artery occlusive disorders. J Neurol Neurosurg Psychiatry 1986;49:510–518.

7 Ringelstein EB, Wulfinghoff F, Bruckmann H, Zeumer H, Hacke W, Buchner H: Transcranial Doppler sonography as a non-invasive guide for the transvascular treatment of an inoperable basilar-artery aneurysm. Neurol Res 1985;7:171–176.

8 Contorni L: The vertebro-vertebral collateral circulation in obliteration of the subclavian artery at its origin. Minerva Chir 1960;15:268–271.

9 Ackermann H, Diener HC, Dichgans J: Stenosis and occlusion of the subclavian artery: Ultrasonographic and clinical findings. J Neurol 1987;234:396–400.

10 von Reutern GM, Budingen HJ: Doppler sonographic study of the vertebral artery in subclavian steal syndrome. Dtsch Med Wochenschr 1977;102:140–141.

11 Seidel E, Eicke BM, Tettenborn B, Krummenauer F: Reference values for vertebral artery flow volume by duplex sonography in young and elderly adults. Stroke 1999;30:2692–2696.

12 Touboul PJ, Bousser MG, LaPlane D, Castaigne P: Duplex scanning of normal vertebral arteries. Stroke 1986;17:921–923.

13 Schoning M, Walter J, Scheel P: Estimation of cerebral blood flow through color duplex sonography of the carotid and vertebral arteries in healthy adults. Stroke 1994;25:17–22.
14 Caplan LR, Wityk RJ, Glass TA, Tapia J, Pazdera L, Chang HM, et al: New England Medical Center Posterior Circulation registry. Ann Neurol 2004;56:389–398.
15 Saito K, Kimura K, Nagatsuka K, Nagano K, Minematsu K, Ueno S, et al: Vertebral artery occlusion in duplex color-coded ultrasonography. Stroke 2004;35:1068–1072.

Dr. Hans-Christian von Büdingen
Department of Neurology, University Hospital
Frauenklinikstrasse 26
CH–8091 Zürich (Switzerland)
Tel. +41 1 255 9782, Fax +41 1 255 4380, E-Mail hc.vonbuedingen@usz.ch

Baumgartner RW (ed): Handbook on Neurovascular Ultrasound.
Front Neurol Neurosci. Basel, Karger, 2006, vol 21, pp 70–84

Ultrasound Diagnosis of Cervical Artery Dissection

D.H. Benninger, Ralf W. Baumgartner

Department of Neurology, University Hospital, Zürich, Switzerland

Abstract

Ultrasound allows the reliable exclusion of spontaneous dissection of the cervical internal carotid artery (sICAD) in patients with carotid territory ischemia. The possibility of falsely positive ultrasound findings indicates that cervical magnetic resonance imaging (MRI) and angiography must confirm ultrasonic suspicion of sICAD. The sensitivity of ultrasound for assessing sICAD which causes no carotid territory ischemia, but headache, neck pain, Horner syndrome, or palsy of the cranial nerves on the side of dissection is about 70%, and for identifying spontaneous dissection of the vertebral artery (sVAD) the sensitivity is 75–86%. The negative predictive value and specificity for ultrasound diagnosis of the latter two types of cervical artery dissection is unknown. Consequently, all patients with clinical suspicion of sICAD causing no ischemic event or sVAD should undergo cervical MRI and angiography. Ultrasound is useful for noninvasive monitoring of vessel recanalization and for determining the duration of antithrombotic therapy.

This chapter will present the examination technique, typical findings, diagnostic pitfalls, follow-up investigation, and the impact of ultrasound findings on the management of patient with spontaneous cervical artery dissection.

Examination Technique of the Anterior Cerebral Circulation

The exploration of the anterior cerebral circulation includes the investigation of (1) the extracranial common, internal, and external carotid artery (chapter by Sitzer, pp. 36–56), (2) the carotid siphon and the ophthalmic artery (OphA) using the orbital window (chapter by Baumgartner, pp. 105–116), and (3) the basal cerebral arteries using the temporal window (chapters by Baumgartner, pp. 105–116 and pp. 117–126). It is mandatory to investigate also the cervical portion of the internal carotid artery (ICA), because spontaneous cervical internal carotid artery dissection (sICAD) may lead to a stenosis with an increased flow velocity in the cervical ICA and normal Doppler spectra at the origin. We routinely insonate also the horizontal segment of the pars petrosa of the ICA using axial and coronal planes [1], because the detection of flow signals allows to distinguish sICAD, causing subtotal stenosis from those leading to carotid occlusion. Furthermore, sICAD may rarely cause increased flow velocity in the pars petrosa, whereas the extracranial ICA shows normal findings.

The proximal portion of the cervical ICA is investigated with high-frequency (4–8 MHz) linear transducers, which enable color Doppler sonography and B-mode imaging of the vessel wall. In the distal portion of the cervical ICA, however, the distance between the vessel and the ultrasound probe progressively increases. Consequently, the examination is performed with low-frequency (1.8–3.6 MHz) sector (or Doppler) probes, which have a lower resolution for color Doppler and B-mode imaging compared to linear probes. Thus, the wall of the distal cervical ICA usually cannot be assessed with B-mode imaging.

B-Mode and Color Doppler Imaging Findings in Acute sICAD

Patients with sICAD have no or at best mild atherosclerosis of the cerebral arteries [2–10]. B-mode and color Doppler imaging may visualize abnormalities in the cervical ICA, suggesting the presence of a dissection, which include a thickened and mainly hypoechogenic vessel wall, an intimal flap, or a pseudoaneurysm (table 1) [4, 6, 11]. In contrast to atherosclerotic carotid artery disease, luminal narrowing and thickening of the wall in patients with sICAD begin distal to the carotid bifurcation and extend over a longer distance (fig. 1) [3]. These ultrasound findings are in accordance with the results of cervical magnetic resonance imaging (MRI), which showed no involvement of the carotid bifurcation by the wall hematoma or the adjacent thrombus [3]. A thickened vessel wall was detected in 25% of an unpublished series of 200 patients with sICAD. The low detection rate is probably due to the fact, as mentioned in 'examination technique', that only the proximal part of the cervical ICA can be studied with high-frequency linear transducers, whereas mural hematomas can be located exclusively in the less-accessible distal part of the vessel. The thickened wall is composed of the hematoma and intraluminal thrombus [4, 6]. Although both portions of the wall cannot be reliably differentiated by color duplex sonography (CDS), the presence of an intima reflex may allow the reliable distinction of the wall hematoma (fig. 1) [4, 6, 8, 9, 12]. The intimal flap is a flat and hyperechogenic structure bordering the presumed intramural

Table 1. Color duplex ultrasound findings in 181 patients with 200 spontaneous carotid dissections with and without ischemic events

	Ischemia (n = 145) [n (%)]	No ischemia (n = 55) [n (%)]	All (n = 200) [n (%)]
Atherosclerotic carotid artery plaque	13 (9)	2 (4)	15 (8)
Cervical ICA			
Vessel wall thickened and hypoechogenic	36 (25)	12 (22)	48 (24)
Second lumen	3 (2)	1 (2)	4 (2)
Dissecting aneurysm	1/10 (10)†	0/7 (0)‡	1/17 (6)#
Normal hemodynamics	7 (5)**	16 (29)**	24 (12)
Stenosis			
≤50%	7 (5)*	9 (16)*	16 (8)
51–80%	10 (7)	8 (15)	18 (9)
>80% or occlusion	120 (83)**	22 (40)**	142 (71)
Intracranial stenosis or occlusion[δ]	43 (30)	2 (4)	45 (23)
Median latency (range) from symptom onset to ultrasonography	2 (0–90) days	10 (0–125) days	10 (0–125) days

ICA = Internal carotid artery.

†10 of 101 dissections showed an aneurysm at catheter or magnetic resonance angiography (MRA).

‡7 of 44 dissections showed an aneurysm at catheter or MRA.

#17 of 145 dissections showed an aneurysm at catheter or MRA.

*/**$p < 0.01/p < 0.0001$ that the difference between carotid dissections with and without ischemia is significant (Wilcoxon signed-rank test).

[δ]Middle and anterior cerebral arteries.

hematoma, floating in the lumen or separating the two lumina with different Doppler signals [4, 7–10, 12, 13]. An aortic dissection extending in the carotid arteries is typically associated with an intimal flap separating the false from the true vessel lumen, which typically show two different flow patterns at spectral Doppler sonography. Conversely, an intimal flap as well as a perfused false lumen are rare findings in sICAD (table 1). An intimal flap must be distinguished from the wall of the adjacent jugular vein. Ultrasound rarely visualizes a pseudoaneurysm [3]. The low detection rate is probably due to the fact that the aneurysms are often located in the depth of the neck and must thus be investigated with low-frequency transducers. In addition, it is difficult to reliably distinguish ICA redundancies of the cervical ICA from an aneurysm.

The above-mentioned B-mode and color Doppler findings have not yet been validated by a standard of reference, such as MRI and MR angiography (MRA). Thus, diagnosis of sICAD is mainly established by hemodynamical criteria such as the delineation of a stenosis or occlusion in the cervical ICA.

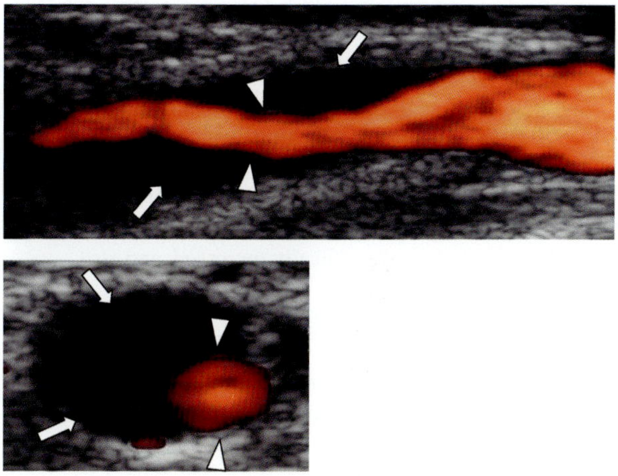

a

b

Fig. 1. Color duplex sonography (power Doppler imaging) with longitudinal (*a*) and axial (*b*) planes shows a spontaneous dissection of the cervical internal carotid artery. Luminal narrowing and the hypoechogenic and thickened vessel wall (white arrows) begin distal to the carotid bulb. The unequivocal depiction of the border between the vessel wall and the lumen including the presence of an intimal reflex (arrowheads) suggests that mural thickening is mainly due to a wall hematoma and not an intraluminal thrombus.

Spectral Doppler Findings in Acute sICAD

The sensitivity of the combined use of extracranial Doppler and duplex sonography and transcranial Doppler sonography (TCD) for diagnosis of sICAD has been reported to be 95–100% [4, 9, 10, 13] and the sensitivity of combined extra- and transcranial CDS for detecting sICAD to be 91% [3]. The corresponding diagnostic criteria are mentioned in table 2. Using the same diagnostic criteria, a recent prospective study investigated the accuracy of CDS to diagnose sICAD in patients with first-time occurrence of carotid territory ischemia [14]. Consecutive patients with first-time occurrence carotid territory stroke, transient ischemic attack (TIA), or retinal ischemia underwent clinical and laboratory examinations, electrocardiography (ECG), CDS of the cerebral arteries, cranial CT in case of stroke or transient ischemic attack (TIA), and echocardiography and 24-h ECG in selected cases. Patients were included in the study, if they were (1) <65 years of age, and (2) CDS showed a probable sICAD (cervical ICA stenosed or occluded) or had no determined etiology of ischemia. All included patients underwent cervical MRI and MRA, with or without cerebral catheter angiography, and the sonographer was blinded to the results of MRI and angiography studies. Out of 1,652 patients who were screened the authors included 177 in the study. Excluded patients (n = 1,475)

Table 2. Color duplex ultrasound criteria for diagnosis of stenosis and occlusion in cervical internal carotid artery dissection

Stenosis	
≤50%	Intrastenotic PSV >90 cm/s in women[†], >80 cm/s in men[†], and PSV quotient of intrastenotic ICA/contralateral cervical ICA >1.12
51–80%	Intrastenotic PSV >120 cm/s and PSV quotient of intrastenotic ICA/CCA on the side of carotid dissection >1.5
>80%	Intrastenotic flow velocities decreased or focally increased, and at least two of the following three criteria (1) Resistance index[‡] quotient of ipsilateral CCA/contralateral CCA >0.15 (2) Reversed flow in the ipsilateral ophthalmic artery (3) Cross-flow through the anterior communicating artery
Occlusion	No flow at color and spectral Doppler, no pulsatile wall motion, and at least two of the following three criteria (1) Resistance index[‡] quotient of ipsilateral CCA/contralateral CCA >0.15 (2) Reversed flow in the ipsilateral ophthalmic artery (3) Cross-flow through the anterior communicating artery

PSV = Peak systolic velocity; ICA = internal carotid artery; CCA = common carotid artery.

[†]Each reference value is higher than the PSV mean value plus 3 standard deviations of healthy volunteers.

[‡]Resistance index = (peak systolic velocity – peak diastolic velocity)/peak systolic velocity

were ≥65 years old (n = 818) and had another determined cause of ischemia (n = 1,485) and intracranial hemorrhage (n = 58). CDS diagnosed sICAD in 77 of 177 patients, while the etiology of ischemia was undetermined in the remaining 100 patients. Cervical MRI and angiography showed 74 sICAD; there were 6 false-positive and 3 false-negative CDS findings. Thus, sensitivity for CDS diagnosis of patients with sICAD causing carotid territory ischemia was 96%, specificity 94%, positive predictive value 92%, and negative predictive value 97%. These findings suggest that CDS allows the reliable exclusion of sICAD in patients with carotid territory ischemia, whereas diagnosis of sICAD must be confirmed with cervical MRI and MRA.

In contrast, a stenosis or occlusion of the cervical ICA was found in just 71% of sICAD, causing no ischemic event [3]. The latter sICADs either presented with local symptoms and signs, such as headache or neck pain, Horner syndrome, or cranial nerve palsy, on the side of the dissection or were clinically asymptomatic [3]. These CDS findings also suggest that most patients with suspicion of sICAD, causing carotid territory ischemia, have a stenosis or

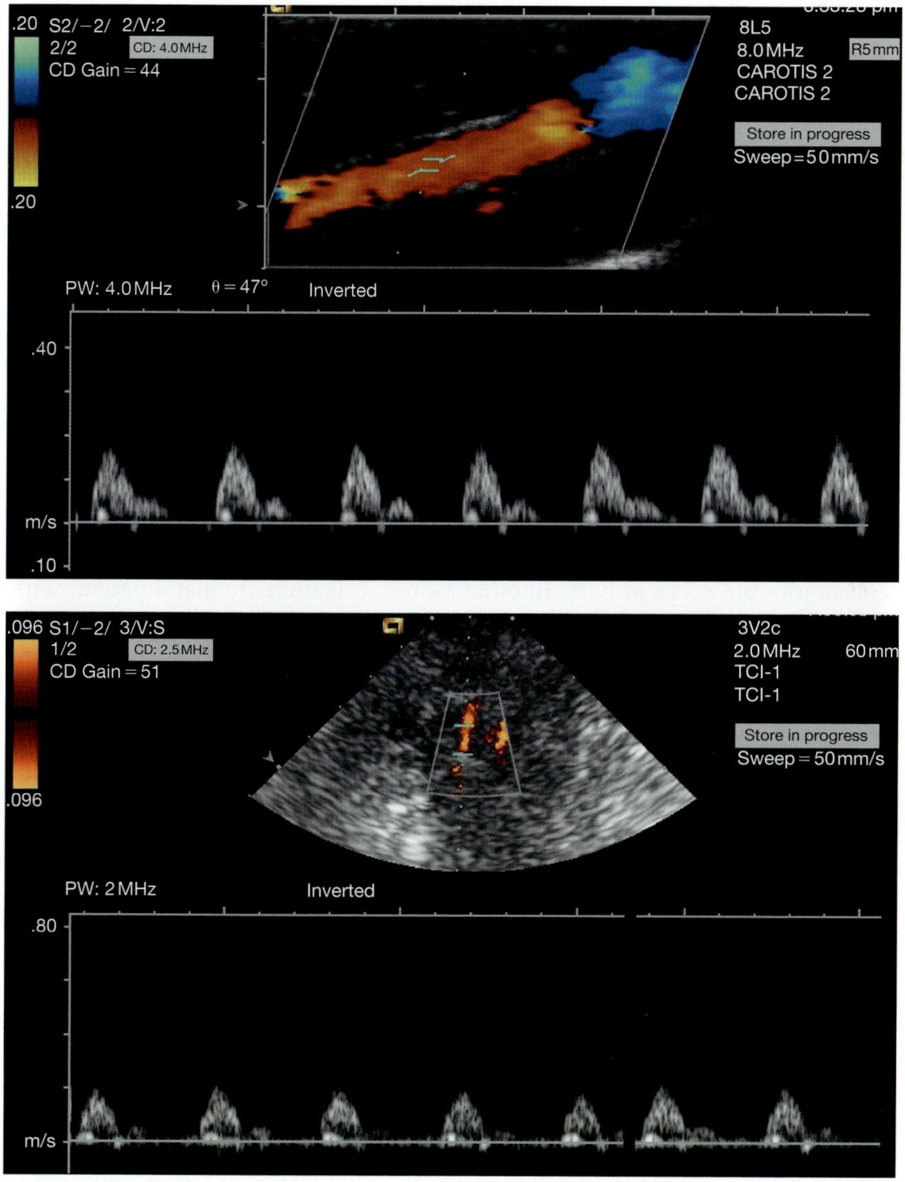

a

b

Fig. 2. Color duplex sonography with longitudinal planes of a spontaneous dissection of the cervical internal carotid artery causing a >80% stenosis shows the carotid bulb and the proximal cervical segment (***a***; linear transducer) and the distal cervical segment prior to the entry in the skull base (***b***; sector scan; power Doppler imaging). Spectral analysis depicts slow systolic and absent end-diastolic velocities, suggesting that carotid stenosis is >80% and long.

Table 3. Color duplex ultrasound findings in 135 patients with 142 spontaneous carotid dissections, causing >80% stenosis or occlusion

	n (%)
Cervical internal carotid artery	
Stenosis	
Intrastenotic flow velocity	
Increased	14 (10)
Decreased	51 (36)
Occlusion	77 (54)
Cross-flow through	
Anterior communicating artery	111 (78)
Posterior communicating artery	75 (53)
Anterior and/or posterior communicating artery	136 (96)
Ophthalmic artery	72 (51)

occlusion in the cervical ICA. In other words, it is unlikely that a patient with carotid territory ischemia and normal cervical ICA findings suffers from sICAD. Thus, it has become our policy that these patients first undergo a search for another cause of carotid territory ischemia. If the latter investigations do not identify the etiology of ischemia, cervical MRI and MRA may be performed.

In contrast to atherosclerotic stenoses of the carotid and other cerebral arteries, >80% stenoses of the cervical ICA lead more often to decreased than increased intrastenotic flow velocities (fig. 2, table 3) [unpubl. data], which is an accordance with the results of previous studies [5]. Decreased intrastenotic flow velocities are according to the law of Hagen-Poiseuille due to the fact that stenoses are much longer in sICAD compared to atherosclerotic disease (fig. 3). Therefore, for diagnosis of >80% stenoses, pre- and poststenotic hemodynamic criteria mentioned in table 2 must be fulfilled.

Pitfalls in Ultrasound Diagnosis of sICAD

As mentioned before, diagnosis of sICAD causing stenosis is based on hemodynamic criteria. Therefore, diseases causing no or mild atherosclerosis and increased or decreased flow velocities in the cervical ICA may lead to the ultrasonic misdiagnosis of sICAD, and are discussed below.

(1) Increased flow velocities in the cervical ICA may result either from a stenosis or a disease with increased blood flow. *Redundancies of the cervical ICA* such as kinking, coiling, and looping may mimic ≤50% stenosis, and it is

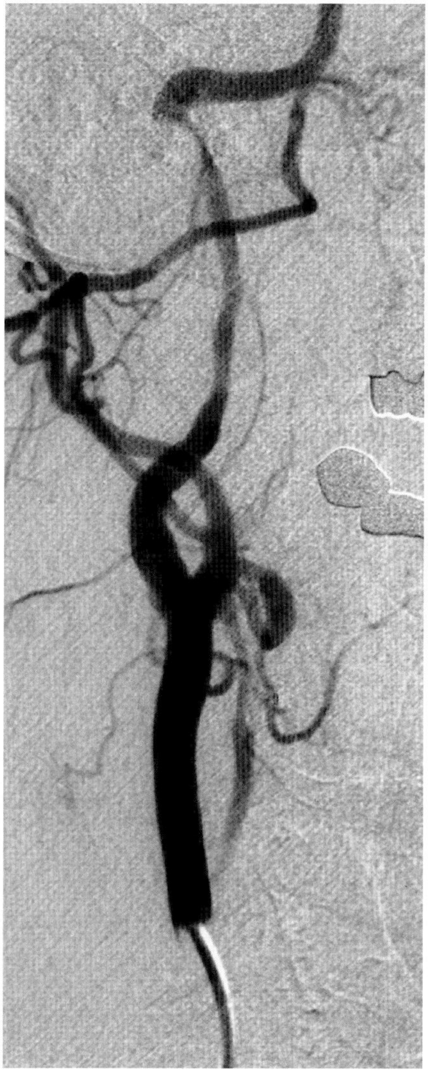

Fig. 3. Catheter angiography of the common carotid artery in antero-posterior projection shows a spontaneous dissection of the cervical internal carotid artery beginning a few centimeters after the origin and ending just beyond the base of the skull with a severe stenosis.

impossible to differentiate whether raised flow velocity in a redundant artery results from the redundancy itself or an additional stenosis. The high prevalence of redundancies in patients with sICAD [15, 16] is an important cause of false-positive ultrasound findings. *Fibromuscular dysplasia* (FMD) may narrow the cervical ICA. In rare cases, CDS depicts irregular stenoses and aneurysmal dilatations ('string of beads') associated with FMD [17–20]. *Vasospasm* is a rare etiology of transient cervical ICA stenosis [21]. Increased blood flow and flow velocities (and sometimes also vessel diameter) in the cervical ICA may be observed in *large* (diameter >4 mm) *arteriovenous-malformations of the brain* [22] and *carotid-cavernous fistulas* [23, 24]. Another cause of increased blood flow and flow velocities in the ICA is a *persistent primitive trigeminal artery*, which connects the intracranial ICA with the basilar artery (BA). The additional presence of hypoplastic vertebral arteries (VA) and direct visualization of the persistent primitive vessel by transcranial CDS may indicate the diagnosis, which must be confirmed by MRA. Tachycardia and increased blood flow and flow velocities in all vessels, including the cerebral arteries, may be observed in anemia and hyperthyreosis.

(2) Decreased flow velocities in the cervical ICA may occur in *severe stenosis or occlusion of the intracranial ICA or MCA*. Patients with occlusion of the lower carotid siphon show slow flow velocities without a diastolic component in the cervical ICA, and in most cases reversed flow direction in the homolateral OphA. Patients with severe intracranial carotid stenosis or occlusion located distal to the origin of the OphA, or M1 MCA occlusion typically present with decreased flow velocities and a preserved diastolic component in the ipsilateral cervical ICA. The antegrade flow direction in the OphA will indicate that carotid obstruction is located in the upper siphon or C1 ICA. Nevertheless, it is not possible to decide in the above-mentioned cases, whether the decreased flow velocities in the cervical ICA are due to the intracranial obstruction alone or the intracranial obstruction and an associated sICAD.

Angiographic findings observed in occlusive sICAD are nonspecific, and the same applies to ultrasound.

We observed in 2 (0.3%) of 315 consecutive patients with 344 sICAD a hypoechogenic wall thickening of the vessel wall, which extended into the carotid bulb, and in one case even to carotid bifurcation [unpubl. observations]. Ultrasound did not allow for the differentiation of the thickening from an atherothrombotic plaque.

Follow-Up Investigation in sICAD

Recanalization of the obstructed ICA results from the resorption of the wall hematoma and resolution of the intraluminal thrombus. Doppler sonography showed recanalization in 34 (68%) of 50 sICAD after an average time interval of 51 days [9]. In another investigation, sICAD recanalization was observed in 63% of 43 patients, whereas occlusion persisted in 37% [10]. We found less favourable data in 188 cases of sICAD examined one year after symptoms onset: complete recanalization was present in 59%, a ≤50% stenosis in 9%,

Table 4. Color duplex ultrasound findings at presentation and 1-year follow-up in 200 spontaneous carotid dissections†

	Presentation (n = 200) [n (%)]	Follow-up (n = 188) [n (%)]
Atherosclerotic carotid artery plaque	15 (8)	19 (10)
Cervical ICA		
Vessel wall thickened and hypoechogenic	48 (24)	0
Second lumen	4 (2)	0
Dissecting aneurysm	1/17 (6)	1/17 (6)
Normal	24 (12)	110 (59)
Stenosis		
≤50%	16 (8)	17 (9)
51–80%	18 (9)	3 (2)
81–99%	75 (38)	17 (9)
Occlusion	77 (34)	41 (22)
Intracranial stenosis or occlusion‡	45 (23)	0

ICA = Internal carotid artery.

†200 dissections occurred in 181 patients; ultrasonic follow-up was obtained in 188 carotid dissections, because 3 dissections had caused letal strokes, 3 dissections had no follow-up, and 6 dissections were excluded for other reasons (thrombolytic therapy for acute stroke, surgical, or endovascular therapy of the dissected carotid artery).

‡Middle and anterior cerebral arteries.

a 51–80% stenosis in 2%, a 81–99% stenosis in 9%, and an occlusion in 22% (table 4) [unpubl. data].

Examination Technique of the Posterior Cerebral Circulation

The examination of the posterior cerebral circulation is described in detail in the chapter by von Büdingen et al., pp. 57–69, and the foramen occipitale magnum window is specially discussed in the chapter by Baumgartner, pp. 105–116. In brief, the investigation of the extracranial VA includes the insonation of the origin (V0), the prevertebral part (V1), the pars transversaria (V2), and the atlas loop (V3). Transforaminal (transnuchal) insonation allows the unequivocal identification of both VA and the distinction of the V3 from the intracranial (V4) segment. Both VA join and form the BA at an insonation depth of 70–71 mm [25, 26]. The BA can often be followed up to the top, located at insonation depth of up to 110 mm. Sagittal insonation planes may prove useful, when the VA and BA are not clearly identified in the axial plane.

Linear probes are used to assess the V0, V1, and V2 segments of the right VA, and the V1 and V2 segments of the left VA, whereas the investigation of V3 may be difficult. Conversely, most left V0 and V1 segments, the V4 segment, and the BA are insonated with sector (or Doppler) probes. Spontaneous dissection of the vertebral artery (sVAD) can affect all segments of the VA [27–32]. Thus, B-mode and color Doppler imaging will detect wall abnormalities, mainly in the right V0 and V1, both V2, and eventually both V3 segments. Conversely, wall abnormalities in the remaining parts of the VA are rarely depicted.

B-Mode and Color Doppler Imaging Findings in Acute sVAD

Imaging abnormalities, which may be detected in patients with sVAD, include an irregular stenosis, a thickened, hypo- or isoechogenic vessel wall (fig. 4), a dissecting membrane, a true and false lumen, a pseudoaneurysm, and a tapering stenosis with distal occlusion [27, 29]. Touboul et al. [32] described the combination of local increase in vessel diameter with hemodynamic signs of stenosis or occlusion at the same level and decreased pulsatility and presence of intravascular echoes in the enlarged vessel as typical findings. A subsequent study using extracranial CDS and TCD observed these signs in 2 of 11 (18%) extracranial sVAD.

Spectral Doppler Findings in Acute sVAD

Pathological hemodynamic findings observed in patients with acute sVAD are nonspecific, and just their location in the V2 or V3 segment, which is rarely affected by atherosclerotic vascular disease, suggests that a dissection might be the underlying cause. The sensitivity of pathological hemodynamics for diagnosis of sVAD has been examined in small monocentric series, including up to 20 patients with 24 sVAD; MRI and angiography were used as standard of reference [27–29, 31, 32]. Sensitivity for detecting patients with extracranial sVAD was 75% in a study examining 20 cases with CDS [27], and 86% in 7 patients examined with extracranial CDS and continuous-wave Doppler, and TCD [28]. The sensitivity for detecting patients with extra- and intracranial sVAD was 86% in 14 patients insonated with extracranial pulsed-wave Doppler and duplex sonography and TCD [31]. The sensitivity for detecting intracranial sVAD was 100% in 9 patients examined with extracranial CDS and continuous-wave Doppler, and TCD [28]. No study has investigated the specificity, positive and negative predictive values of ultrasound assessment of sVAD.

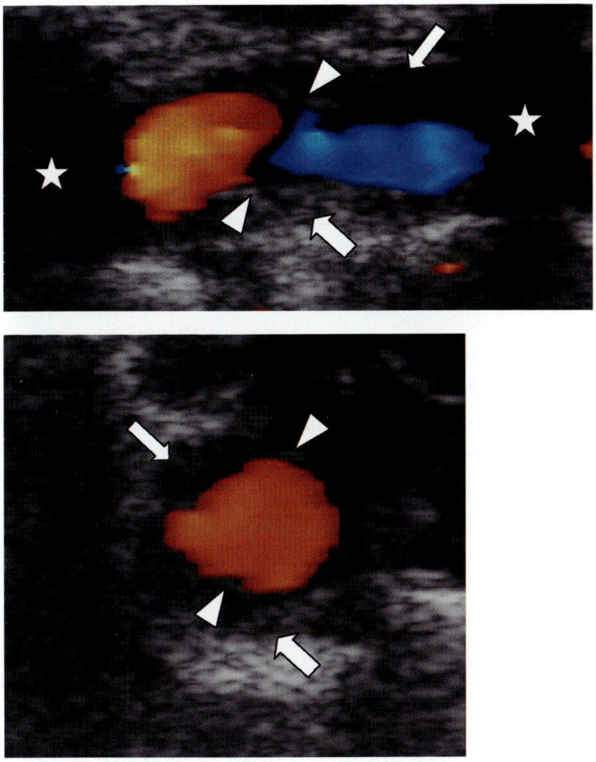

a

b

Fig. 4. Color duplex sonography with longitudinal (***a***) and axial (***b***) scanning planes shows the pars transversaria (V2) of a spontaneously dissected vertebral artery. The thickened hypo- and isoechogenic wall (white arrows) narrows the vessel lumen. The clear depiction of the boundary between the vessel wall and the lumen, including the presence of an intima reflex (arrowheads), insinuates that the mural thickening is mainly due to the wall hematoma and not an intraluminal thrombus. The white stars indicate the position of the transverses processes.

The hemodynamic criteria used for diagnosis of VA stenosis and occlusion in patients with sVAD and atherosclerotic VA disease are identical, although they vary somewhat between different authors [27–36]. VA stenosis is defined by a focal increase of flow velocity, and a severe stenosis leads to intrastenotic, bi-directional, low frequency and high-intensity Doppler signals, as well as prestenotic (increased resistance index) and poststenotic (decreased resistance index) hemodynamic abnormalities [28]. However, a severe stenosis extending over several centimeters may also cause decreased intrastenotic flow velocities [unpubl. data]. In VA occlusion there are neither intraluminal spectral and color Doppler signals nor wall motion during the heart cycle, and B-mode imaging may disclose intraluminal echoes resulting from the fresh thrombus [27–36]. Occlusion of the proximal (V0 or V1) VA is regularly associated with cervical collaterals, which enter V2 or V3 and lead to undulating or antegrade flow in V4 [34, 36]. Occlusion of V4 before the origin of the posterior inferior cerebellar artery (PICA) is associated with abnormally slow systolic, but no diastolic flow velocities, and often reversal of flow direction is found in the distal V4, which irrigates the PICA [28, 33–35]. Occlusion of V4 located distal to the origin of the PICA is associated with slow systolic and slow, but preserved, diastolic flow velocities, whereas the distal V4 is not detected by transforaminal insonation [28, 33–35]. Occlusion of V3 may lead to the same pre- and postocclusional hemodynamic findings, as in occlusion of V4 before the origin of the PICA, or the whole V4 may show a high-resistance profile with no diastolic flow velocities and reversed flow direction [unpubl. data].

Pitfalls of Ultrasound Diagnosis of Acute sVAD

It may be difficult to differentiate V4 occlusion from VA hypoplasia. A hypoplastic VA shows slow systolic and diastolic flow velocities, and may disclose undulating flow in the V4 segment. The connection with the BA will be absent in a hypoplastic VA, which ends in the PICA [37]. The differentiation from a V4 occlusion is feasible by detection of a small vessel diameter, the preserved diastolic velocities in preocclusional VA, and reversed flow in postocclusional VA in case of VA occlusion located proximal to the origin of the PICA. Nevertheless, the diagnosis of sVAD in a hypoplastic vessel is difficult, especially when the occlusion is located distal to the origin of the PICA.

Follow-Up Investigation in sVAD

There are few available data about recanalization of sVAD. Recanalization of extracranial sVAD, causing stenosis, was reported in 8 of 10 (80%) cases, and in 2 of 7 (29%) occlusions after a mean follow-up of 8 months [27]. Another investigation found recanalization of the obstructed sVAD in 3 of 6 (50%) extracranial stenoses and 1 of 3 (33%) extracranial occlusions [28].

Recanalization of intracranial sVAD causing stenosis was observed in 6 of 11 (55%) cases, and in 1 of 3 (33%) occlusions [28].

References

1 Baumgartner RW, Mattle HP, Aaslid R: Transcranial color-coded duplex sonography, magnetic resonance angiography, and computed tomography angiography: Methods, applications, advantages, and limitations. J Clin Ultrasound 1995;23:89–111.

2 Houser OW, Mokri B, Sundt TMJ, Baker HL, Reese DF: Spontaneous cervical cephalic arterial dissection and its residuum: Angiographic spectrum. AJNR Am J Neuroradiol 1984;5:27–34.

3 Baumgartner RW, Arnold M, Baumgartner I, Mosso M, Gönner F, Studer A, Schroth G, Schuknecht B, Sturzenegger M: Carotid dissection with and without ischemic events: Local symptoms and cerebral artery findings. Neurology 2001;57:827–832.

4 de Bray JM, Lhoste P, Dubas F, Emile J, Saumet JL: Ultrasonic features of extracranial carotid dissections: 47 cases studied by angiography. J Ultrasound Med 1994;13:659–664.

5 Hennerici M, Steinke W, Rautenberg W: High resistance flow pattern in extracranial carotid artery dissection. Arch Neurol 1989;46:670–672.

6 Logason K, Hardemark HG, Barlin T, Bergqvist D, Ahlstom H, Karacagil S: Duplex scan findings in patients with spontaneous cervical artery dissections. Eur J Vasc Endovasc Surg 2002;23:295–298.

7 Mullges W, Ringelstein EB, Leibold M: Non-invasive diagnosis of internal carotid artery dissections. J Neurol Neurosurg Psychiatry 1992;55:98–104.

8 Sidhu PS, Jonker ND, Khaw KT, Patel N, Blomley MJ, Chaudhuri KR, Frackowiak RS, Cosgrove DO: Spontaneous dissections of the internal carotid artery: Appearances on colour Doppler ultrasound. Br J Radiol 1997;70:50–57.

9 Steinke W, Rautenberg W, Schwartz A, Hennerici M: Noninvasive monitoring of internal carotid artery dissection. Stroke 1994;25:998–1005.

10 Sturzenegger M, Mattle HP, Rivoir A, Baumgartner RW: Ultrasound findings in carotid artery dissection: Analysis of 43 patients. Neurology 1995;45:691–698.

11 Sturzenegger M: Spontaneous internal carotid artery dissection. Early diagnosis and management in 44 patients. J Neurol 1995;242:231–238.

12 Clevert DA, Rupp N, Reiser M, Jung EM: Improved diagnosis of vascular dissection by ultrasound B-flow: A comparison with color-coded Doppler and power Doppler sonography. Eur Radiol 2005;151:342–347.

13 Treiman GS, Treiman RL, Foran RF, Levin PM, Cohen JL, Wagner WH, Cossmann DV: Spontaneous dissection of the internal carotid artery: A nineteen-year clinical experience. J Vasc Surg 1996;24:597–607.

14 Benninger DH, Georgiadis D, Gandjour J, Baumgartner RW: Accuracy of color duplex ultrasound diagnosis of spontaneous carotid dissection causing ischemia. Stroke 2006;37:377–381.

15 Barbour PJ, Castaldo JE, Rae-Grant AD, Gee W, Reed JF 3rd, Jenny D, Longennecker J: Internal carotid artery redundancy is significantly associated with dissection. Stroke 1994;25:1201–1206.

16 Ozdoba C, Sturzenegger M, Schroth G: Internal carotid artery dissection: MR imaging features and clinical-radiologic correlation. Radiology 1996;199:191–198.

17 Arning C, Grzyska U: Color Doppler imaging of cervicocephalic fibromuscular dysplasia. Cardiovasc Ultrasound 2004;20:1–7.

18 Edell SL, Huang P: Sonographic demonstration of fibromuscular hyperplasia of the cervical internal carotid artery. Stroke 1981;12:518–520.

19 Perren F, Urbano L, Rossetti AO, Ruchat P, Uske A, Meuli R, Lobrinus JA, Bogousslavsky J, Devuyst G: Ultrasound image of a single symptomatic carotid stenosis disclosed as fibromuscular dysplasia. Neurology 2004;62:1023–1024.

20 Winter R, Ringleb P, Hacke W: Color-coded duplex ultrasound imaging of intimal fibromuscular dysplasia of the carotid artery. Nervenarzt 1998;69:905–908.

21 Arning C, Schrattenholzer A, Lachenmayer L: Cervical carotid artery vasospasms causing cerebral ischemia. Detection by immediate vascular ultrasonographic investigation. Stroke 1998;29: 1063–1066.

22 Baumgartner RW, Mattle HP, Schroth G: Transcranial color-coded duplex sonography of cerebral arteriovenous malformations. Neuroradiol 1996;38:734–737.

23 Chen YW, Jeng JS, Liu HM, Hwang BS, Lin WH, Yip PK: Carotid and transcranial color-coded duplex sonography in different types of carotid-cavernous fistula. Stroke 2000;31:701–706.

24 Lin HJ, Yip PK, Liu HM, Hwang BS, Chen RC: Noninvasive hemodynamic classification of carotid-cavernous sinus fistulas by duplex carotid sonography. J Ultrasound Med 1994;13: 105–113.
25 Kaps M, Seidel G, Bauer T, Behrmann B: Imaging of the intracranial vertebrobasilar system using color-coded ultrasound. Stroke 1992;23:1577–1582.
26 Schöning M, Walter J: Evaluation of the vertebrobasilar-posterior system by transcranial color duplex sonography in adults. Stroke 1992;23:1280–1286.
27 Bartels E, Flügel KA: Evaluation of extracranial vertebral artery dissection with duplex color-flow imaging. Stroke 1996;27:290–295.
28 De Bray JM, Penisson-Besnier I, Dubas F, Emile J: Extracranial and intracranial vertebrobasilar dissections: Diagnosis and prognosis. J Neurol Neurosurg Psychiatry 1997;63:46–51.
29 Lu CJ, Sun Y, Jeng JS, Huang KM, Hwang BS, Lin WH, Chen RC, Yip PK: Imaging in the diagnosis and follow-up evaluation of vertebral artery dissection. J Ultrasound Med 2000;19:263–270.
30 Röther J, Schwartz A, Rautenberg W, Hennerici M: Magnetic resonance angiography of spontaneous vertebral artery dissection suspected on Doppler ultrasonography. J Neurol 1995;242: 430–436.
31 Sturzenegger M, Mattle HP, Rivoir A, Rihs F, Schmid C: Ultrasound findings in extracranial vertebral artery dissection. Stroke 1993;24:1910–1921.
32 Touboul PJ, Mas JL, Bousser MG, Laplane D: Duplex scanning in extracranial vertebral artery dissection. Stroke 1987;18:116–121.
33 Kimura K, Yasaka M, Moriyasu H, Tsuchiya T, Yamaguchi T: Ultrasonographic evaluation of vertebral artery to detect vertebrobasilar axis occlusion. Stroke 1994;25:1006–1009.
34 Ringelstein EB, Zeumer H, Poeck K: Non-invasive diagnosis of intracranial lesions in the vertebrobasilar system – a comparison of Doppler sonographic and angiographic findings. Stroke 1985;16:848–855.
35 Saito K, Kimura K, Nagatsuka K, Nagano K, Minematsu K, Ueno S, Naritomi H: Vertebral artery occlusion in duplex color-coded ultrasonography. Stroke 2004;35:1068–1072.
36 Von Reutern GM, Von Büdingen HJ: Ultrasound Diagnosis of Cerebrovascular Disease. Stuttgart, Thieme, 1993.
37 Baumgartner RW, Siebler M: Ultraschalldiagnostik beim Schlaganfall. München, Ecomed-Verlag, 2002.

David H. Benninger, MD
Department of Neurology, University Hospital
Frauenklinikstrasse 26
CH–8091 Zürich (Switzerland)
Tel. +41 1 255 56 86, Fax +41 1 255 88 64, E-Mail david.benninger@usz.ch

Baumgartner RW (ed): Handbook on Neurovascular Ultrasound.
Front Neurol Neurosci. Basel, Karger, 2006, vol 21, pp 85–95

Intracranial Dural Arteriovenous and Carotid-Cavernous Fistulae and Paragangliomas

Joubin Gandjour, Ralf W. Baumgartner

Department of Neurology, University Hospital Zürich, Zürich, Switzerland

Abstract

This chapter summarizes the diagnostic criteria and reliability of ultrasound detection of intracranial dural arteriovenous fistulae (DAVF), carotid-cavernous fistulae (CCF), and paragangliomas. In arteries feeding DAVF ultrasound shows increased blood flow, systolic and, especially, end-diastolic velocities causing a decreased resistance index (RI), and an increased diameter. The RI of the external carotid artery (ECA; cutoff: right, 0.72; left, 0.71) yielded a sensitivity of 74%, a specificity of 89%, a positive predictive value of 79%, and a negative predictive value of 86%, for detecting DAVF. Preliminary data suggest that contrast-enhanced transtemporal color duplex sonography (CDS) may be useful for screening patients with clinical suspicion of DAVF of the transverse/sigmoid sinus. Most patients with CCF show a dilated superior ophthalmic vein with reversed blood flow direction. Decreased RI and increased blood flow and flow velocities are found in internal carotid arteries supplying the cavernous sinus directly through a fistula (type A CCF) at extracranial CDS, and sometimes in the cavernous sinus of CCF at transtemporal CDS. Definite diagnosis of DAVF and CCF is performed with catheter angiography. Typical CDS findings observed in paragangliomas of the head and neck include their solid, well-defined, and hypoechoic appearance, hypervascularity, intratumoral flow direction, displacement of the internal carotid artery (ICA) and ECA as well as the internal jugular vein. Whereas carotid body tumors can be visualized completely in most patients, other paragangliomas, for example, of the vagal nerve, are at best partially depicted due to their location in the upper neck. Confirmation of ultrasound suspicion of paraganglioma by magnetic resonance imaging or computed tomography of the neck is mandatory.

Intracranial Dural Arteriovenous and Carotid Cavernous Fistulae

Intracranial dural arteriovenous (DAVF) and carotid cavernous (CCF) fistulae are abnormal arteriovenous shunts, which can occur anywhere within the dura mater [1–4]. DAVF involve most commonly the transverse/sigmoid or cavernous sinus [1, 5]. The presumed causes include sinovenous thrombosis, infection, trauma, and surgery [5]. Patients may be clinically asymptomatic or experience mild symptoms up to fatal hemorrhage, depending on the location, size, and venous drainage pattern of the lesion [4]. Symptoms and signs of DAVF include pulsatile tinnitus, bruit, headache, proptosis, papilledema, visual decline, epileptic seizures, and transient or permanent neurological deficits [1, 5, 6]. Catheter angiography remains the gold standard for diagnosis of DAVF. The actual therapy of choice is catheter embolization, although stereotactic irradiation may be an alternative, and surgery is still the preferred option in some cases [4].

DAVF to the transverse/sigmoid sinus are predominantly irrigated by the occipital artery (OA) and meningeal branches of the external carotid artery (ECA). Less frequently, tentorial and dural branches of the internal carotid (ICA) and vertebral artery contribute to the blood supply [1]. The pattern of venous drainage allows classifying DAVF into five types, which are shown in table 1 [5, 7].

CCF differ in several aspects from DAVF. First, the cavernous sinus is sited outside of the dura, whereas other dural sinuses are located between two dural walls. Second, not all CCF are irrigated by dural arteries, as there may be a fistula between the ICA and the cavernous sinus. CCF are commonly classified into four types according to the arterial supply, which is given in table 2 [3, 5, 7, 8]. Suh et al. [9] reported a new classification of CCF into three different angiographic types, which are associated with the presenting clinical symptoms and venous drainage patterns. No study has yet examined the ability of ultrasound to assess the aforementioned three types of CCF. The symptoms and signs of CCF include chemosis, exophthalmus, orbital and periorbital pain, eyelid swelling, anisocoria, paresis of the second and the ocular motor cranial nerves, glaucoma, and retinal hemorrhage [8, 9]. Type A CCF is mainly of traumatic origin, rarely resolves spontaneously, and requires treatment if there are progressive neurological deficits. Type B, C, and D CCF occur and often resolve spontaneously, and produce less severe symptoms than type A.

Ultrasound Findings in DAVF

Arteries feeding DAVF, CCF and arteriovenous malformations (AVM) of the brain have a low peripheral resistance due to the presence of an abnormal

Table 1. Revised classification of intracranial dural arteriovenous fistula [7]

	Drainage	Main location	Frequency and pathomechanism
Type I	Sinus; antegrade flow	Transverse/sigmoid or cavernous sinus	Most frequent type; benign clinical course, rarely intracranial hypertension
Type II	Sinus; retrograde flow with reflux	Transverse/sigmoid or cavernous sinus	
IIa	Reflux into the sinus		Intracranial hypertension (20%)
IIb	Reflux into cortical veins		Hemorrhage (10%)
IIa + b	Reflux into sinus and cortical veins		Intracranial hypertension, hemorrhage
Type III	Cortical veins; no venous ectasia	Tentorium cerebelli, anterior cranial fossa, major sinuses	Hemorrhage (40%)
Type IV	Cortical veins, venous ectasia (cortical vein >5 mm in diameter and three times larger than the diameter of the draining vein	Tentorium cerebelli, anterior cranial fossa, major sinuses	Hemorrhage (65%)
Type V	Spinal perimedullary veins	Spinal cord	Rare; progressive myelopathy (50%)

Table 2. Classification of carotid-cavernous fistula

	Arterial supply	Dural shunts supplied by meningeal branches
Type A	Internal carotid artery	No
Type B	Internal carotid artery	Yes
Type C	External carotid artery	Yes
Type D	Internal and external carotid artery	Yes

arteriovenous communication. Feeding arteries of DAVF, CCF, and AVM thus show the same hemodynamic abnormalities, which include increased blood flow, systolic and, especially, end-diastolic velocities, and a decreased resistance index (RI) [10–12]. High-flow and large fistulae and AVM will show higher shunt volumes and flow velocities in the feeders, and are thus easier detected as they cause more hemodynamic abnormalities. Furthermore, the diameter of the feeding arteries is increased. Conversely, the nidus of fistulae and AVM cannot be detected reliably. Draining veins and sinus will also show increased blood flow, flow velocities, and lumen, which may be difficult to detect due to the interindividual variability of normal flow velocities in cerebral veins and sinus [13]. In addition, draining veins may reveal pseudoarterialized flow patterns [10, 14, 15].

Ultrasound assessment before and after interventional therapy of intracranial DAVF. To validate the diagnostic accuracy of extracranial color duplex sonography (CDS) in diagnosis of intracranial DAVF, 35 patients with and 64 patients without DAVF, confirmed by catheter angiography, were investigated [16]. Four CDS parameters, including RI, flow volume, peak systolic and end-diastolic velocity, were evaluated [16]. Abnormal CDS findings were defined as values above the 95th or below 5th percentile of 180 control subjects [16]. The RI of the ECA (cutoff: right, 0.72; left, 0.71) yielded the highest sensitivity (74%), specificity (89%), positive predictive value (79%), negative predictive value (86%), and accuracy (84%) for predicting DAVF [16]. All other ECA-related parameters produced sensitivity values below 70%, and those related to the ICA were below 30% [16]. The sensitivity of RI of the ECA was 54% (7/13 patients) for detecting CCF and 86% (19/22 patients) for identifying non-cavernous sinus DAVF [16]. These data suggest that CDS of the ECA is a reliable screening tool for detecting DAVF.

Another study investigated flow direction, waveform, and velocity of the superior ophthalmic vein (SOV) using transorbital CDS in 20 patients with intracranial DAVF [17]. Fourteen patients were symptomatic, and retrograde cortical venous filling occurred in 14 patients at catheter angiography. The average SOV diameter was 2.95 mm, which is larger ($p < 0.05$) than the values of the control subjects, and flow direction was reversed in 2 of 20 (10%) patients. The average SOV diameter and RI were higher ($p < 0.05$) in patients with clinical symptoms, angiographic retrograde cortical venous filling, or large DAVF compared to their counterparts [17]. In the absence of reliable cut-off values for diameter and RI of the SOV, reversed SOV flow direction is the only criterion, suggesting the presence of intracranial DAVF after the exclusion of other more likely causes such as severe stenosis or occlusion of the homolateral ICA. The low sensitivity and specificity of retrograde flow in the SOV limit the use of this criterion in clinical routine.

Several prospective studies have shown that endovascular or surgical therapy of DAVF will reduce or normalize flow velocities of the feeders and increase the RI of the ECA [10, 18].

The additional assessment of the global cerebral circulation time by using Doppler echo contrast-bolus tracking may prove useful for screening and follow-up of DAVF [15]. Measurement of flow velocities in draining veins and sinuses using contrast-enhanced transcranial Doppler sonography is another technique, which allows the assessment of hemodynamic changes occurring after the occlusion of DAVF [19].

In *DAVF of the transverse/sigmoid sinus*, hemodynamic abnormalities are most frequently detected in the homolateral OA, less often in the ECA, contralateral OA, and vertebral arteries (fig. 1–3) [10]. In addition, CDS may show proximally in the OA one or several spots with focally increased systolic and, in particular, end-diastolic velocities, which derive from at least one fistula (fig. 3). Harrer et al. [19] investigated 24 patients with transverse/sigmoid sinus DAVF using contrast-enhanced transtemporal CDS before and after catheter embolization. Four (17%) of the twenty-four patients could not be studied because of an insufficient temporal bone window. In the remaining 20 patients, draining veins/sinuses were identified by increased peak systolic flow velocities of >50 cm/s. Transtemporal CDS identified 25 (93%) of 27 draining vessels, which included the basal vein (n = 3), the straight sinus (n = 3), the superior sagittal sinus (1/3 vessels), the transverse sinus (n = 9), the sigmoid sinus (n = 4), and the superior petrosal sinus (n = 5). As expected, CDS failed to detect cortical draining veins. After endovascular therapy mean flow velocity was reduced by 44% ($p < 0.01$). These findings suggest that contrast-enhanced transtemporal CDS may be useful for screening patients with clinical suspicion of DAVF of transverse/sigmoid sinus and assessing the results of interventional therapy.

Ultrasound Findings in CCF

Few studies reported ultrasound criteria for hemodynamic classification of CCF [14, 20, 21]. One study compared RI and flow volume in the extracranial ICA and ECA assessed with duplex sonography in 14 patients with CCF classified by catheter angiography as shown in table 2 [20]. Type A CCF showed reduced RI with increased flow volume in the ICA, type B CCF normal RI and flow volume in the ICA and ECA, and type C and D CCF reduced RI with or without increased flow volume in the ECA [20]. RI and flow volume normalized after endovascular therapy [20]. A limitation of ultrasound assessment of CCF is that small fistulae may be missed, and the limited capability of ultrasound to differentiate types B, C, and D, in particular, the inability to differentiate type C

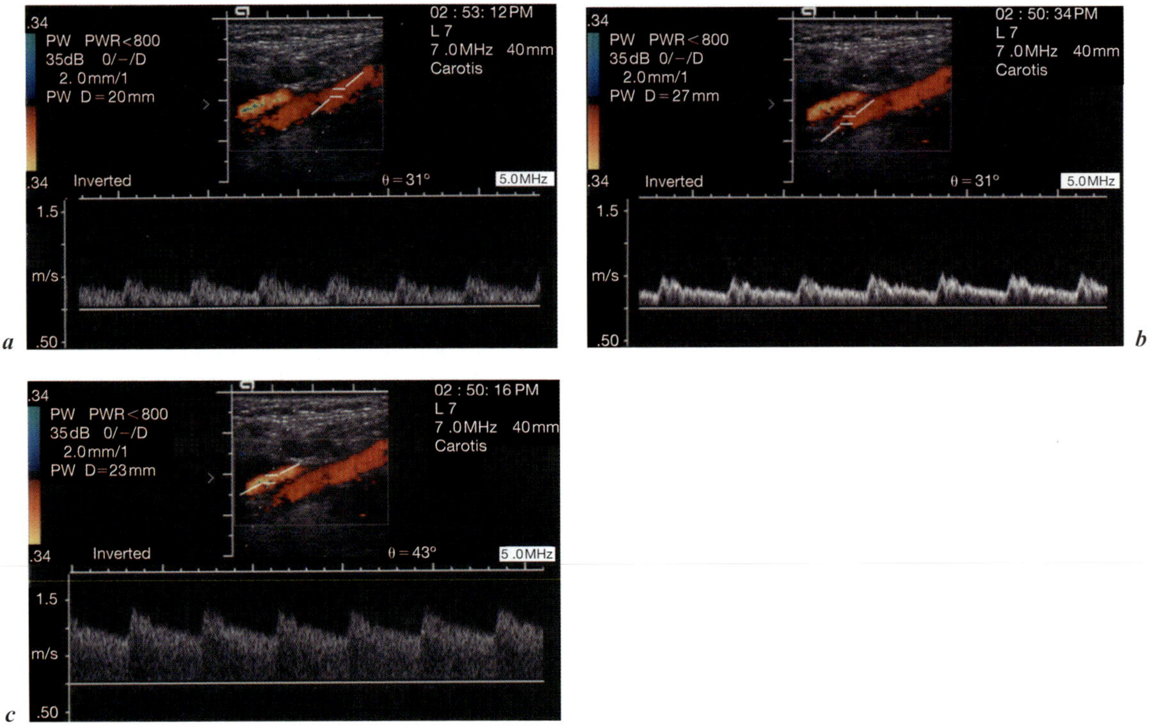

Fig. 1. Extracranial color duplex sonography findings in a patient with a dural fistula to the transverse sinus. The common (***a***) and internal (***b***) carotid arteries show normal Doppler spectra, whereas the external carotid artery (***c***) shows increased systolic and, particularly, diastolic flow velocities.

from type D lesions as both show the same hemodynamic abnormalities. Further, transtemporal CDS may directly visualize the cavernous sinus with or without a surrounding 'mosaic flash' at CDS, and high-flow velocities with turbulence at Doppler spectral analysis (fig. 3) [14, 21]. In one study, these structures were visualized in type A CCF [14].

Mainly the anterior draining vessels of the cavernous sinus, in particular, the SOV, are visualized by CDS [14]; most importantly, dilated SOV with reversed flow direction were detected in all ultrasound studies [14, 21, 22].

In conclusion, patients with suspicion of CCF should undergo extra- and transcranial CDS, including an investigation of the extracranial ICA and ECA, transorbital insonation of the SOV, and transtemporal assessment of the cavernous sinus and all draining veins and sinus, as described in the chapter by Stolz, pp. 182–193.

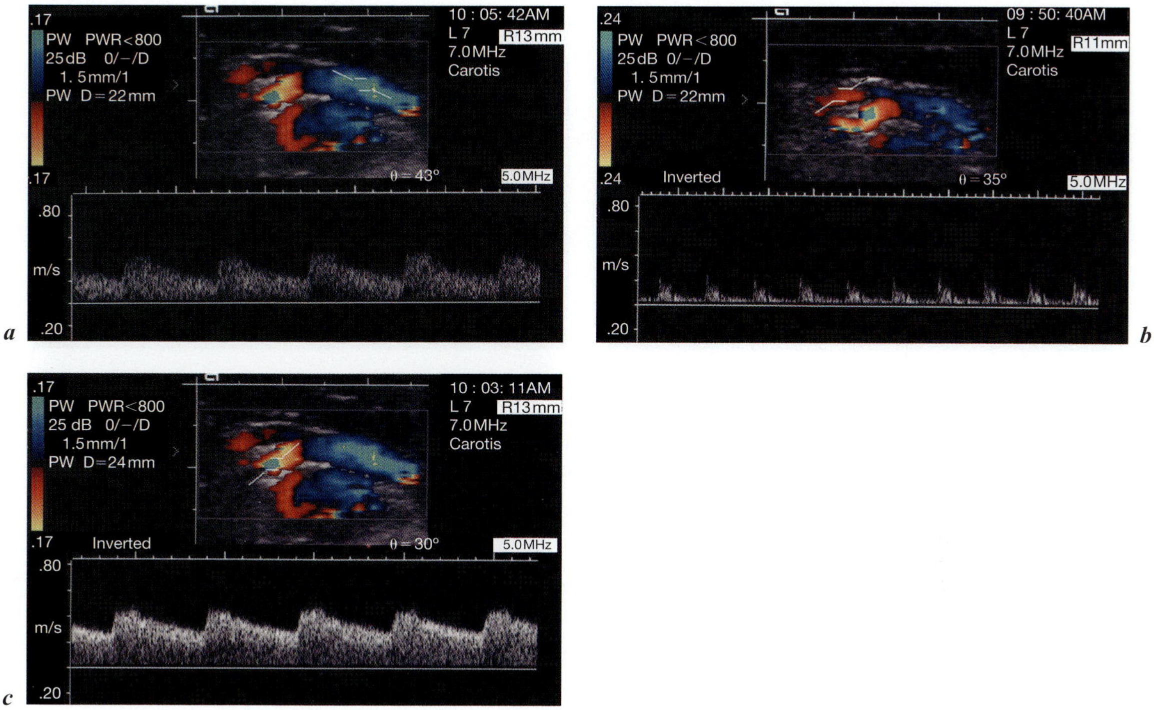

Fig. 2. Extracranial color duplex sonography findings in a patient with a dural fistula to the transverse/sigmoid sinus. The feeding occipital artery is dilated and shows an abnormal Doppler spectrum with increased systolic and, especially, diastolic flow velocities (***a***), divides into two branches with normal (***b***) and abnormal (***c***) Doppler spectra supplying the dural fistula.

Paragangliomas of the Head and Neck

Paragangliomas are derived from the extra-adrenal paraganglia of the autonomic nervous system [23–25]. Those occurring within the head and neck are most often located in the carotid bifurcation (carotid body tumor; CBT), followed by the jugulotympanic paragangliomas located in the jugular fossa and tympanic cavity. The rarest forms are situated along the nodose ganglia of the vagal nerve (vagal paraganglioma) [23]. These tumors generally exhibit a slow rate of growth (median, 1.0 mm/year) with a median tumor doubling time of 4.2 years. Patients most often present with an asymptomatic, space occupying mass noted clinically or radiographically [26]. Diagnosis is generally established by a combination of clinical findings and magnetic resonance imaging or computed tomography of the neck [25]. Treatment depends on the size,

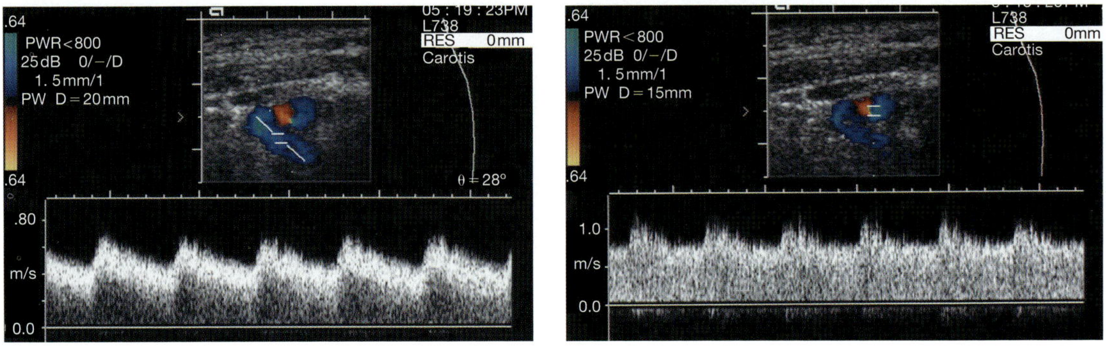

a b

Fig. 3. Extracranial color duplex sonography findings in a patient with a dural fistula to the sigmoid sinus shows the dilated feeding occipital artery with an abnormal Doppler spectrum consisting of increased systolic and, in particular, diastolic flow velocities (***a***), and Doppler spectra from a small feeding artery issueing from the occipital artery (***b***).

location, biological activity, and presence of local infiltration of the tumor as well as on the medical condition of the patient. Therapeutic options include observation of tumor growth ('wait and scan'), endovascular, or, in some cases, percutaneous embolization, surgery, and radiotherapy [24, 25, 27, 28].

Ultrasound Findings in Paragangliomas of the Head and Neck

Several small-scale studies examined ultrasound, including CDS findings in paragangliomas of the neck and head [23, 29–36]. Paragangliomas present in B-mode sonography as solid, well-defined, and hypoechoic tumors [23, 31]. Color Doppler imaging revealed hypervascularity throughout the entire tumor in 82–95% of cases [23, 30–32, 34, 35]. Flow is mainly detected in small blood vessels that cannot be visualized with B-mode imaging. Spectral analysis shows a low-resistance flow pattern with a decreased RI. A small number of paragangliomas show no hypervascularity or only peripheral hypervascularity with central hypovascularity [23, 31]. Intratumoral thrombosis, embolization, or regressive changes are possible explanations.

Ultrasound Findings in Carotid Body Tumors

CDS detected CBT in 93–100% of cases [23, 31]. Due to the favorable anatomical location, the whole tumor can be depicted (fig. 4) [31]. The shape

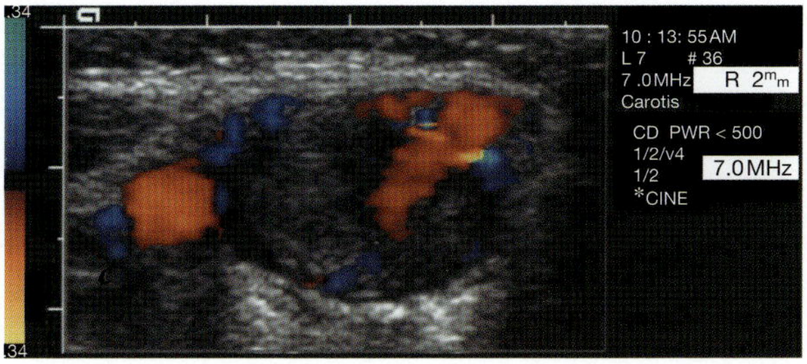

Fig. 4. Extracranial color duplex sonography using a transverse plane in a patient with a carotid body tumor shows the hypo- and isoechogenic, ovale tumor. The internal carotid artery and the jugular vein are displaced posteriorly and laterally, and the external carotid artery anteriorly and medially. Hypervascularity is mainly located in the periphery of the tumor, which is irrigated by a branch of the external carotid artery.

of CBT is round or ovoid, and the size ranges from 1.2 to 5.0 cm [23, 31, 32]. Although no capsule is depicted, the border of the tumor is well defined in most cases [32, 37]. CBT typically displace the ECA anteriorly and medially, the ICA posteriorly and laterally, and the internal jugular vein posteriorly [31, 34]. The tumor may cause mild compression of the ICA or ECA, but does not invade the vessel wall [23]. Intratumoral blood flow is mostly directed upwards, which is in accordance with the direction of vascular supply and growth of the tumor. CBT must mainly be differentiated from other tumorous structures, which include mainly lymph nodes. Hypovascularized lymph node metastases showed no flow signals at Doppler sonography [36], and a sympathetic neuroma caused neither hypervascularization nor displaced the ICA and ECA [34]. In another patient, CBT could not be differentiated from surrounding enlarged lymph nodes, resulting from thyroid cancer [32]. Taking into account that no study has evaluated the diagnostic accuracy of ultrasound diagnosis of CBT, confirmation by magnetic resonance imaging or computed tomography of the neck is mandatory.

Ultrasound Findings in Other Paragangliomas

Vagal paragangliomas were identified in 55% (6/11 cases) [23] up to 100% (all 3 cases) [31]. Vagal paragangliomas are just partially detected, because the tumor is at best partially located below the mandibular angle [31]. Blood flow in the tumor is predominantly directed caudally [31]. The ICA and ECA are displaced anteriorly and the internal jugular vein posteriorly [23, 31].

Caudal extension of 2 *temporal paragangliomas* was recognized within the expanded lumen of the internal jugular vein [31]. Intratumoral blood flow was mainly directed downwards.

References

1 Newton TH, Cronqvist S: Involvement of dural arteries in intracranial arteriovenous malformations. Radiology 1969;93:1071–1078.
2 Aminoff MJ: Vascular anomalies in the intracranial dura mater. Brain 1973;96:601–602.
3 Borden JA, Wu JK, Shucart WA: Correction: Dural arteriovenous fistulous malformations. J Neurosurg 1995;82:705–706.
4 Kiyosue H, Hori Y, Okahara M, Tanoue S, Sagara Y, Matsumoto S, Nagatomi H, Mori H: Treatment of intracranial dural arteriovenous fistulas: Current strategies based on location and hemodynamics, and alternative techniques of transcatheter embolization. Radiographics 2004;24: 1637–1653.
5 Cognard C, Gobin YP, Pierot L, Bailly AL, Houdart E, Casasco A, Chiras J, Merland JJ: Cerebral dural arteriovenous fistulas: Clinical and angiographic correlation with a revised classification of venous drainage. Radiology 1995;194:671–680.
6 Corrin LS, Sandok BA, Houser OW: Cerebral ischemic events in patients with carotid artery fibromuscular dysplasia. Arch Neurol 1981;38:616–618.
7 Djindjian R, Merland JJ, Théron J: Superselective Arteriography of the External Carotid Artery. New York, Springer, 1977.
8 Barrow DL, Spector RH, Braun IF, Landman JA, Tindall SC, Tindall GT: Classification and treatment of spontaneous carotid-cavernous sinus fistulas. J Neurosurg 1985;62:248–256.
9 Suh DC, Lee JH, Kim SJ, Chung SJ, Choi CG, Kim HJ, Kim CJ, Kook M, Ahn HS, Kwon SU, Kim JS: New concept in cavernous sinus dural arteriovenous fistula. Correlation with presenting symptom and venous drainage patterns. Stroke 2005;36:1134–1139.
10 Arning C, Grzyska U, Lachenmayer L: Lateral cranial dural fistula. Detection with Doppler and duplex ultrasound. Nervenarzt 1997;68:139–146.
11 Tsai LK, Jeng JS, Liu HM, Wang HJ, Yip PK: Intracranial dural arteriovenous fistulas with or without cerebral sinus thrombosis: Analysis of 69 patients. J Neurol Neurosurg Psychiatry 2004;75:1639–1641.
12 Baumgartner RW, Mattle HP, Schroth G: Transcranial color-coded duplex sonography of cerebral arteriovenous malformations. Neuroradiol 1996;38:734–737.
13 Baumgartner RW, Gönner F, Arnold M, Müri RM: Transtemporal power- and frequency-based color-coded duplex sonography of cerebral veins and sinuses. AJNR Am J Neuroradiol 1997;18: 1771–1781.
14 Chen YW, Jeng JS, Liu HM, Yip PK, Hwang BS, Lin WH, Chang YC, Tu YK: Diagnosis and follow-up of carotid-cavernous fistulas by carotid duplex sonography and transcranial color Doppler imaging. Ultrasound Med Biol 1996;22:1155–1162.
15 Schreiber SJ, Diehl RR, Weber W, Henkes H, Nahser HC, Lehmann R, Doepp F, Valdueza JM: Doppler sonographic evaluation of shunts in patients with dural arteriovenous fistulas. AJNR Am J Neuroradiol 2004;25:775–780.
16 Tsai LK, Jeng JS, Wang HJ, Yip PK, Liu HM: Diagnosis of intracranial dural arteriovenous fistulas by carotid duplex sonography. J Ultrasound Med 2004;23:785–791.
17 Kawaguchi S, Sakaki T, Uranishi R: Color doppler flow imaging of the superior ophthalmic vein in dural arteriovenous fistulas. Stroke 2002;33:2009–2013.
18 Tsai LK, Liu HM, Lu CJ, Jeng JS, Yip PK: Carotid duplex sonography in the follow-up of intracranial dural arteriovenous fistulae. AJNR Am J Neuroradiol 2005;26:625–629.
19 Harrer JU, Popescu O, Henkes HH, Klotzsch C: Assessment of dural arteriovenous fistulae by transcranial color-coded duplex sonography. Stroke 2005;36:976–979.

20 Lin HJ, Yip PK, Liu HM, Hwang BS, Chen RC: Noninvasive hemodynamic classification of carotid-cavernous sinus fistulas by duplex carotid sonography. J Ultrasound Med 1994;13: 105–113.
21 Chen YW, Jeng JS, Liu HM, Hwang BS, Lin WH, Yip PK: Carotid and transcranial color-coded duplex sonography in different types of carotid-cavernous fistula. Stroke 2000;31:701–706.
22 Muttaqin Z, Arita K, Uozumi T, Kuwabara S, Oki S, Ohba S, Kurisu K, Nakahara T, Kohno H, Satoh H: Transcranial doppler sonography in carotid-cavernous fistulas: Analysis of five cases. Surg Neurol 1992;38:179–185.
23 Jansen JC, Baatenburg de Jong RJ, Schipper J, van der Mey AG, van Gils AP: Color Doppler imaging of paragangliomas in the neck. J Clin Ultrasound 1997;25:481–485.
24 Axmann C, Dorenbeck U, Reith W: [Glomus tumors of the head-neck-region]. Radiologe 2004;44:389–399.
25 Pellitteri PK, Rinaldo A, Myssiorek D, Gary Jackson C, Bradley PJ, Devaney KO, Shaha AR, Netterville JL, Manni JJ, Ferlito A: Paragangliomas of the head and neck. Oral Oncol 2004;40: 563–575.
26 Jansen JC, van den Berg R, Kuiper A, van der Mey AG, Zwinderman AH, Cornelisse CJ: Estimation of growth rate in patients with head and neck paragangliomas influences the treatment proposal. Cancer 2000;88:2811–2816.
27 Van der Mey AG, Frijns JH, Cornelisse CJ, Brons EN, van Dulken H, Terpstra HL, Schmidt PH: Does intervention improve the natural course of glomus tumors? A series of 108 patients seen in a 32-year period. Ann Otol Rhinol Laryngol 1992;101:635–642.
28 Harman M, Etlik O, Unal O: Direct percutaneous embolization of a carotid body tumor with n-butyl cyanoacrylate: An alternative method to endovascular embolization. Acta Radiol 2004;45: 646–648.
29 Raby N: Ultrasonographic appearances of glomus vagale tumour. Br J Radiol 1988;61:246–249.
30 Steinke W, Hennerici M, Aulich A: Doppler color flow imaging of carotid body tumors. Stroke 1989;20:1574–1577.
31 Stoeckli SJ, Schuknecht B, Alkadhi H, Fisch U: Evaluation of paragangliomas presenting as a cervical mass on color-coded Doppler sonography. Laryngoscope 2002;112:143–146.
32 Derchi LE, Serafini G, Rabbia C, De Albertis P, Solbiati L, Candiani F, Musante F, Bertoglio C, Rizzatto G: Carotid body tumors: US evaluation. Radiology 1992;182:457–459.
33 Gooding GA: Gray-scale ultrasound detection of carotid body tumors: Report of 2 cases. Radiology 1979;132:409–410.
34 Schreiber J, Mann W, Ringel K: The role of color duplex ultrasound in diagnosis and differential diagnosis of carotid body tumors. Laryngorhinootologie 1996;75:100–104.
35 Trattnig S, Hubsch P, Schwaighofer B, Karnel F, Eilenberger M: Vascular space-occupying lesions of the carotid artery – Detection with color-coded Doppler sonography. Comparison with duplex sonography and angiography. Ultraschall Med 1991;12:70–73.
36 Gritzmann N, Herold C, Haller J, Karnel F, Schwaighofer B: Duplex sonography of tumors of the carotid body. Cardiovasc Intervent Radiol 1987;10:280–284.
37 Koch T, Vollrath M, Berger T, Reimer P, Milbradt H, Heintz P: Diagnosis of carotid body tumor by imaging procedures. HNO 1990;38:148–153.

Joubin Gandjour, MD
Department of Neurology, University Hospital
Frauenklinikstrasse 26
CH–8091 Zürich (Switzerland)
Tel. +41 1 255 56 48, Fax +41 1 255 88 64, E-Mail joubin.gandjour@usz.ch

Baumgartner RW (ed): Handbook on Neurovascular Ultrasound.
Front Neurol Neurosci. Basel, Karger, 2006, vol 21, pp 96–104

Takayasu and Temporal Arteritis

Wolfgang A. Schmidt

Medical Center for Rheumatology Berlin-Buch, Berlin, Germany

Abstract

Takayasu and temporal arteritis are primary large-vessel vasculitides. Ultrasound directly depicts the inflamed vessel wall, which is homogenously and circumferentially thickened. Furthermore, stenoses and occlusions occur. Ultrasound almost completely depicts the whole length of the common superficial temporal arteries, including the frontal and parietal ramus. Inflammation is often segmental. This may lead to a false-negative histology. The wall swelling is hypoechoic in acute temporal arteritis. It disappears within 2–3 weeks with corticosteroid treatment. Sonographers should use 8–15 MHz linear probes. The pulse repetition frequency should be about 2.5 kHz. Color box steering and beam steering should be maximal. It is essential that the color covers the artery lumen exactly. Sensitivities and specificities with regard to clinical diagnosis and histology are high. Large-vessel giant cell arteritis is a subset of temporal arteritis, with involvement of the subclavian, axillary, and proximal brachial arteries. The wall swelling resolves much slower with treatment. In Takayasu arteritis ultrasound is a valuable diagnostic tool to investigate particularly the common carotid, subclavian, and vertebral arteries. The echogenicity of the arterial wall thickening is, in general, higher than in giant cell arteritis, as the nature of Takayasu arteritis is more chronic, with less wall edema.

Temporal arteritis (giant cell arteritis) and Takayasu arteritis are primary vasculitides that affect large arteries. Patients often present with malaise, weight loss, and signs of inflammation.

Temporal arteritis is the most common primary vasculitis in white populations. According to data from several clinical studies, including a total of 1,740 patients with temporal arteritis, more than 99% of them are ≥50 years old at disease onset. Localized headache in the temporal region occurs in 74% of patients. Sixty-four percent of patients have swollen, tender, and firm temporal arteries, perhaps with reduced pulse. Jaw claudication occurs in 37% of patients, and 32% of patients have eye involvement. Most commonly this is anterior ischemic optic neuropathy with blindness of the involved eye. The ESR is ≥50 mm/h in 85% of patients, and nearly all patients have an ESR of >20 mm/h. Temporal artery histology is positive in 85% of patients with temporal arteritis [1].

Takayasu arteritis occurs less frequently. Eighty to ninety-seven percent of patients with Takayasu arteritis are females. The age at disease onset is between 10 and 40 years in most patients. In contrast to temporal arteritis, many patients have a longer prodromal phase with malaise before they present with symptoms of stenosis or occlusion of large arteries. The subclavian arteries are most commonly involved (93%), followed by the aorta (65%) and carotid arteries (58%). Renal arteries are involved in 38%, and vertebral arteries in 32%. Nevertheless, nearly all other large arteries may be affected [2].

With increasing use of imaging studies, two other forms of large-vessel involvement become more frequently recognized. Large-vessel giant cell arteritis is a subgroup of temporal arteritis in at least 17% of cases with temporal arteritis [1]. In these cases inflammation occurs at the axillary, the distal subclavian, and the proximal brachial arteries. Furthermore, isolated primary aortitis ('idiopathic aortitis') is increasingly diagnosed mainly with positron emission tomography (PET), magnetic resonance imaging (MRI), and computed tomography.

Ultrasound in Temporal Arteritis

With improving ultrasound technology it is possible to reach both axial and lateral resolutions of about 0.1 mm and to easily delineate the temporal arteries.

The common superficial temporal artery derives from the external carotid artery. In most cases, it divides into the frontal and parietal ramus in front of the ear. The distal common superficial temporal artery and the rami are localized between the two layers of the temporal fascia that can be easily depicted by ultrasound as a bright band. Both the diameter of the lumen and each layer of the temporal fascia, including the wall of the temporal arteries, is about 0.7 mm, respectively.

Three findings are important for the diagnosis of temporal arteritis [3, 4] (fig. 1):

- Dark (hypoechoic), circumferential wall thickening ('halo') around the lumen of an inflamed temporal artery, which represents vessel wall edema.
- Stenoses are present if blood-flow velocity is more than twice the rate recorded in the area of stenosis compared with the area before the stenosis,

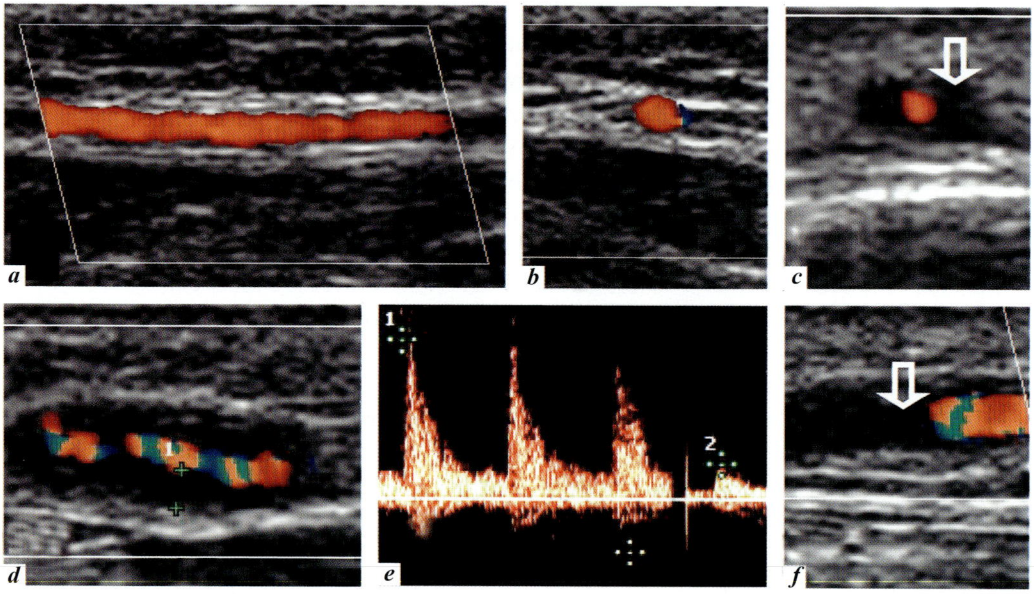

Fig. 1. Duplex ultrasound of the temporal arteries: ***a*** longitudinal view of a normal frontal ramus; ***b*** transverse view of a normal frontal ramus; ***c*** transverse view of a frontal ramus in active temporal arteritis. The arrow shows the hypoechoic wall swelling ('halo'). ***d*** Longitudinal view of a frontal ramus in active temporal arteritis. The sagittal diameter of the hypoechoic wall swelling is 0.9 mm (++). The colored area delineates increased blood flow velocity, which is suspicious for a stenosis. ***e*** pw-Doppler ultrasound of a frontal ramus in active temporal arteritis. Peak flow velocity is 86 cm/s in the stenosis (1+) and 19 cm/s behind the stenosis (2+). ***f*** Inflammatory occlusion (↓) of a parietal ramus in active temporal arteritis.

perhaps with wave forms demonstrating turbulence and reduced velocity behind the area of stenosis.

- Acute occlusions in which the ultrasound image is similar to that of acute embolism in other vessels, showing hypoechoic material in the former artery lumen with absence of color signals.

Furthermore, pulsation of temporal arteries is reduced. This feature is typical, but more difficult to define than the other features.

With corticosteroid therapy the halo disappears in most patients within 2–3 weeks [4]. Temporal artery ultrasound should be performed within the first 7 days of treatment, preferably as early as possible. Nevertheless, diagnostic assessment should not delay the start of therapy. Ultrasound may also detect inflamed temporal arteries in patients with clinically normal temporal arteries. Some patients with occult temporal arteritis and the clinical image of 'pure' polymyalgia rheumatica may be diagnosed by ultrasonography [5].

Technical Requirements. High-quality ultrasound equipment is mandatory to both adequately depict small superficial structures, like the temporal arteries, and to provide a good color signal that exactly covers the perfused artery lumen. One should use linear probes with a minimum gray scale frequency of 8 MHz. Excellent color Doppler probes are available with frequencies between 10 and 15 MHz. Color frequency should be about 10 MHz. Higher frequencies sometimes lead to decreased color sensitivity. Gray scale equipment has been used to up to 50 MHz (ultrasound biomicroscopy) with encouraging results [6, 7]. This equipment does not provide any information on flow characteristics, and it is difficult to handle the probes to investigate the complete distance of the temporal arteries, as it has been primarily designed to depict the anterior compartments of the eyes.

Machine Adjustments. The pulse repetition frequency should be about 2.5 kHz as maximum systolic velocities are rather high (20–100 cm/s). Steering of the color box and the Doppler beam should be maximal as the rami are parallel to the probe. It is essential that the color covers the artery lumen exactly. If it only covers the center of the artery lumen, the uncovered area may be misinterpreted as inflammatory wall swelling. If the color covers too much of the vessel wall, minor or moderate inflammation may be overlooked.

Sonographer Training. The sonographer should be experienced in vascular ultrasound. He or she should perform at least 50 scans of subjects without temporal arteritis to be sure about the appearance of normal temporal arteries before starting to evaluate patients with suspected temporal arteritis.

Sequence of the Sonographic Investigation. The investigation should start at the left common superficial temporal artery using a longitudinal scan. Thus, the patient can see the monitor as examination commences. The probe should then be moved along the course of the temporal artery to the parietal ramus as distal as possible. On the way back one should delineate the temporal artery in transverse scans. When applying the transverse scan, one can find the frontal ramus, which should then be delineated both in longitudinal and transverse scans to an area as distal as possible. Afterwards, one should repeat the investigation in the same way on the right temporal artery. If the color signals show localized aliasing and persistent diastolic flow, one should use the pw-Doppler mode to confirm the presence of stenoses [8].

Sensitivity and Specificity of Temporal Artery Ultrasound. Sensitivity of temporal artery ultrasound with the clinical diagnosis of temporal arteritis is comparable with that of histology. Histology can also detect minor degrees of inflammation, but ultrasound investigates nearly the whole length of the temporal arteries. The most important reason for a false-negative temporal artery biopsy is the occurrence of inflammation only in segments of the temporal arteries ('skip lesions'). In our own series of 751 cases, 101 of whom had active temporal arteritis, the sensitivity of duplex ultrasound is 88% with regard to clinical diagnosis and 95% with regard to positive temporal artery histology. The specificity is 99.5% for a halo and 96% for the occurrence of stenoses with regard to diagnosis [9]. A meta-analysis of twenty-three studies on temporal artery ultrasound including 2,036 cases arrives at sensitivities of 87% and specificities of 96% with regard to 'halo', stenoses and occlusions [10]. Both positive and negative temporal artery ultrasound results considerably influence post-test probabilities for the diagnosis of temporal arteritis. In cases with a pretest probability of 10%, the post-test probability is 71% with positive ultrasound and 2% with negative ultrasound. A pretest probability of 50% correlates with post-test probabilities of 96 and 12% with positive and negative ultrasound, respectively. In cases with a pretest probability of 90%, the post-test probabilities are 99 and 55%, respectively. Centers with experienced sonographers who are sure about the normal appearance of a temporal artery, and thus provide high specificities for the diagnosis of temporal arteritis, may, in our mind, replace temporal artery biopsy by ultrasound investigation in patients with typical clinical (hard, tender, swollen temporal arteries) and typical sonographic features ('halo').

Other Imaging Studies. Studies with arteriography that had been performed in the 1970s showed stenoses and occlusions in temporal arteritis [11]. As arteriography does not delineate the artery wall, findings were unspecific. Furthermore, the invasiveness of arteriography does not justify its clinical use for the diagnosis of temporal arteritis. A pilot study describes positive findings with scintigraphy of the temporal arteries in 9 patients with active temporal arteritis [12]. Larger studies are needed before this method can be introduced as a routine diagnostic test. PET only depicts arteries with a diameter of >4 mm [13]. Promising results have been recently published with regard to gadolinium-enhanced MRI [14]. As resolution is improving, MRI shows wall swelling of temporal and occipital arteries in giant cell arteritis as described by ultrasound.

Ultrasound in Large-Vessel Giant Cell Arteritis

Giant cell arteritis may appear in several vessels other than the temporal arteries. The ultrasound image is similar in other arteries like the occipital, vertebral, facial, and several other arteries [15, 16]. The wall swelling is hypoechoic with or without smooth stenoses or occlusions [17]. The axillary, distal subclavian, and proximal brachial arteries are most frequently involved (fig. 2). Thus, we recommend bilateral auscultation of the subclavian and axillary regions and bilateral measurement of blood pressure. We also perform ultrasound at least of the axillary region in all patients with suspected giant cell

a

b

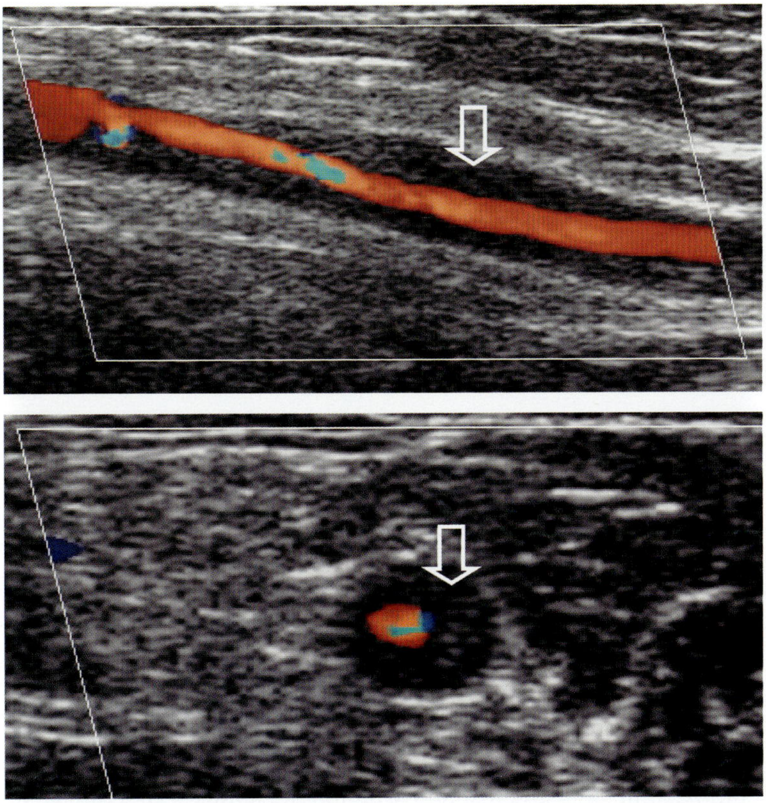

Fig. 2. Color Doppler ultrasound in large-vessel giant cell arteritis. ***a*** Longitudinal view of an axillary artery. The arrow shows the hypoechoic wall swelling. ***b*** Transverse view of an axillary artery. The arrow shows the hypoechoic wall swelling.

(temporal) arteritis, in patients with polymyalgia rheumatica, and in patients with fever of unknown origin. Wall swelling and stenoses of larger arteries usually remain for months and years despite corticosteroid treatment. The thickened wall becomes brighter with treatment because of decreasing amount of edema. Patients often develop collateral flow in the course of the disease.

Ultrasound in Takayasu Arteritis

In Takayasu arteritis, homogenous swelling of the arterial wall is observed, and may be associated with stenoses or occlusions like in temporal arteritis. The wall swelling is usually midechoic. Thus, it is brighter than in temporal arteritis

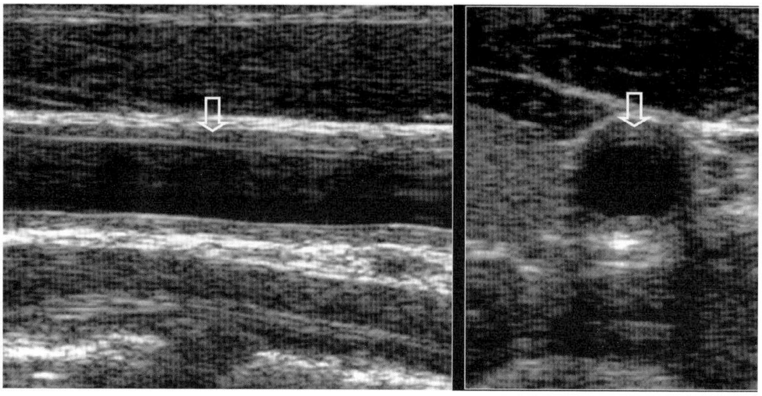

a *b*

Fig. 3. Gray scale ultrasound in Takayasu arteritis. ***a*** Longitudinal view of a common carotid artery. The arrow shows the midechoic wall swelling. ***b*** Transverse view of a common carotid artery. The arrow shows the midechoic wall swelling.

[18] (fig. 3). Takayasu arteritis has a more chronic course in most cases. The homogenous wall thickening has been described as 'macaroni phenomenon' [19]. The stiffness of the wall is increased in most cases [20]. The sonographic appearance of vasculitis is fundamentally different from that of arteriosclerosis. Arteriosclerotic lesions are irregular and usually contain calcified (hyperechoic) plaques.

Equipment, machine adjustments, and scanning techniques are equivalent to that of ultrasound investigations of these arteries for other indications. The ultrasound image of the common carotid, subclavian, and femoral arteries is excellent, except for the left proximal subclavian artery. The image of the iliac, renal, mesenteric arteries, the celiac truncus, and the abdominal aorta is moderate. Most parts of the thoracic aorta can only be analyzed by transesophageal ultrasound. The common carotid artery is much more frequently involved than the carotid bulb and internal and external carotid arteries. As Takayasu arteritis almost always involves either the subclavian or carotid arteries; ultrasound of these vessels is adequate in the search for vasculitis in young patients with chronic inflammation of unknown origin [21]. It is difficult to determine with ultrasound if a lesion is active or inactive. Activity can be suspected if artery wall swelling increases [22]. In most cases wall diameters change significantly only within months.

Several other imaging studies have been performed for the diagnosis of large artery vasculitis [23]. The greatest experience exists with arteriography, which provides a good overview, including that of small arteries, and interventions are also possible. The drawbacks of arteriography are invasiveness, with complications at the arterial injection site, high iodinated contrast load, and high-dose radiation exposure. Arteriography does not delineate the vessel wall. Therefore, it misses minor findings with slight wall swelling that do not yet cause major stenoses, particularly in the early phase of Takayasu arteritis which can last up to 3 years [21].

MRI, magnetic resonance angiography and computed tomography delineate artery wall swelling, but fail to depict very small arteries. Computed tomography is superior to MRI for detection of calcifications. PET displays inflamed areas, and thus provides a good overview, and it is probably the most sensitive method for follow-up investigations of small arteries. On the other hand, it is very expensive, does not depict details of the artery wall, and is unable to provide any information on vessels with a diameter of <4 mm [13]. In one study ultrasound and PET showed complete agreement in the anatomical distribution of patients with large-vessel giant cell arteritis [24]. In Takayasu arteritis, both magnetic resonance angiography and color Doppler flow imaging showed a substantial correlation in the ability to detect obstructive lesions in supra-aortic vessels compared with arteriography. Ultrasound displayed common carotid artery wall thickening in five vessels that were considered normal by arteriography [25].

Costs for ultrasound investigations are reasonably low. Equipment is widely available. There is no radiation, and follow-up investigations are easily possible. The resolution is excellent, and it provides additional information on arteriosclerotic plaques, blood flow characteristics, and pulsatility of the artery walls. On the other hand, ultrasound fails to delineate the thoracic aorta unless performed endoscopically, and it does not provide a good overview on a larger anatomical area.

In conclusion, color duplex ultrasound is an excellent new imaging technique for diagnosis and follow-up of temporal arteritis, large-vessel giant cell arteritis, and Takayasu arteritis.

References

1 Schmidt WA, Gromnica-Ihle E: What is the best approach to diagnose large-vessel vasculitis? Best Pract Res Clin Rheumatol 2005;19:223–242.

2 Kerr GS, Hallahan CW, Giordano J, et al: Takayasu arteritis. Ann Intern Med 1994;120:919–929.

3 Schmidt WA, Kraft HE, Völker L, et al: Colour Doppler sonography to diagnose temporal arteritis. Lancet 1995;345:866.

4 Schmidt WA, Kraft HE, Vorpahl K, et al: Color duplex ultrasonography in the diagnosis of temporal arteritis. N Engl J Med 1997;337:1336–1342.

5 Schmidt WA, Gromnica-Ihle E: Incidence of temporal arteritis in patients with polymyalgia rheumatica: A prospective study using colour Doppler sonography of the temporal arteries. Rheumatology 2002;41:46–52.

6 Wenkel H, Michelson G: Korrelation der Ultraschallbiomikroskopie mit histologischen Befunden in der Diagnostik der Riesenzellarteriitis. Klin Monatsbl Augenheilkd 1997;210:48–52.

7 Roters S, Szurman P, Engels BF, et al: The suitability of the ultrasound biomicroscope for establishing texture in giant-cell arteritis. Br J Ophthalmol 2001;85:946–948.
8 Schmidt WA: Doppler sonography in rheumatology. Best Pract Res Clin Rheumatol 2004;18: 827–846.
9 Schmidt WA, Gromnica-Ihle E: Duplex ultrasonography in temporal arteritis. Ann Intern Med 2003;138:609.
10 Karassa FB, Matsagas MI, Schmidt WA, et al: Diagnostic performance of ultrasonography for giant-cell arteritis: A meta-analysis. Ann Intern Med 2005;142:359–369.
11 Hunder GG, Baker HL Jr, Rhoton AL, et al: Superficial temporal arteriography in patients suspected of having temporal arteritis. Arthritis Rheum 1972;15:561–570.
12 Reitblat T, Ben-Horin C, Reitblat A: Gallium-67 SPECT scintigraphy may be useful in diagnosis of temporal arteritis. Ann Rheum Dis 2003;62:257–260.
13 Schmidt WA, Blockmans D: Use of ultrasonography and positron emission tomography in the diagnosis and assessment of large-vessel vasculitis. Curr Opin Rheumatol 2005;17:9–15.
14 Bley TA, Wieben O, Uhl M, et al: High-resolution MRI in giant cell arteritis: Imaging of the wall of the superficial temporal artery. AJR Am J Roentgenol 2005;184:283–287.
15 Schmidt WA, Natusch A, Möller DE, et al: Involvement of peripheral arteries in active giant cell arteritis: A study using color Doppler sonography. Clin Exp Rheumatol 2002;20:309–318.
16 Pfadenhauer K, Weber H: Duplex sonography of the temporal and occipital artery in the diagnosis of temporal arteritis: A prospective study. J Rheumatol 2003;30:2177–2181.
17 Schmidt WA, Kraft HE, Borkowski A, et al: Colour duplex ultrasonography in large-vessel giant cell arteritis. Scand J Rheumatol 1999;28:374–376.
18 Schmidt WA: Use of imaging studies in the diagnosis of vasculitis. Curr Rheumatol Rep 2004;6: 203–211.
19 Maeda H, Handa N, Matsumoto M, et al: Carotid lesions detected by B-mode ultrasonography in Takayasu's arteritis: 'Macaroni sign' as an indicator of the disease. Ultrasound Med Biol 1991;17: 695–701.
20 Raninen RO, Kupari MM, Hekali PE: Carotid and femoral artery stiffness in Takayasu's arteritis. An ultrasound study. Scand J Rheumatol 2002;31:85–88.
21 Schmidt WA, Nerenheim A, Seipelt E, et al: Early diagnosis of Takayasu arteritis by colour Doppler ultrasonography. Rheumatology 2002;41:496–502.
22 Park S, Chung J, Lee J: Carotid artery involvement in Takayasu's arteritis: Evaluation of the activity by ultrasonography. J Ultrasound Med 2001;20:371–378.
23 Kissin EY, Merkel PA: Diagnostic imaging in Takayasu arteritis. Curr Opin Rheumatol 2004;16: 31–37.
24 Brodmann M, Lipp RW, Passath A, et al: The role of 2-18F-fluoro-2-deoxy-*D*-glucose positron emission tomography in the diagnosis of giant cell arteritis of the temporal arteries. Rheumatology 2004;43:241–242.
25 Cantu C, Pineda C, Barinagarrementeria F, et al: Noninvasive cerebrovascular assessment of Takayasu arteritis. Stroke 2000;31:2197–2202.

Wolfgang A. Schmidt, MD
Medical Center for Rheumatology Berlin-Buch
Karower Strasse 11
DE–13125 Berlin (Germany)
Tel. +49 30 94792335, Fax +49 30 94792555, E-Mail w.schmidt@immanuel.de

Baumgartner RW (ed): Handbook on Neurovascular Ultrasound.
Front Neurol Neurosci. Basel, Karger, 2006, vol 21, pp 105–116

Transcranial Insonation

Ralf W. Baumgartner

Department of Neurology, University Hospital of Zürich, Zürich, Switzerland

Abstract

Insonation of the intracranial cerebral arteries, veins, and sinus is performed with transcranial Doppler or color duplex sonography. The orbital window is mainly used to identify the ophthalmic artery and carotid siphon, which can be detected in most patients. The temporal window allows the investigation of the anterior, middle, and posterior cerebral and the terminal (C1) segment of the internal carotid arteries, and the deep middle cerebral and basal veins in 80–84% of cases. Intracranial vessels located in the periphery of the temporal insonation field [postcommunicating (A2) anterior cerebral artery, the carotid siphon and more proximal parts of the internal carotid artery, the insular (M2) and opercular (M3) parts of the middle cerebral artery, the quadrigeminal (P3) part of the posterior cerebral artery, the great cerebral vein, the straight and transverse sinus] will be missed more often, particularly in patients who are older, of female gender, or Black or Asiatic ethnicity. The foraminal window is used to assess the intracranial (V4) vertebral and basilar arteries, which are detected in 79–94% and 89–96%, respectively. Echo contrast agents increase the detection rate and diagnostic confidence of transtemporal and -foraminal insonation. The frontal and occipital bony windows are rarely used to insonate the basal cerebral arteries and the internal cerebral vein, and the straight sinus, respectively.

Transcranial insonation of the intracranial cerebral arteries, veins, and sinus is mainly performed through the orbital (fig. 1), temporal (fig. 2), and foraminal (fig. 3) windows. Further insonation windows, which may be used for special purposes, include the frontal (fig. 4) and occipital (fig. 5) windows.

Orbital Window

Already in the seventies transorbital insonation with A- and B-mode imaging was used to assess dilated superior ophthalmic veins [1]. In the late eighties,

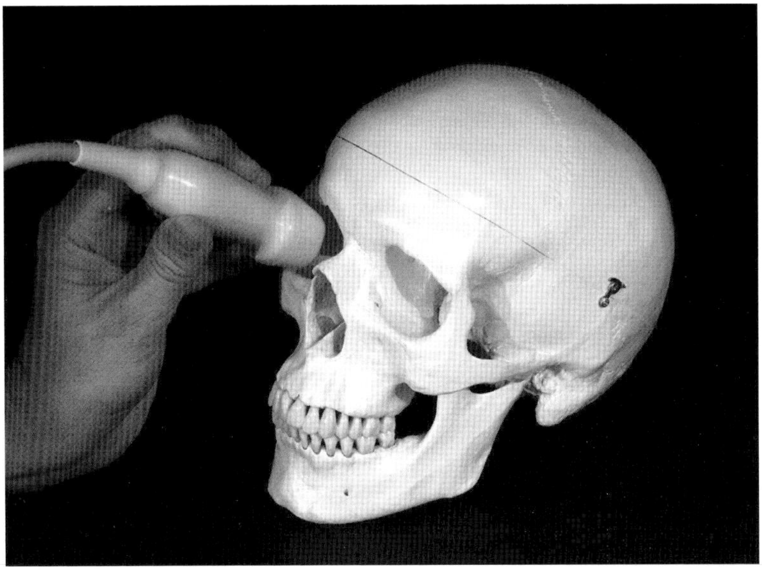

Fig. 1. The orbital ultrasound window.

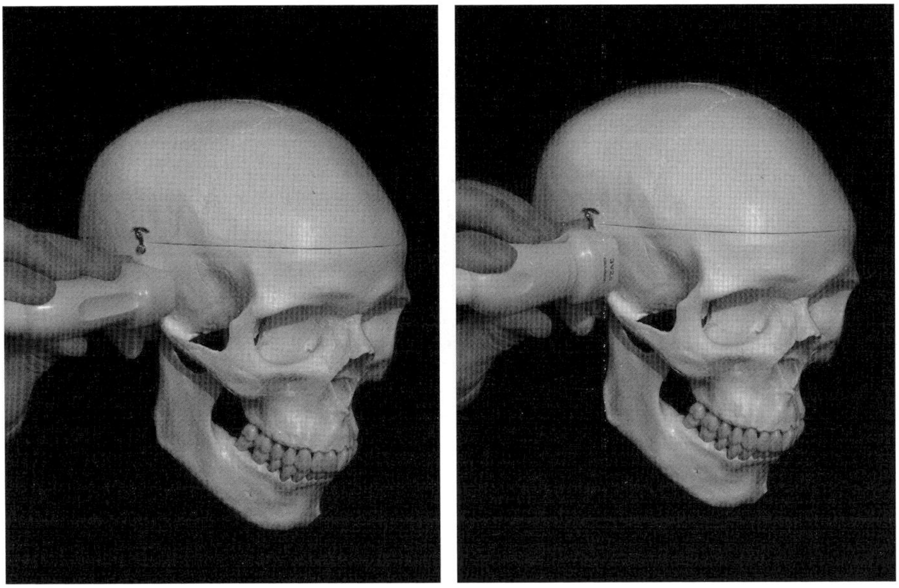

a *b*

Fig. 2. The temporal ultrasound window using axial (***a***) and coronal (***b***) scanning planes.

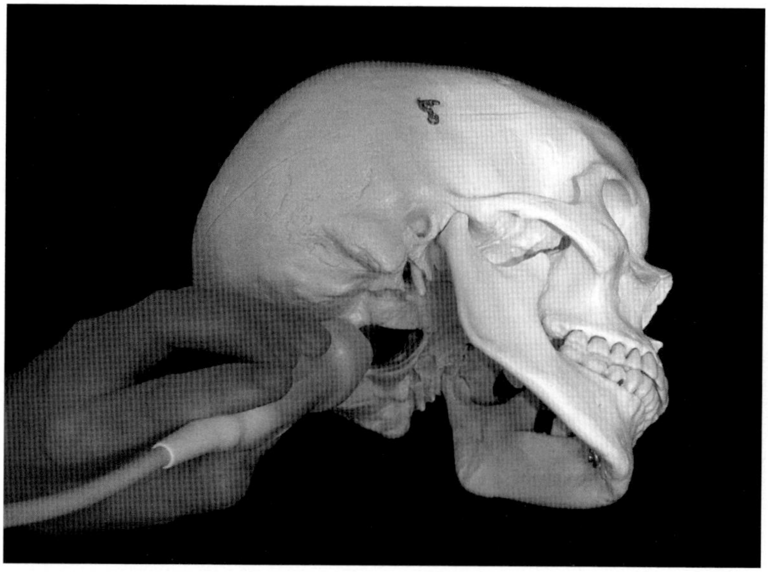

Fig. 3. The foraminal ultrasound window.

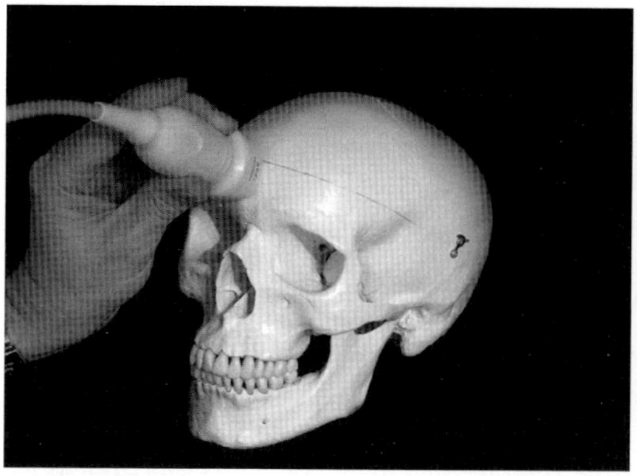

a

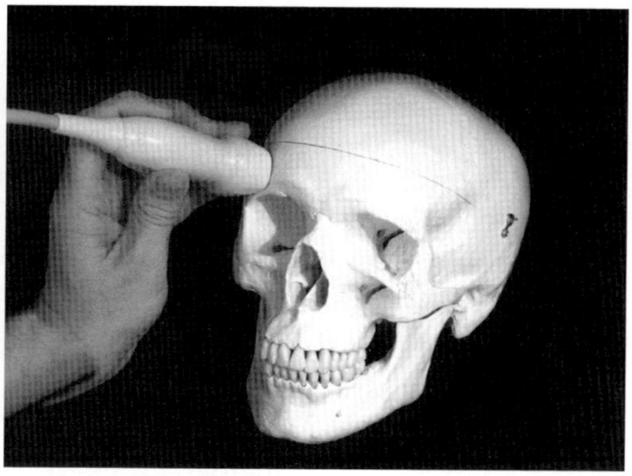

b

Fig. 4. The paramedian (***a***) and lateral (***b***) frontal ultrasound windows.

transorbital color duplex sonography (CDS) was added to investigate intraorbital arteries [ophthalmic (OphA) and central retinal artery, posterior ciliary branches, terminal lacrimal branch] and veins (superior ophthalmic and central retinal vein, venae vorticosae) [2]. With the exception of the OphA the abovementioned vessels are not insonated during a neurovascular examination, and will thus not be discussed in this book.

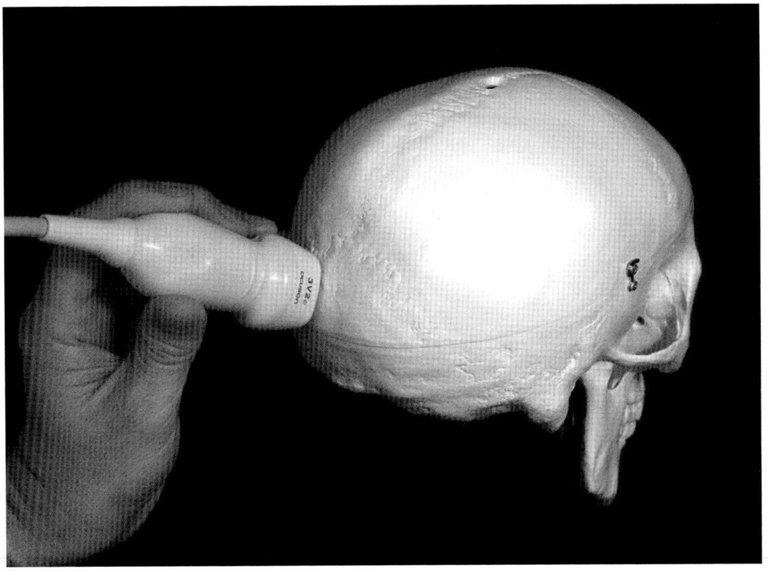

Fig. 5. The occipital ultrasound window using a sagittal scanning plane.

Transorbital Doppler sonography is used for investigating the OphA and the carotid siphon [3–6]. The patient is in the supine position, and the vessels are identified by the depth of insonation and direction of blood flow. Flow towards the probe is assumed to come from the OphA or C4 segment of the internal carotid artery (ICA; lower carotid siphon), whereas the upper carotid siphon (C2 segment of the ICA) leads to Doppler signals being directed away from the probe. The distance between the ultrasound transducer and the ICA as well as the neighboring anterior (ACA) and middle (MCA) cerebral and posterior communicating (PCoA) arteries differ between subjects, and the course of the vessels may be tortuous. Thus, it may become necessary to use common carotid artery compression (CCA) for the identification of the insonated vessel. ICA flow velocities disappear during ipsilateral CCA compression and augment, while the opposite CCA is compressed. In contrast, flow velocity in the PCoA is reduced but not annihilated during compression of the ipsilateral CCA. Flow velocities in the ACA are reduced or reversed during ipsilateral CCA compression, and increased during contralateral CCA compression. Flow velocities in the MCA decrease during compression of the ipsilateral CCA, and remain unchanged or show a slight increase during contralateral CCA compression. The detection rate of the OphA, the upper and lower carotid siphon was either not reported or 100% in small-scale transcranial Doppler sonography (TCD) series [3–6] (table 1).

Table 1. Transorbital insonation – detection rates of cerebral arteries [3–6, 10] and veins [7]

		Doppler sonography (%)	Color duplex sonography (%)
Artery	Ophthalmic	100	85
	Internal carotid		
	supraclinoid portion	100	79
	cavernous sinus portion	100	67
	Middle cerebral	ne	74
	Anterior cerebral		
	precommunicating portion	ne	83
	postcommunicating portion	ne	80
	Posterior cerebral	ne	32
Vein	Parasellar	84	ne

ne = Not examined.

Parasellar venous TCD spectra were detected in 72 of 86 (84%) examinations performed in 43 subjects with a mean age of 32 ± 10 (range, 18–56) years [7]. The flow was always directed away from the probe and considered to derive from in- and outflow vessels of the cavernous sinus.

Transorbital ultrasound is assumed to be safe when the lowest emission energies are used, and the insonation time is as short as possible [8, 9]. For safety reasons, the use of echo contrast agents is prohibited.

In a Chinese study, transorbital CDS (fig. 1) was used to insonate the OphA, supraclinoid and cavernous sinus portion of the ICA, pre- (A1) and postcommunicating (A2) ACA, MCA, and posterior cerebral artery (PCA) in 50 volunteers (32 men) with a men age of 56 ± 12 (range, 38–79) years [10]. The arteries were mainly identified using color Doppler and B-mode imaging, whereas CCA compression was just needed in a few cases. The subjects had to turn their eyes away from the probe to avoid the refraction of the lens [10]. The ultrasound beam was directed at the apex of the orbit in either an anteroposterior direction through the superior orbital fissure and optic canal or in an oblique direction through the roof of the orbit [10]. The output energy was <25 mW/cm^2 (maximum estimated in situ spatial peak temporal average intensity: 9.7 mW/cm^2 for color Doppler imaging, 9.1 mW/cm^2 for pulsed Doppler ultrasound) or <50 mW/cm^2 (maximum estimated in situ spatial peak temporal average intensity: 29 mW/cm^2 for both color and spectral Doppler ultrasound) [10]. The maximum estimated in situ spatial peak temporal average intensity at 26 dB was 14.5 mW/cm^2 for B-mode imaging [10]. The detection rates of the insonated arteries are given in table 1. Poor transorbital acoustic windows were found in 24% (men, 20%; women, 33%) of subjects younger than 60 years of age, and in 42% (men, 42%; women, 44%) of subjects with at least 60 years of age. Transorbital CDS detected the ACA (80–83% vs. 68–70%) more often than transtemporal CDS ($p < 0.05$). Furthermore, in 5 subjects without temporal acoustic windows, the ICA, MCA, and ACA were successfully investigated using transorbital CDS. Because the temporal window is significantly worse in Asian subjects [11–14], it is unclear whether the aforementioned advantage applies also for white subjects. Furthermore, echo contrast agents will improve the diagnostic accuracy of transtemporal CDS, whereas safety concerns prohibit their use for transorbital studies.

Temporal Bony Window

Transtemporal insonation is performed using axial (fig. 2a) and coronal (fig. 2b) planes. The axial mesencephalic plane depicts the midbrain, which is hypoechogenic and shaped like a butterfly, the sphenoidal (M1) and insular (M2) parts of the MCA, A1 ACA, the terminal segment (C1) of the ICA, and post-communicating (P2) PCA [15]. The deep middle cerebral vein is examined above and posterior to the MCA, the basal vein in its middle segment above P2 PCA, the great cerebral vein just posterior to the pineal gland, the straight sinus in the middle of its course, and the contralateral transverse sinus in the lateral part of its horizontal section (sino-venous flow is directed away from the transducer) [16, 17]. By tilting the transducer somewhat caudally, the carotid siphon, P1 PCA and in up to 75% the PCoA are identified [15, 18, 19]. By further tilting the transducer caudally, the ganglionic (C5) portion and the horizontal segment of the pars petrosa of the ICA [18] and adjacent most distal part of the sigmoid sinus and or bulb of the jugular vein [unpubl. observations] are detected. A more detailed description of transtemporal insonation of the aforementioned and further cerebral veins and sinuses is provided in the chapter by Stolz, pp. 182–193. The axial ventricular plane is obtained by tilting the transducer 10° upwards with respect to the mesencephalic plane [20]. It shows the hypoechogenic third ventricle surrounded by bright margins, the hyperechogenic pineal gland and choroid plexus of the trigonum, insular (M2) and opercular (M3) MCA, post-communicating (A2) ACA, and quadrigeminal (P3) PCA [15]. This plane is used to determine the position and displacement (midline shift) of the third ventricle, for example, in space-occupying MCA infarcts [21, 22]. The *anterior coronal plane* shows M1 MCA, A1 ACA, C1 ICA, parts of the carotid siphon, and C5 ICA. The posterior coronal plane depicts the PCA, distal basilar artery (BA), M2 and M3 MCA, and horizontal segment of the petrosal part of the ICA [15, 18].

Table 2. Transtemporal color duplex sonography – detection rates of cerebral arteries [19, 35, 47]

Artery	Detected/Examined vessels, n (%)
Anterior cerebral	515/620 (83)
Middle cerebral	563/620 (91)
Posterior cerebral	557/620 (90)
precommunicating (P1) segment	243/264 (92)
postcommunicating (P2) segment	248/264 (94)
Posterior communicating	
normal	65/100 (65)
collateral	43/69 (62)

Table 3. Transtemporal color duplex sonography – detection rates of cerebral veins and sinuses [16, 17, 48]

		Both sexes (%)	Women (%)	Men (%)	Age 20–59 years	Age 60–79 years
Vein	Deep middle cerebral	76–78	71	81	87–88	53–55
	Basal	89–93	92	95	93–97	86–85
	Internal cerebral	23	ne	ne	ne	ne
	Great cerebral (Galen)	89–91	ne	ne	94	84
Sinus	Straight	48–72	47	48	60–79	23–57
	Transverse	35–71	35	34	42–77	20–46
	Distal superior sagittal	52–55	ne	ne	61	38

ne = Not examined.

With advancing age, and especially in postmenopausal women, the temporal bone window becomes smaller or may even disappear, and the frequency of ultrasonic detection of intracranial vessels decreases. Consequently, vascular structures located in the periphery of the insonation field, such as the petrosal part, C5 and the siphon of the ICA, A2 ACA, M3 and M2 MCA, P3 PCA, the straight-, and transverse sinus will be missed in older patients. The detection rates of intracranial cerebral arteries, veins, and sinus reported in different studies are given in tables 2 and 3.

The temporal window is better in men than women [23], and in white compared to black and Asiatic patients [11–14].

In a transtemporal CDS study, the temporal window of 33 moribund patients was classified as excellent, intermediate, or poor [24]. At autopsy, a rectangular sample of 37 temporal bones was removed, which corresponded to the area of the in vivo acoustic window. High-resolution CT was used to determine the thickness, density and homogeneity of the temporal bone, its cortical part, and the diploe. The authors observed that the thickness of the cortical parts was quite constant, but the thickness of the diploe increased with increasing width of the temporal bone. Thus, quality of transtemporal CDS imaging is mainly influenced by the diploe, which is known to scatter the ultrasound beam [25]. The authors found that the quality of the CDS image mainly depends on the thickness of the diploe. A retrospective in vivo investigation correlated the quality of the TCD Doppler signal with the thickness of 99 temporal bones in its thinnest portion at cranial CT. Temporal squama thickness of ≥5 mm had a sensitivity of 86%, a specificity of 90%, a positive predictive value of 70%, and a positive likelihood ratio of 8.6 for predicting an insufficient temporal bony window [26]. Conversely, bone thickness of 2.7 mm was associated with a good window, and values of 5.0 mm permitted just a partial transcranial study [26].

Two studies have shown that 1-MHz probes increase the diagnostic yield of transcranial ultrasound in patients presenting with absent or insufficient temporal bone windows at transtemporal insonation with 2-MHz probes [27, 28].

Many studies have shown that the administration of echo contrast agents increase diagnostic confidence by improving the detection rate of the basal cerebral arteries [29–32].

Foramen Magnum Window

Transforaminal (transnuchal) insonation is performed with an axial scanning plane (fig. 3), and allows the distinction of the atlas loop (V3) and the intracranial segment (V4) of both vertebral arteries (VA), and the BA [33, 34]. Useful anatomical landmarks include the hyperechogenic processus transversus and clivus [33, 34]. Due to the higher insonation depth necessary for the assessment of the BA, it is detected less often (79–94%) [33–36] than V4 VA (89–98%) [33, 35, 36]. The VA, and in particular, the BA are less often detected in men compared to women [23, 37]. The cause for the gender difference in quality of the foramen magnum window is not clear, and several hypotheses have been proposed. One theory is that men have larger and thicker neck tendons compared to women [23]. Another assumption is that elderly women are assumed to have short, stiff, arthritic necks, preventing appropriate inclination of the head, which is necessary to detect the BA [37]. Finally, the smaller cross-sectional area of the foramen magnum in women could explain the lower detection rate of BA [37, 38].

Table 4. Transfrontal color duplex sonography – detection rates of cerebral arteries and internal cerebral vein [44]

		All (%)	Age ≤60 years (%)	Age >60 years (%)
Artery	Anterior cerebral			
	precommunicating (A1)	49	60	18
	postcommunicating (A2)	60	74	23
	Middle cerebral	43	53	15
	Posterior cerebral	41	49	18
	Posterior communicating	40	40	15
Vein	Internal cerebral	52	60	30

Several studies have shown that the administration of echo contrast agents increase diagnostic confidence by improving the detection rate of V4 VA and BA [39–42].

The inferior petrosal sinus can be found in a depth of 9–10 cm lateral to the BA with a flow directed towards the probe [43]. The inferior petrosal sinus was investigated using TCD in 80 healthy volunteers and patients without central nervous system disorders with a mean age of 38 ± 15 (range, 15–84) years. It was detected in 96% at least on one side, bilaterally in 60%, on the right and left side in 93% and 64%, respectively.

Frontal Bony Windows

Stolz et al. [44, 45] have described the paramedian (fig. 4a) and lateral (fig. 4b) frontal bony windows for insonation of the ACA, MCA, PCA, PCoA, and internal cerebral vein. The corresponding detection rates are given in table 4. The paramedian window is located slightly lateral of the midline, and the lateral window above the lateral aspect of the eyebrow.

Occipital Bony Window

Transoccipital insonation is performed with the patient in a sitting position and the head bent slightly forward. The transducer is positioned approximately 1 cm above the external occipital protuberance using sagittal scanning planes (fig. 5). Transoccipital CDS allows the assessment of the straight sinus in the midline and laterally the calcarine branches of both PCA, and anteriorly the great cerebral and internal cerebral vein [46]. The clivus and the frontal skull are used as anatomic landmarks. The aforementioned vessels are identified according to their anatomic location and the strong velocity changes occurring during Valsalva's maneuver, which are only observed in sinuses and veins. In our experience it is not possible to distinguish both internal cerebral veins, because the length of both vessels is just a few millimeters, which is below the resolution of the transcranial probe. Transoccipital CDS detected the straight sinus in 81% and great cerebral vein and internal cerebral vein in 34% of subjects aged 20–59 years [46]. In subjects aged 60–79 years, detection rates were about 50% for the straight sinus, and 13–20% for the great cerebral and internal cerebral vein [46].

References

1 Moster MR, Kennerdell JS: B-scan ultrasonic evaluation of a dilated superior ophthalmic vein in orbital and retro-orbital arteriovenous anomalies. J Clin Neuroophthalmol 1983;3:105–108.
2 Erickson SJ, Hendrix LE, Massaro BM, Harris GJ, Lewandowski MF, Foley WD, Lawson TL: Color Doppler flow imaging of the normal and abnormal orbit. Radiology 1989;173:511–516.
3 Ley-Pozo JA, Ringelstein EB, Willmes K: Noninvasive detection of occlusive disease of the carotid siphon and middle cerebral artery. Ann Neurol 1990;28:640–647.
4 Lindegaard K, Bakke S, Aaslid R, Nornes H: Doppler diagnosis of intracranial artery occlusive disorder. J Neurol Neurosurg Psychiatr 1986;49:510–518.
5 Schneider PA, Rossman ME, Bernstein EF, Ringelstein EB, Otis SM: Noninvasive assessment of cerebral collateral blood supply through the ophthalmic artery. Stroke 1991;22:31–36.
6 Spencer MP, Whisler G: Transorbital Doppler diagnosis of intracranial arterial stenosis. Stroke 1986;17:916–921.
7 Valdueza JM, Hoffmann O, Doepp F, Lehmann R, Einhäupl KM: Venous Doppler ultrasound assessment of parasellar region. Cerebrovasc Dis 1998;8:113–117.
8 Lie WE, Cohen SM, Merton DA, Shields JA, Mitchell DG, Golderg BB: Color Doppler imaging of the eye and orbit: Technique and normal vascular anatomy. Arch Ophthalmol 1991;109:527–531.
9 Lizzi FL, Mortimer AJ: Bioeffects considerations for the safety of diagnostic ultrasound. J Ultrasound Med 1988;7(suppl):1–38.
10 Hu HH, Luo CL, Sheng WY, Teng MM, Wong WJ, Luk YO: Transorbital color Doppler flow imaging of the carotid siphon and major arteries at the base of the brain. AJNR Am J Neuroradiol 1995;16:591–598.
11 Eden A: Transcranial Doppler ultrasonography and hyperostosis of the skull. Stroke 1988;19: 1445–1446.
12 Halsey JH: Effect of emitted power on waveform intensity in transcranial Doppler. Stroke 1990;21:1573–1578.
13 Nakatani S, Wakayama A, Ozaki H, Kumura E, Shimizu K, Mogami H: Proc Conf Jpn Acad Neuroson 1986;5:58–59.
14 Hansberg T, Wong KS, Droste DW, Ringelstein EB, Kay R: Effects of the ultrasound contrast-enhancing agent Levovist on the detection of intracranial arteries and stenoses in Chinese by transcranial Doppler ultrasound. Cerebrovasc Dis 2002;14:105–108.
15 Bogdahn U, Becker G, Winkler J, Greiner K, Perez J, Meurers B: Transcranial color-coded real-time sonography in adults. Stroke 1990;21:1680–1688.
16 Baumgartner RW, Gönner F, Arnold M, Müri RM: Transtemporal power- and frequency-based color-coded duplex sonography of cerebral veins and sinuses. AJNR Am J Neuroradiol 1997;18: 1771–1781.

17 Stolz E, Kaps M, Kern A, Babacan SS, Dorndorf W: Transcranial color-coded duplex sonography of intracranial veins and sinuses in adults. Reference data from 130 volunteers. Stroke 1999;30: 1070–1075.

18 Baumgartner RW, Mattle HP, Aaslid R: Transcranial color-coded duplex sonography, magnetic resonance angiography, and computed tomography angiography: Methods, applications, advantages, and limitations. J Clin Ultrasound 1995;23:89–111.

19 Klötzsch C, Popescu O, Berlit P: Assessment of the posterior communicating artery by transcranial color-coded duplex sonography. Stroke 1996;27:486–489.

20 Seidel G, Kaps M, Gerriets T, Hutzelmann T: Evaluation of the ventricular system in adults by transcranial duplex sonography. J Neuroimaging 1995;5:105–108.

21 Gerriets T, Stolz E, Modrau B, Fiss I, Seidel G, Kaps M: Sonographic monitoring of midline shift in hemispheric infarctions. Neurology 1999;52:45–49.

22 Gerriets T, Stolz E, König S, Babacan SS, Fiss I, Jauss M, Kaps M: Sonographic monitoring of midline shift in space occupying stroke: An early outcome predictor. Stroke 2001;32:442–446.

23 Marinoni M, Ginanneschi A, Forleo P, Amaducci L: Technical limits in transcranial Doppler recording: Inadequate acoustic windows. Ultrasound Med Biol 1997;23:1275–1277.

24 Kollar J, Schulte-Altedorneburg G, Sikula J, Fulesdi B, Ringelstein EB, Mehta V, Csiba L, Droste DW: Image quality of the temporal bone window examined by transcranial Doppler sonography and correlation with postmortem computed tomography measurements. Cerebrovasc Dis 2004;17: 61–65.

25 Grolimund P: Transmission of Ultrasound Through the Temporal Bone. Vienna, Springer, 1986.

26 Jarquin-Valdivia AA, McCartney J, Palestrant D, Johnston SC, Gress D: The thickness of the temporal squama and its implication for transcranial sonography. J Neuroimaging 2004;14: 139–142.

27 Klotzsch C, Popescu O, Berlit P: A new 1-MHz probe for transcranial Doppler sonography in patients with inadequate temporal bone windows. Ultrasound Med Biol 1998;24:101–103.

28 Georgiadis D, Karatschei R, Uhlmann F, Lindner A: Diagnostic yield of a 1-MHz transducer in evaluation of the basal cerebral arteries. J Neuroimaging 1999;9:15–18.

29 Baumgartner RW, Mattle HP, Aaslid R, Kaps M: Transcranial color-coded duplex sonography in arterial cerebrovascular disease. Cerebrovasc Dis 1997;7:57–63.

30 Görtler M, Kross R, Bäumer M, Jost S, Grote R, Weber S, Wallesch C-W: Diagnostic impact and prognostic relevance of early contrast-enhanced transcranial color-coded duplex sonography in acute stroke. Stroke 1998;29:955–962.

31 Postert T, Federlein J, Braun B, Köster O, Börnke C, Przuntek H, Büttner T: Contrast-enhanced transcranial color-coded real-time sonography: A reliable tool for the diagnosis of middle cerebral artery trunk occlusion in patients with insufficient temporal bone window (letter). Stroke 1998;29:1070–1073.

32 Gerriets T, Seidel G, Fiss I, Modrau B, Kaps M: Contrast-enhanced transcranial color-coded duplex sonography. Neurology 1999;52:1133–1137.

33 Kaps M, Seidel G, Bauer T, Behrmann B: Imaging of the intracranial vertebrobasilar system using color-coded ultrasound. Stroke 1992;23:1577–1582.

34 Schöning M, Walter J: Evaluation of the vertebrobasilar-posterior system by transcranial color duplex sonography in adults. Stroke 1992;23:1280–1286.

35 Baumgartner RW, Mattle HP, Schroth G: Assessment of 50 and <50% intracranial stenoses by transcranial color-coded duplex sonography. Stroke 1999;30:87–92.

36 Martin PJ, Evans DH, Naylor AR: Transcranial color-coded sonography of the basal cerebral circulation. Stroke 1994;25:390–396.

37 Hoksbergen AW, Legemate DA, Ubbink DT, Jacobs MJ: Success rate of transcranial color-coded duplex ultrasonography in visualizing the basal cerebral arteries in vascular patients over 60 years of age. Stroke 1999;30:1450–1455.

38 Catalina-Herrera CJ: Study of the anatomic metric values of the foramen magnum and its relation to sex. Acta Anat (Basel) 1987;130:344–347.

39 Droste DW, Nabavi DG, Kemény V, Schulte-Altedorneburg G, Ritter MA, Weber S, Ringelstein EB: Echocontrast enhanced transcranial colour-coded duplex offers improved visualization of the vertebrobasilar system. Acta Neurol Scand 1998;98:193–199.

40 Brunner-Beeg F, von Reutern GM: Farbduplexsonograpie des intrakraniellen vertebrobasilaren systems: Verbesserung der Darstellung durch Echosignalverstärker. Ultraschall Med 1999;20:83–86.
41 Iglseder B, Huemer M, Staffen W, Ladurner G: Imaging the basilar artery by contrast-enhanced color-coded ultrasound. J Neuroimaging 2000;10:195–199.
42 Stolz E, Nuckel M, Mendes I, Gerriets T, Kaps M: Vertebrobasilar transcranial color-coded duplex ultrasonography: Improvement with echo enhancement. AJNR Am J Neuroradiol 2002;23: 1051–1054.
43 Doepp F, Hoffmann O, Lehmann R, Einhäupl KM, Valdueza JM: The inferior petrosal sinus: Assessment by transcranial Doppler ultrasound using the suboccipital approach. J Neuroimaging 1999;9:193–197.
44 Stolz E, Kaps M, Kern A, Dorndorf W: Frontal bone windows for transcranial color-coded duplex sonography. Stroke 1999;30:814–820.
45 Stolz E, Mendes I, Gerriets T, Kaps M: Assessment of intracranial collateral flow by transcranial color-coded duplex sonography using a temporal and frontal axial insonation plane. J Neuroimaging 2002;12:136–143.
46 Baumgartner RW, Nirkko AC, Müri RM, Gönner F: Transoccipital power-based color-coded duplex sonography of cerebral sinuses and veins. Stroke 1997;28:1319–1323.
47 Baumgartner RW, Baumgartner I, Mattle HP, Schroth G: Transcranial color-coded duplex sonography in the evaluation of collateral flow through the circle of Willis. AJNR Am J Neuroradiol 1997;18:127–133.
48 Stolz E, Kaps M, Dorndorf W: Assessment of intracranial venous hemodynamics in normal individuals and patients with cerebral venous thrombosis. Stroke 1999;30:70–75.

Ralf W. Baumgartner, MD
Department of Neurology, University Hospital
Frauenklinikstrasse 26
CH–8091 Zürich (Switzerland)
Tel. +41 1 255 56 86, Fax +41 1 255 88 64, E-Mail ralf.baumgartner@usz.ch

Baumgartner RW (ed): Handbook on Neurovascular Ultrasound.
Front Neurol Neurosci. Basel, Karger, 2006, vol 21, pp 117–126

Intracranial Stenoses and Occlusions, and Circle of Willis Collaterals

Ralf W. Baumgartner

Department of Neurology, University Hospital of Zürich, Zürich, Switzerland

Abstract

Stenoses and occlusions of the anterior, middle, pre- and postcommunicating posterior cerebral, and basilar and intracranial vertebral arteries are reliably detected by transcranial Doppler (TCD) and transcranial color duplex sonography (TCCS). Diagnosis of carotid siphon stenosis is consistently obtained by transorbital Doppler sonography. Internationally accepted criteria for diagnosing intracranial arterial obstructions are lacking. Both TCD and TCCS reliably identify collateral flow through the anterior and posterior communicating arteries. It is unclear whether TCCS is more accurate than TCD for detecting intracranial obstructions and collaterals, as no study has examined this issue.

Intracranial Stenosis

Intracranial stenosis is characterized by the presence of a focal increase of flow velocities, which is associated in most cases with high-intensity and low-frequency Doppler signals (fig. 1). Several transcranial Doppler sonography (TCD) [1–7] and transcranial color duplex sonography (TCCS) [8] studies used catheter angiography as 'gold' standard and described criteria for detecting intracranial stenoses. There are no internationally accepted criteria for diagnosing intracranial stenosis. Furthermore, the diagnostic accuracy of predefined TCD and TCCS criteria for assessing intracranial stenosis has not yet been investigated. A TCCS study evaluated peak systolic velocity cutoff values for the assessment of ≥50 and <50% stenoses of the intracranial cerebral arteries (table 1) [8]. For TCCS diagnosis of ≥50% stenoses, the sensitivity, specificity and positive predictive values (PPV) were 100%, and the negative predictive values (NPV) 91–100%. For TCCS diagnosis of <50% stenoses, the

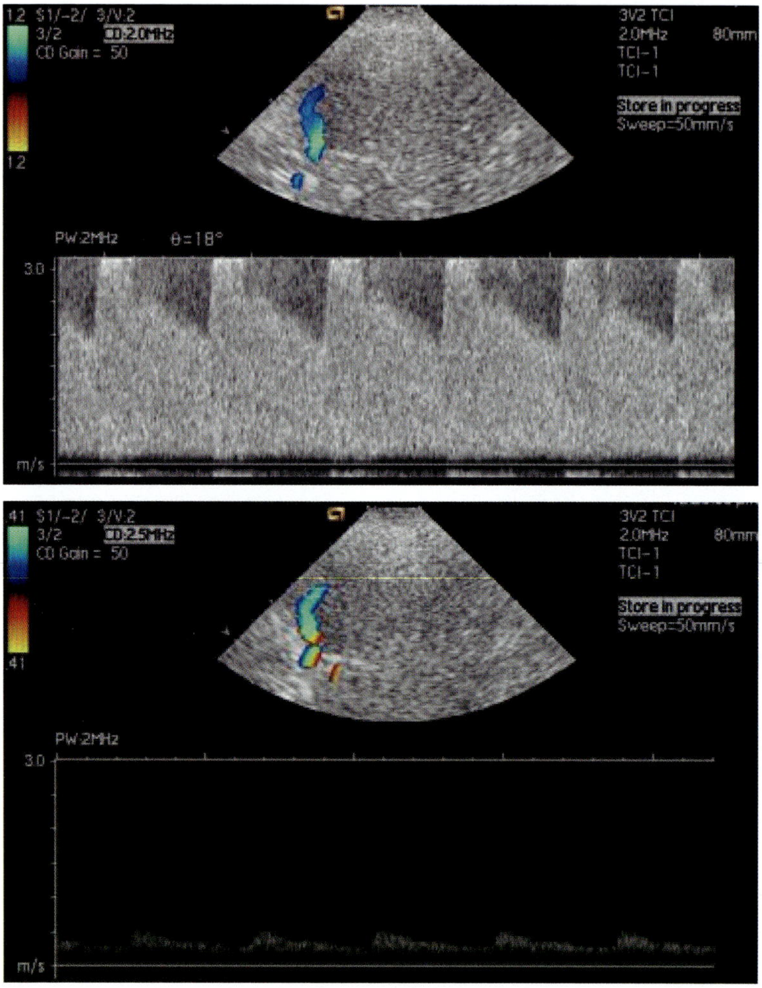

a

b

Fig. 1. Transtemporal color duplex sonography with an axial plane shows a ≥50% stenosis of the sphenoidal segment of the middle cerebral artery with increased intrastenotic flow velocities (***a***), and decreased flow velocities and pulsatility distal to the stenosis (***b***).

sensitivity was 94–100%, the specificity 99–100%, the PPV 73–100%, and the NPV 100%. Peak mean flow velocity (MFV) values of >120 cm/s were shown to be consistent predictors of carotid siphon stenosis investigated with transorbital TCD [5]. The use of absolute velocities for diagnosis of intracranial stenosis has several limitations: (1) false-positive stenoses may be diagnosed in patients with disturbed autoregulation (e.g., subarachnoid hemorrhage,

Table 1. Criteria for diagnosis of intracranial cerebral artery stenosis

	Peak systolic flow velocity, cm/s	
	<50%	≥50%
Anterior cerebral artery	≥155	≥220
Middle cerebral artery	≥120	≥155
Posterior cerebral artery	≥100	≥145
Vertebral artery	≥100	≥140
Basilar artery	≥90	≥120

trauma), after the inappropriate use of the angle corrector or administration of ultrasound contrast agents, which better detect the fastest erythrocytes, and thus lead to the detection of higher flow velocities [9], (2) intracranial stenoses can be missed in hypoplastic vessels such as the precommunicating (A1) anterior (ACA) and precommunicating (P1) posterior (PCA) cerebral and intracranial vertebral (VA) arteries, in the presence of additional downstream obstructions, which is frequent in patients with acute stroke, and after the inappropriate use of the angle corrector. Increased blood flow and velocity may also occur in cerebral arteries supplying Willisian collaterals, arteriovenous malformations (see chapter by Klötzsch and Harrer, pp. 171–181) and dural arteriovenous fistula (see chapter by Gandjour and Baumgartner, pp. 85–95), and anemia and hyperthyreosis. Thus, transcranial ultrasound cannot diagnose stenoses in the latter diseases [10].

Severe middle cerebral artery (MCA) stenoses may also be suspected in the presence of increased velocities in the ACA, which are related to leptomeningeal collaterals [11]. Preliminary data using angiography as standard of reference indicate that contrast-enhanced (CE) TCCS may reliably detect intracranial stenosis [12, 13], and that CE TCCS using the power Doppler mode improves the visualization of intra- and poststenotic flow [14].

It is not possible to differentiate cerebral artery narrowing due to a vasospasm and stenosis as well as embolic from atherosclerotic stenoses. Vasospasm and stenoses due to cerebral embolism typically recanalize within days, weeks, or months. In contrast, atherosclerotic stenoses are assumed to show no recanalization, although no study has investigated this issue. Thus, recurrent transcranial ultrasound studies are needed to differentiate these causes of intracranial cerebral artery narrowing.

No study has evaluated diagnostic criteria for diagnosing a stenosis in the terminal segment (C1) of the internal carotid artery (ICA), the insular (M2) and more distal segments of the MCA, the postcommunicating (A2) ACA and the quadrigeminal (P3) PCA.

The therapeutic consequence of quantifying symptomatic intracranial stenoses by ultrasound has diminished, because the investigators of the Warfarin-Aspirin Symptomatic Intracranial Disease study [15] recommend that aspirin should be used instead of warfarin also in patients with ≥50% intracranial stenoses, since warfarin was associated with higher rates of adverse events and provided no benefit over aspirin. However, quantification of intracranial stenosis is still useful for guiding the blood pressure management in patients with acute stroke, assessing recanalization, and in the follow-up of intracranial stents.

Intracranial Occlusion

TCD diagnosis of intracranial cerebral artery occlusion is established by the absence of Doppler signals in a cerebral artery of a patient with an appropriate acoustic window proven by the detection of at least one ipsilateral cerebral artery [6, 11, 16]. TCCS diagnosis of intracranial occlusion is based on the absence of color and spectral Doppler signals in the occluded vessel, whereas the adequate insonation window can also be demonstrated by depicting adjacent intracranial veins or structures [17, 18]. It has also been shown that the detection of associated hemodynamic abnormalities is helpful. Occlusion of M1 MCA is frequently associated with increased velocities in the ipsilateral ACA due to the presence of leptomeningeal collaterals [11, 16]. Occluded intracranial ICA, VA, and basilar artery (BA) cause reduced velocities and increased pulsatility in the preocclusional vessels, although this may not occur in the BA when adequate cerebellar cross-flow is present [6, 19, 20]. Downstream to these occlusions collateral pathways may develop. These collaterals include, in ICA occlusion, the ophthalmic artery and the circle of Willis, in BA occlusion the posterior communicating artery (PCoA), and in intracranial VA occlusion located before the origin of the posterior inferior cerebellar artery, the ipsilateral distal VA [6, 19–21].

Occluded intracranial arteries recanalize in most cases, which can be detected by ultrasound and confirms the diagnosis of previous occlusion [22, 23].

Another TCD study has evaluated the accuracy of TCD diagnosis of intracranial occlusion using predefined ultrasound criteria [24]. The corresponding sensitivities were 93% for M1 MCA, 56% for the intracranial VA, and 60% for the BA; specificities ranged from 96 to 98%. The same group determined 5 years later the yield and accuracy of combined carotid/vertebral duplex and TCD in patients with acute cerebral ischemia to identify lesions amenable for interventional treatment (LAIT) [25]. LAIT was defined by digital subtraction angiography as an occlusion or near-occlusion, or ≥50% stenosis or thrombi in the symptomatic artery, and were located in M1 or M2 MCA, the ICA, BA, or VA. Thirty patients were included, and DSA was performed on average 230 min after ultrasound. The location and details of LAIT were not reported. The sensitivity of TCD for detecting a LAIT was 96%, the specificity 75%, the PPV 96%, and the NPV 75%. The corresponding values for the combined carotid/vertebral duplex and TCD assessment were 100%. It is questionable whether it is not preferable to restrict the definition of LAIT to occlusions, because intra-arterial and mechanical thrombolysis is just performed in occluded, but not stenosed, cerebral arteries.

The accuracy of TCD to diagnose stenosis and occlusion of C1 ICA was investigated in 22 patients [26]. Angiography was used as standard of reference. Four patients had abnormal TCD findings that were not confirmed by angiography, and 2 patients with normal TCD findings showed <50% stenoses of the C1 and cavernous ICA segments at angiography. Thus, sensitivity for TCD diagnosis of C1 ICA stenosis or occlusion was 90%, specificity 83%, PPV 82%, and NPV 86%.

The ability of a TCD MFV ratio using reciprocal MCA depths bilaterally, i.e., affected MCA-to-contralateral MCA MFV ratio (aMCA/cMCA MFV ratio), to identify a proximal arterial occlusion that requires local intra-arterial thrombolysis was investigated in 29 of 80 patients enrolled in the Interventional Management of Stroke study [27]. No temporal window was found in 3 of 29 patients. Cerebral angiography was performed after a mean delay of 174 ± 36 min after the onset of stroke symptoms, and TCD after a median time interval of 93.5 min from onset. The aMCA/cMCA MFV ratio <0.6 had a sensitivity of 94%, a specificity of 100%, a PPV of 100%, and a NPV of 86% for identifying proximal occlusion in the anterior circulation that require local intra-arterial thrombolsyis.

Another TCD study has shown that the occlusion of more than three MCA branches is associated with decreased velocities in M1 MCA [28].

A TCCS study using predefined criteria for diagnosis of M1 MCA occlusion (fig. 2) showed a sensitivity, specificity, PPV, and NPV of 100% in 30 patients with ischemic stroke of duration less than 24 h and appropriate temporal bony windows [29]. Another study using predefined criteria but no ‘gold standard’ found that CE TCCS enabled within 5–7 min the diagnosis of MCA occlusions located in the main stem or branches in 20 of 23 patients with acute ischemic stroke of duration less than 5 h [30]. Other studies confirmed that CE TCCS may reliably detect M1 MCA occlusion [12, 31]. CE TCCS without spectral Doppler confirmation identified M1 MCA occlusions with a sensitivity of 94% and a specificity of 93% in a study, which evaluated 30 patients with

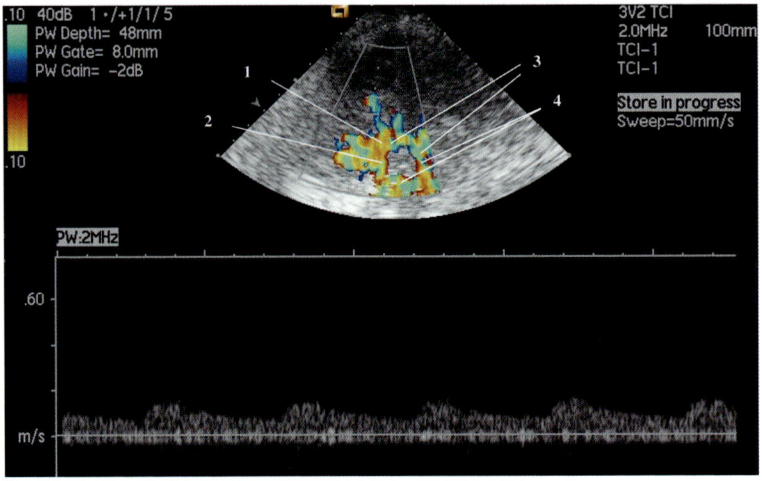

Fig. 2. Transtemporal color duplex sonography with an axial plane using an echo-contrast agent shows an occlusion of the distal sphenoidal segment of the middle cerebral artery with slow flow velocities at spectral Doppler sonography of the preocclusional portion of the vessel. (1) denotes the ipsilateral anterior cerebral, (2) the contralateral anterior cerebral, (3) the ipsilateral posterior cerebral, and (4) the contralateral posterior cerebral artery.

ischemic stroke and insufficient acoustic windows within 12 h after symptom onset [32].

Cross-Flow through the Circle of Willis

The reliability of TCCS assessment of collateral flow through the circle of Willis using predefined criteria [33] was investigated in 132 patients with ≥70%, uni- or bilateral stenosis or occlusion of the carotid artery [10]. Cross-flow through the anterior communicating artery (fig. 3) was diagnosed in the presence of reversed flow in the ACA located on the side of the obstructed carotid artery. If this ACA was missed, decrease of flow velocity in the homolateral MCA during digital compression of the contralateral common carotid artery was used for diagnosis. The corresponding sensitivity was 98%, specificity 100%, PPV 100%, and NPV 98%. Thus, carotid compression for the assessment of cross-flow through the anterior communicating artery is no more justified because of the well-known risks of this maneuver [34, 35]. Furthermore, most ipsilateral ACA are detected by using ultrasound contrast agents. TCCS was less reliable for detecting cross-flow through the PCoA (fig. 4), and the sensitivity

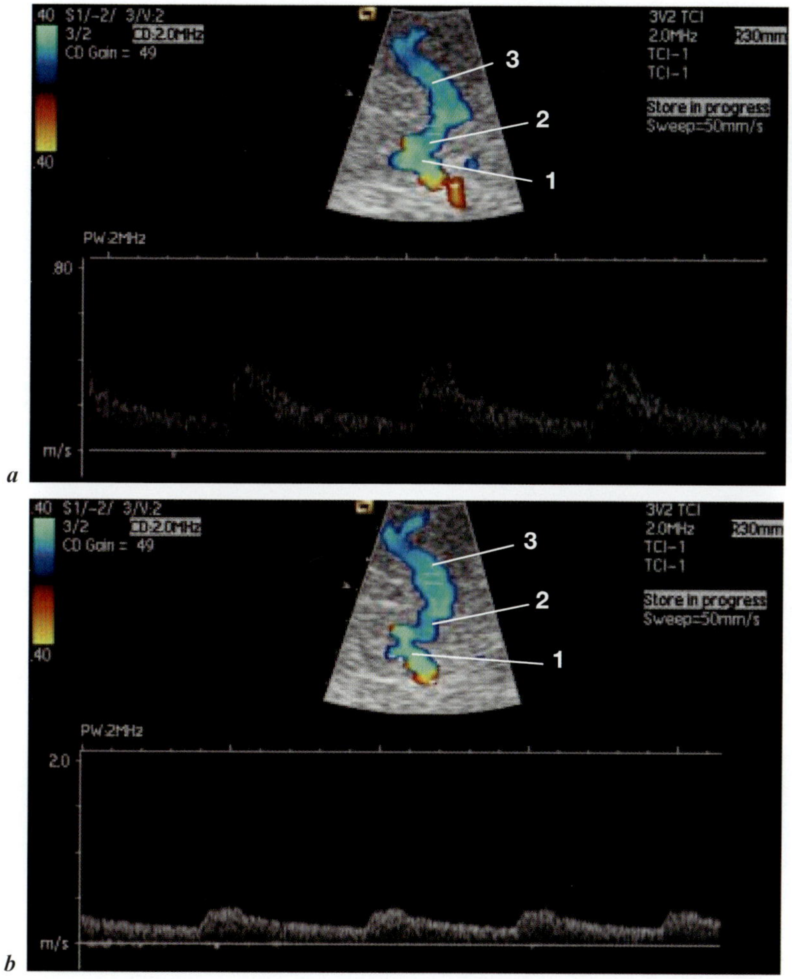

Fig. 3. Transtemporal color duplex sonography with an axial plane shows cross-flow through the anterior communicating artery to the middle cerebral artery distal to a severe carotid stenosis. The contralateral (1) and ipsilateral (2) anterior cerebral and the ipsilateral middle cerebral (3) arteries are colored in blue, indicating cross-flow from the contralateral through the ipsilateral anterior cerebral to the middle cerebral artery. The Doppler spectra in the ipsilateral anterior (***a***) and middle (***b***) cerebral arteries confirm the color duplex findings.

was 84%, the specificity 94%, the PPV 94%, and the NPV 84%. Cross-flow through the PCoA was diagnosed, when the PCoA was detected or peak systolic velocities in P1 PCA were higher than the mean value plus two standard deviations of normals.

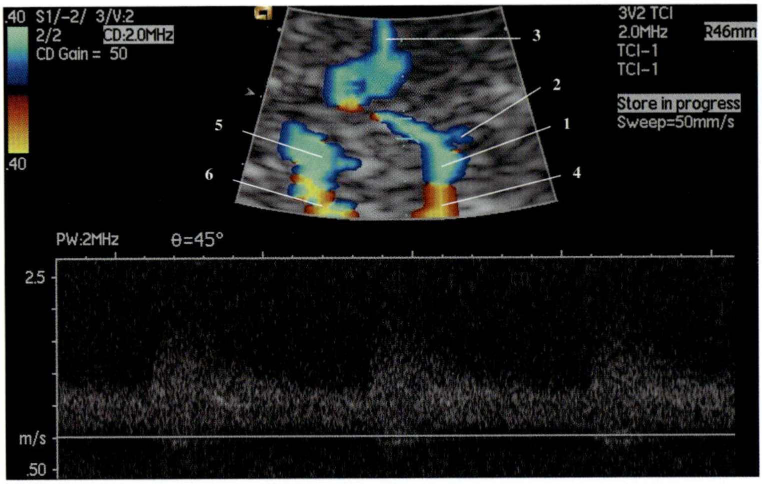

Fig. 4. Transtemporal color duplex sonography with an axial plane shows cross-flow through the posterior communicating artery to the intracranial carotid artery distal to a severe extracranial carotid stenosis. The posterior communicating artery containing the volume sampled by spectral Doppler sonography, the pre- (1) and postcommunicating (2) posterior, and the middle (3) cerebral arteries are colored in blue, indicating cross-flow from the vertebrobasilar to the carotid system through the posterior communicating artery. The Doppler spectra obtained in the posterior communicating artery confirm the color duplex findings. (4) denotes the contralateral precommunicating posterior cerebral artery, (5) the ipsilateral, and (6) the contralateral anterior cerebral artery.

Ultrasound contrast agents increase the detection rate of Willisian collaterals compared to nonenhanced TCCS [9, 13], and preliminary data indicate that power Doppler imaging may better visualize the PCoA [36]. Two studies suggest that the amount of cross-flow through the circle of Willis is better assessed using extracranial [37] than transcranial [38] ultrasound.

Collateral flow through the PCoA to the BA and contralateral PCA in case of BA occlusion may be assessed by detecting reversed flow in P1 PCA [10].

References

1 Babikian V, Sloan MA, Tegeler CH, DeWitt LD, Fayad PB, Feldmann E, Gomez CR: Transcranial Doppler validation pilot study. J Neuroimag 1993;3:242–249.

2 De Bray J, Joseph P, Jeanvoine H, Maugin D, Dauzat M, Plassard F: Transcranial Doppler evaluation of middle cerebral artery stenosis. J Ultrasound Med 1988;7:611–616.

3 Felberg RA, Christou I, Demchuk AM, Malkoff M, Alexandrov AV: Screening for intracranial stenosis with transcranial Doppler: The accuracy of mean flow velocity thresholds. J Neuroimag 2002;12:9–14.

4 Hennerici M, Rautenberg W, Schwartz A: Transcranial Doppler ultrasound for the assessment of intracranial arterial flow velocity. II. Evaluation of intracranial artery disease. Surg Neurol 1987;27:523–532.

5 Ley-Pozo JA, Ringelstein EB, Willmes K: Noninvasive detection of occlusive disease of the carotid siphon and middle cerebral artery. Ann Neurol 1990;28:640–647.

6 Lindegaard K, Bakke S, Aaslid R, Nornes H: Doppler diagnosis of intracranial artery occlusive disorder. J Neurol Neurosurg Psychiatr 1986;49:510–518.

7 Röther J, Schwartz AS, Wentz KU, Rautenberg W, Hennerici M: Middle cerebral artery stenoses: Assessment by magnetic resonance angiography and transcranial Doppler ultrasound. Cerebrovasc Dis 1994;4:273–279.

8 Baumgartner RW, Mattle HP, Schroth G: Assessment of ≥50% and <50% intracranial stenoses by transcranial color-coded duplex sonography. Stroke 1999;30:87–92.

9 Baumgartner RW, Arnold M, Gönner F, Staikow I, Herrmann C, Rivoir A, Müri RM: Contrast-enhanced transcranial color-coded duplex sonography in ischemic cerebrovascular disease. Stroke 1997;28:2473–2478.

10 Baumgartner RW, Baumgartner I, Mattle HP, Schroth G: Transcranial color-coded duplex sonography in the evaluation of collateral flow through the circle of Willis. AJNR Am J Neuroradiol 1997;18:127–133.

11 Mattle HP, Grolimund P, Huber P, Sturzenegger M, Zurbrügg H: Transcranial Doppler sonographic findings in middle cerebral artery disease. Arch Neurol 1988;45:289–295.

12 Nabavi DG, Droste DW, Kemeny V, Schulte-Altedorneburg G, Weber S, Ringelstein EB: Potential and limitations of echocontrast-enhanced ultrasonography in acute stroke patients. Stroke 1998;29:949–954.

13 Droste DW, Jürgens R, Weber S, Tietje R, Ringelstein EB: Benefit of echocontrast-enhanced transcranial color-coded duplex ultrasound in the assessment of intracranial collateral pathways. Stroke 2000;31:920–923.

14 Griewing B, Schminke U, Motsch L, Brassel F, Kessler C: Trancranial duplex sonography of middle cerebral artery stenosis: A comparison of colour-coding techniques – Frequency- or power-based Doppler and contrast enhancement. Neuroradiol 1998;40:490–495.

15 Chimowitz MI, Lynn MJ, Howlett-Smith H, Stern BJ, Hertzberg VS, Frankel MR, Levine SR, Chaturvedi S, Kasner SE, Benesch CG, Sila CA, Jovin TG, Romano JG: Warfarin-Aspirin Symptomatic Intracranial Disease Trial Investigators: Comparison of warfarin and aspirin for symptomatic intracranial arterial stenosis. N Engl J Med 2005;252:1305–1316.

16 Kaps M, Damian MS, Teschendorf U, Dorndorf W: Transcranial Doppler ultrasound findings in middle cerebral artery occlusion. Stroke 1990;21:532–537.

17 Baumgartner RW, Mattle HP, Aaslid R: Transcranial color-coded duplex sonography, magnetic resonance angiography, and computed tomography angiography: Methods, applications, advantages, and limitations. J Clin Ultrasound 1995;23:89–111.

18 Seidel G, Kaps M, Gerriets T: Potential and limitation of transcranial color-coded sonography in stroke patients. Stroke 1995;26:2061–2066.

19 Ringelstein EB, Zeumer H, Poeck K: Non-invasive diagnosis of intracranial lesions in the vertebrobasilar system. A comparison of Doppler sonographic and angiographic findings. Stroke 1985;16:848–855.

20 Demchuk AM, Christou I, Wein TH, Felberg RA, Malkoff M, Grotta JC, Alexandrov AV: Specific transcranial Doppler flow findings related to the presence and site of arterial occlusion. Stroke 2000;31:140–146.

21 Saito K, Kimura K, Nagatsuka K, Nagano K, Minematsu K, Ueno S, Naritomi H: Vertebral artery occlusion in duplex color-coded ultrasonography. Stroke 2004;35:1068–1072.

22 Ringelstein EB, Biniek R, Weiller C, Ammeling B, Nolte PN, Thron A: Type and extent of hemispheric brain infarctions and clinical outcome in early and delayed middle cerebral artery recanalization. Neurology 1992;42:289–298.

23 Fieschi C, Bozzao L: Transient embolic occlusion of the middle cerebral and internal carotid arteries in cerebral apoplexy. J Neurol Neurosurg Psychiatr 1969;32:236–240.

24 Demchuk AM, Christou I, Wein TH, Felberg RA, Malkoff M, Grotta JC, Alexandrov AV: Accuracy and criteria for localizing arterial occlusion with transcranial Doppler. J Neuroimaging 2000;10:1–12.

25 Chernyshev OY, Garami Z, Calleja S, Song J, Campbell MS, Noser EA, Shaltoni H, Chen C-I, Iguchi Y, Grotta JC, Alexandrov AV: Yield and accuracy of urgent combined carotid/transcranial ultrasound testing in acute cerebral ischemia. Stroke 2005;36:32–37.
26 Navarro JC, Mikulik R, Garami Z, Alexandrov AV: The accuracy of transcranial Doppler in the diagnosis of stenosis or occlusion of the terminal internal carotid artery. J Neuroimaging 2004;14:314–318.
27 Saqqur M, Shuaib A, Alexandrov AV, Hill MD, Calleja S, Tomsick T, Broderick J, Demchuk AM: Derivation of transcranial Doppler criteria for rescue intra-arterial thrombolysis: Multicenter experience from the Interventional Management of Stroke study. Stroke 2005;36:865–868.
28 Zanette EM, Roberti C, Mancini G, Pozzilli C, Bragoni M, Toni D: Spontaneous middle cerebral artery reperfusion in ischemic stroke: A follow-up study with transcranial Doppler. Stroke 1995;26:430–433.
29 Kenton A, Martin P, Abbott R, Moody A: Comparison of transcranial color-coded duplex sonography and magnetic resonance angiography in acute stroke. Stroke 1997;28:1601–1606.
30 Görtler M, Kross R, Bäumer M, Jost S, Grote R, Weber S, Wallesch C-W: Diagnostic impact and prognostic relevance of early contrast-enhanced transcranial color-coded duplex sonography in acute stroke. Stroke 1998;29:955–962.
31 Gerriets T, Seidel G, Fiss I, Modrau B, Kaps M: Contrast-enhanced transcranial color-coded duplex sonography. Neurology 1999;52:1133–1137.
32 Postert T, Federlein J, Braun B, Köster O, Börnke C, Przuntek H, Büttner T: Contrast-enhanced transcranial color-coded real-time sonography: A reliable tool for the diagnosis of middle cerebral artery trunk occlusion in patients with insufficient temporal bone window (letter). Stroke 1998;29:1070–1073.
33 Baumgartner RW, Baumgartner I, Schroth G: Diagnostic criteria for transcranial colour-coded duplex sonography evaluation of cross-flow through the circle of Willis in unilateral obstructive carotid artery disease. J Neurol 1996;243:516–521.
34 Khaffaf N, Karnik R, Winkler WB, Valentin A, Slany J: Embolic stroke by compression maneuver during transcranial Doppler sonography. Stroke 1994;25:1056–1057.
35 Nelson DA, Mahru MM: Death following digital arterial occlusion. Arch Neurol 1963;8:640–643.
36 Postert T, Meves S, Bornke C, Przuntek H, Büttner T: Power Doppler compared to color-coded duplex sonography in the assessment of the basal cerebral circulation. J Neuroimag 1997;7:221–226.
37 Ho SS, Metreweli C, Yu CH: Color velocity imaging quantification in the detection of intracranial collateral flow. Stroke 2002;33:1795–1798.
38 Schulte-Altedorneburg G, Becker T: Extent of spontaneous cross-flow via the anterior communicating artery in steno-occlusive carotid artery disease. Neurol Res 2005;27:441–445.

Ralf W. Baumgartner, MD
Department of Neurology University Hospital
Frauenklinikstrasse 26
CH–8091 Zürich (Switzerland)
Tel. +41 1 255 56 86, Fax +41 1 255 88 64, E-Mail ralf.baumgartner@usz.ch

Baumgartner RW (ed): Handbook on Neurovascular Ultrasound.
Front Neurol Neurosci. Basel, Karger, 2006, vol 21, pp 127–139

Acute Stroke: Perfusion Imaging

Günter Seidel, Karsten Meyer-Wiethe

Neurologische Universitätsklinik, Lübeck, Germany

Abstract

Ultrasound perfusion imaging of the human brain is a bedside technique based on the detection of ultrasound contrast agent (UCA) in the cerebral microcirculation. In the last decade, ultrasound technology improved from single-pulse harmonic imaging to multiple-pulse technologies (pulse inversion or power modulation harmonic imaging as well as contrast pulse sequencing), with a further dramatic increase of the contrast-agent-to-tissue ratio. Different kinetic models for the qualitative assessment of brain perfusion have been evaluated so far in healthy subjects as well as in patients suffering from acute ischemic stroke. The analysis of the contrast bolus kinetics yields robust time-intensity curve parameters, which qualitatively describe regional brain perfusion. In the acute phase of ischemic stroke, the peak signal increase and the time-to-peak intensity are the most valuable curve parameters to predict the area of definite infarction and the outcome of the patient. Color-coded parametric imaging of these parameters facilitates the interpretation of contrast kinetics in analyzing brain perfusion. UCA-specific kinetic models, such as replenishment and diminution kinetics, are new modalities for the qualitative visualization of brain perfusion. The latter is more promising for acute ischemic stroke patients because of the faster imaging and processing time, leading to a lower vulnerability to movement artifacts.

Physical Background of Ultrasound Perfusion Imaging

Ultrasound perfusion imaging of the human brain is a new semi-invasive bedside technique based on the detection of ultrasound contrast agent (UCA) in the brain tissue to evaluate brain perfusion. Current UCAs consist of microbubbles composed of a gas that is associated with various types of shells for stabilization. Because of their small size, they can pass through the microcirculation several times, thus representing optimum blood pool tracers.

As a measure of energy impinging on the tissue, the mechanical index (MI) is defined as the peak pressure of a longitudinal ultrasound wave propagating in a uniform medium divided by the square root of the center frequency of the transmitted ultrasound pulse [1].

Depending on the applied energy, various interactions between ultrasound and microbubbles can be observed: at low ultrasound energies, UCA microbubbles show resonance phenomena, emitting ultrasound waves at multiples of the insonated fundamental frequency [2]. In contrast, the insonated tissue mainly yields responses at the fundamental frequency. These higher harmonic frequencies can be selectively received, leading to a high sensitivity for the detection of UCA (low-MI imaging). Increase of the ultrasound energy (high-MI imaging) causes microbubble destruction, leading to a final ultrasound energy emission that can be detected and used for image generation. Apart from harmonic oscillation and disruption, UCA microbubbles can respond with translation, coalescence, fragmentation, sonic cracking, or jetting [3]. The threshold between 'low MI' and 'high MI' is not clearly defined and depends on the organ of interest. For transcranial applications, a high MI must be observed because of the ultrasound absorption of the skull.

In the last few years, ultrasound technology improved from single-pulse conventional harmonic imaging to multiple-pulse technologies (pulse inversion or power modulation harmonic imaging as well as contrast pulse sequencing) with a further dramatic increase of the contrast-agent-to-tissue ratio. Multiple-pulse technologies receive contrast-agent-specific signals in the fundamental frequency band (so-called nonlinear fundamental signals) with a higher sensitivity than conventional single-pulse approaches.

Kinetic Models for the Analysis of Cerebral Perfusion

Considerable difficulties are implicit in using conventional ultrasound technology to analyze cerebral microcirculation. Because of the slow blood flow velocity – between 1 and 10 mm/s – cerebral blood flow cannot be assessed by conventional Doppler techniques. This limitation can be overcome by analyzing the interaction between ultrasound energy and UCA microbubbles.

Perfusion is defined as flow (amount of blood passing per unit time) per volume of tissue. As a result of physical limitations, such as depth dependence and shadowing phenomena, performing a noninvasive *quantitative* cerebral perfusion measurement with contrast ultrasound is not possible, as of yet. Thus, ultrasound contrast methods seek to offer a simple bedside approach for *qualitative* description of cerebral perfusion.

Three kinetic models (bolus, destruction, and replenishment) are used to evaluate cerebral perfusion with contrast ultrasound. The first two models have been tested in ischemic stroke patients.

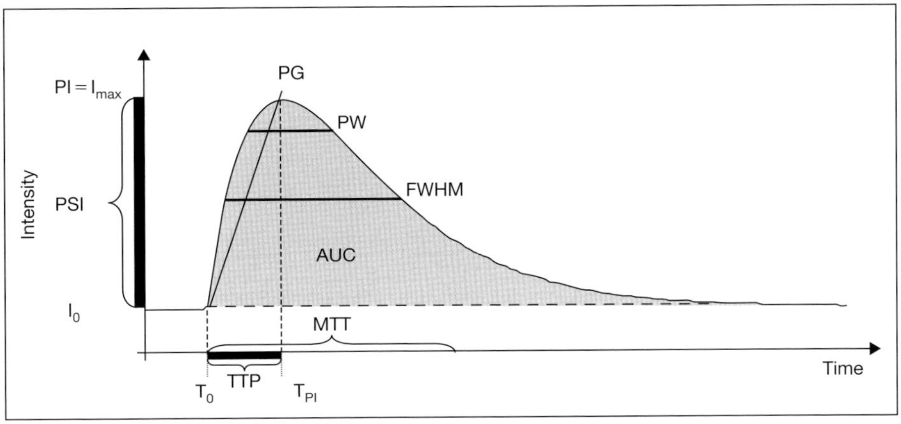

Fig. 1. Schematic representation of different parameters of the time-intensity curve after ultrasound contrast agent bolus injection. PI = Peak intensity (maximum intensity (I_{max})); PSI = peak signal increase; I_0 = baseline intensity; PG = positive gradient; T_0 = time at peak onset; T_{PI} = time to peak intensity; TTP = time to peak; PW = peak width at 90% of maximum; FWHM = full width at half maximum; AUC = area under the curve; MTT = mean transit time.

Bolus Kinetics

After UCA bolus injection, microbubbles entering the insonation field are destroyed by ultrasound energy. To allow inflow into the parenchyma, the slow blood flow velocity in the cerebral microcirculation must be considered. Thus, a frame rate of 0.25–1 Hz must be observed, leading to deterioration in time resolution. In most clinical studies, the wash-in and -out information of the time-intensity curves or image sequences after UCA bolus injection have been analyzed to qualitatively assess regional cerebral blood flow (fig. 1). Different parameters of these curves can be extracted, such as the time-to-peak intensity, time to peak (TTP), mean transit time, peak intensity, peak signal increase, peak width (full width at 90% of the maximum intensity), full width at half of the maximum intensity, area under the curve, and positive gradient (slope of the wash-in phase).

Diminution or Destruction Kinetics

Diminution kinetics is based on the destruction of contrast agent at a constant frame rate with a high MI. The TIC decreases to a new steady state, determined by a balance between destruction and reperfusion of contrast agent.

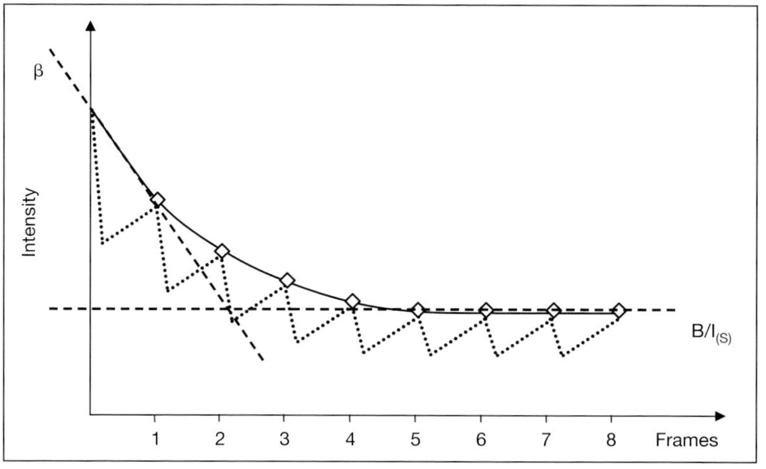

Fig. 2. Scheme of contrast diminution kinetics for brain perfusion assessment. β = ln2/half life, B = baseline intensity (exponential model), equivalent to $I_{(s)}$ = intensity at the steady state (linear model). The dotted line indicates the two components (destructive and reperfusion phase) of the complex exponential model [5].

Three mathematical models for analyzing the diminution curve have been applied: an exponential decay model; a complex exponential model, which separates the curve into destruction and reperfusion phases, thus providing a perfusion and a destruction coefficient, respectively; and a simple linear model [4, 5, 22] (fig. 2).

Because of the short sampling time needed (1–10 s), diminution kinetics can be analyzed using either bolus injection or infusion.

Analysis of Brain Perfusion in Patients with Acute Stroke

In clinical studies on stroke patients, only one of thirteen studies used diminution kinetics (table 1). In all other studies, UCA bolus kinetics was analyzed using different harmonic imaging modalities. Levovist, Optison, and, in more recent studies, SonoVue were used as contrast agents. In elderly stroke patients with intact skull and sufficient insonation conditions for fundamental color-coded duplex sonography, a successful perfusion study could be generated in 76–93% of these patients using Levovist and in up to 100% using SonoVue [6–8]. In such patients, optimum results were achieved with high-MI gray scale harmonic imaging using a low receiving frequency (2.6 MHz [9]). With the introduction of more sensitive ultrasound technologies for the

Table 1. Synopsis of studies on ultrasound perfusion imaging in ischemic stroke patients until March 2005

No. of patients, type of disease (time between symptom onset and ultrasound)	Ultrasound system, ultrasound method, depth, insonation plane	Ultrasound contrast agent (UCA)	Perfusion parameters	Reference method/ Parametric imaging (parameters)	Sufficient acoustic bone window	Authors, year, ref.
Bolus Kinetics						
2 patients, acute ischemic stroke (<48 h)	SONOS 5500, harmonic imaging (HI), gray scale, 10 cm, axial	Bolus: Levovist™ 10 ml (400 mg/ml)	Semiquantitative area of hypoperfusion (cine loop, TIC)	CT/–	Craniectomy	Postert et al. 1999 [19]
25 patients, intact skull, acute ischemic stroke (<24 h), follow-up (<24 h, day 2, within 1 week) + 14 control subjects	SONOS 5500 HI, 10 cm, axial	Bolus: Levovist™ 10 ml 400 mg/ml)	Semiquantitative area of hypoperfusion (cine loop), TIC from infarcted area	CT/–	21/25 (84%) (patients)/ 13/14 (92.9%) (healthy subjects)	Federlein et al. 2000 [6]
1 patient, Moya-Moya syndrome, chronic stage	HDI 5000, pulse inversion HI, gray scale	Bolus: Levovist™ 12.5 ml	Semiquantitative area of hypoperfusion (cine loop), TIC from symptomatic area vs. asymptomatic side (arrival time of UCA)	Xenon-CT, TCD (CVR)/–	Craniectomy	Meairs et al. 2000 [16]
3 patients, after hemicraniectomy	Sequoia 512, loss-of-correlation imaging, fundamental TCCS, 1. frame rate: 6 Hz, 2. freeze–defreeze (3 s), 16 cm, axial	Infusion: Levovist™ 90 ml/h (300 mg/ml)	Semiquantitative area of hypoperfusion	CT/–	Craniectomy	Schlachetzki et al. 2001 [12]

Table 1. (continued)

No. of patients, type of disease (time between symptom onset and ultrasound)	Ultrasound system, ultrasound method, depth, insonation plane	Ultrasound contrast agent (UCA)	Perfusion parameters	Reference method/ Parametric imaging (parameters)	Sufficient acoustic bone window	Authors, year, ref.
2 patients (Moya-Moya syndrome/internal cerebral vein thrombosis) + 10 control subjects	SONOS 5500, HI (power modulation), 11 cm, axial	Bolus: Optison™ 2 ml	Quantitative: MTT (mean transit time), TTP (time to peak), PI (peak increase), AUC (area under the curve), R-T (rise-time)	CT, MRI, angiography/–	2/2	Stolz et al. 2002 [18]
1 patient, acute middle cerebral artery occlusion (12 h)	SONOS 5500, HI, integrated backscatter (IBS), gray scale, 10 cm, axial	Bolus: Levovist™ 5 ml (400 mg/ml)	Semiquantitative area of: TTP, PPI (pixelwise peak intensity)	MRI (PWI, DWI, MRA)/ Ultrasound (TTP, PPI)	–	Meyer et al. 2003 [17]
24 patients, intact skull, acute ischemic stroke (<12 h), follow-up 72 ± 6 h	SONOS 5500, HI, IBS, gray scale, 10 cm, axial	Bolus: Levovist™ 5 ml (400 mg/ml)	Quantitative area of hypoperfusion (cine loop), AUC of TIC from infarcted area vs. asymptomatic side	CT/–	19/24 (79.2%)	Seidel et al. 2003 [7]
10 patients, stroke (hemorrhagic (n = 2) and ischemic (n = 8)), 48 h after craniectomy	Sequoia 512, HI (single-pulse transmission technology), gray scale, unknown depth, axial	Bolus: SonoVue™	Quantitative area of hypoperfusion (TIC)	CT or MRI/ ultrasound (average peak average)	Craniectomy	Bartels and Bittermann 2004 [11]

4 patients, acute ischemic stroke (<12 h)	Sonoline Elegra, pulse inversion HI, gray scale, 15 cm ('bilateral approach'), axial	Bolus: SonoVue™ 2.5 ml	TTP and PW (peak width), fitted model function	CT/Ultrasound (peak intensity)	4/4	Eyding et al. 2004 [10]
23 patients, intact skull, acute ischemic stroke (<40 h)	SONOS 5500, HI, IBS, gray scale, 10 cm, axial	Bolus: SonoVue™ 2.4 ml	Quantitative area of: TTP, PPI	CT/Ultrasound (TTP, PPI)	23/23 (100%)	Seidel et al. 2004 [8]
14 patients, subacute stroke (n = 6) and other diseases (n = 8), 4 with and 10 without temporal skull defect	SONOS 5500, HI with S3 transducer (second HI (SHI2.6 [1.3/2.6]), ultra harmonics (UHI [1.3/3.6 MHz]), power harmonics (PHI2.6 [2.6 MHz] and PHI3.2) and two imaging procedures with S4 transducer (SHI3.6 [1.8/3.6 MHz] and PHI3.6 [3.6 MHz]), gray scale and power Doppler, 12 cm, axial	Bolus: Levovist™ 7 ml (300 mg/ml)	Semiquantitative area of hypoperfusion (cine loop)	CT or MRI/–	Intact skull: best result SHI2.6: 80% Without temporal skull: best result PHI3.6: 100%	Shiogai et al. 2004 [9]

Table 1. (continued)

No. of patients, type of disease (time between symptom onset and ultrasound)	Ultrasound system, ultrasound method, depth, insonation plane	Ultrasound contrast agent (UCA)	Perfusion parameters	Reference method/ Parametric imaging (parameters)	Sufficient acoustic bone window	Authors, year, ref.
23 patients, intact skull, acute ischemic stroke (<12 h)	SONOS 5500, HI, IBS, gray scale, 10 cm, axial	Bolus: Levovist™ 5 ml (400 mg/ml)	Quantitative area of : TTP, PPI, cine loop gray scale	CT/Ultrasound (TTP, PPI)	23/30 (76.7%)	Wiesmann et al. 2004 [15]
Diminution Kinetics						
15 patients, acute ischemic stroke (<24 h)	HDI 5000, power pulse inversion contrast HI, power Doppler, destruction sequence: 20 frames (MI 1.2), 14 Hz, axial	Bolus: SonoVue™ 2.5 ml	Semiquantitative area of hypoperfusion (cine loop, TIC)	MRI/–	15/15 (100%)	Kern et al. 2004 [20]

TCCS = Transcranial color-coded sonography; TCD = transcranial Doppler; CVR = cerebrovascular reserve; PWI = perfusion-weighted imaging; DWI = diffusion-weighted imaging; MRA = magnetic resonance angiography; TIC = time-intensity curve. – = Not done.

detection of contrast agents (pulse inversion harmonic imaging), it might be possible to analyze brain perfusion not only in the ipsilateral but also in the contralateral hemisphere within one investigation [10]. The problem with this approach is that additional artifacts occur (shadowing artifacts caused by calcified pineal gland and/or choroid plexus) besides the depth-dependent signal decrease because of ultrasound attenuation.

Few studies have been performed on ultrasound perfusion imaging in patients after hemicraniectomy [9, 11, 12]. In these cases, Doppler-based harmonic technologies with higher receiving frequencies seem to be superior to gray scale harmonic imaging [9]. When using high-MI imaging, the direct contrast-enhanced insonation of the brain without the skull (which reduces the actual energy in the tissue) could be harmful because of cavitation and capillary rupture [13, 14].

Different parameters of the bolus kinetics curve acquired from ischemic brain regions were compared with computed tomography (CT) in the acute phase of stroke. A combination of the peak intensity and TTP seems appropriate in characterizing the area-of-infarction-to-be in follow-up CT.

Time-intensity data of all pixels under evaluation can be displayed as a color-coded parametric image, which facilitates the visualization of the perfusion state [8, 15] (fig. 3). In 13–14% of acute ischemic stroke patients, a perfusion deficit in the middle cerebral artery territory could be found with parametric imaging, although the supplying artery was found not occluded [6, 8]. The areas of disturbed perfusion in the parametric images correlate with the area of infarction in follow-up CT and the severity-of-stroke symptoms in the early phase as well as after 4 months [8]. Parametric imaging is, however, susceptible to movement artifacts. In studies on restless patients with movement artifacts in the imaging study, it is useful to re-evaluate the original cine loop of the parametric image [15].

Other investigations based on UCA bolus injection were performed on smaller patient populations using Xenon-CT [13], magnetic resonance imaging (MRI) [17, 18] or CT [10, 12, 19] as reference methods. These case reports demonstrated the potential of different contrast-specific modalities, such as power modulation imaging, pulse-inversion harmonic imaging, loss-of-correlation imaging, or conventional harmonic imaging, for the assessment of pathological brain perfusion using contrast ultrasound imaging.

In one study, diminution imaging was evaluated in the very early phase of ischemic stroke (<24 h) and compared with perfusion-weighted MRI [20]. This study showed the diagnostic potential of this fast imaging technique to obtain information on regions of reduced perfusion in the very early phase of ischemic stroke [20]. Disturbed perfusion can be displayed as a parametric image encoding the perfusion coefficient (fig. 4).

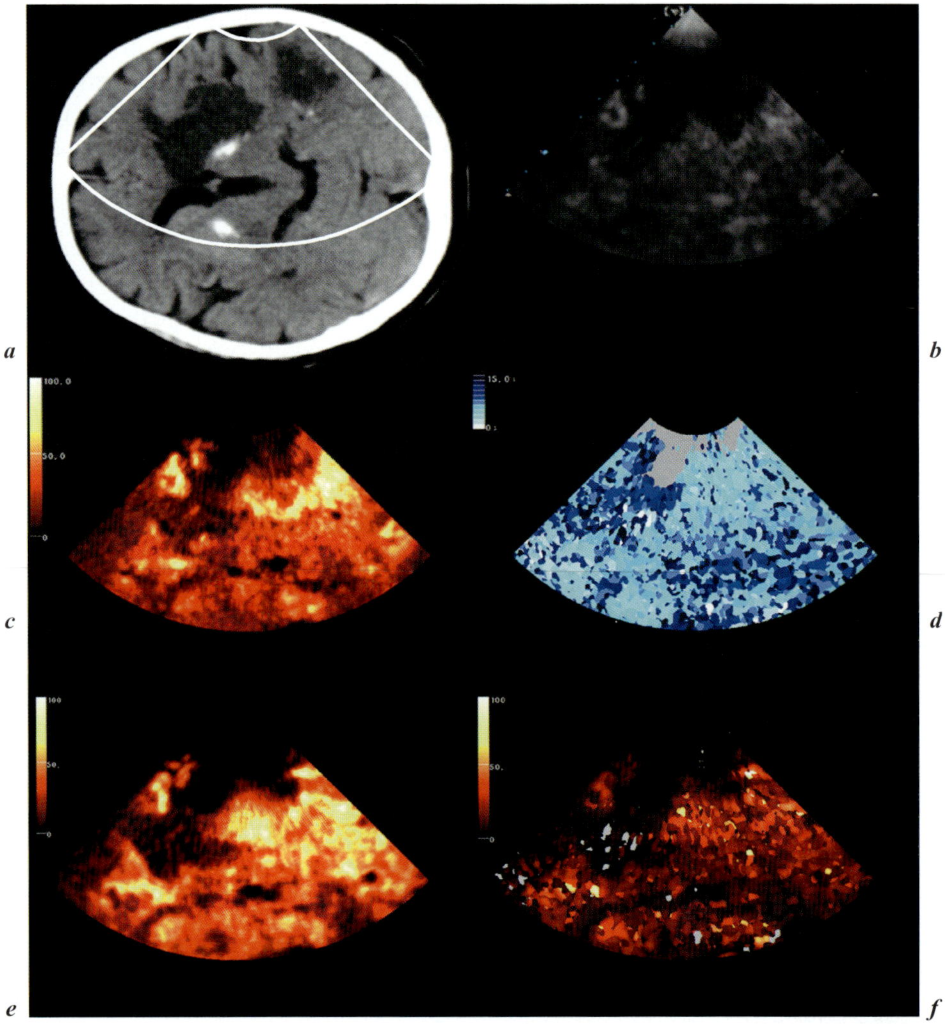

Fig. 3. ***a*** Follow-up CT, 48 h after symptom onset, of a 67-year-old woman suffering from middle cerebral artery occlusion. Ultrasound perfusion imaging (Harmonic imaging 1.8/3.6 MHz, MI 1.6, 2.4 ml SonoVue™ bolus injection, investigation depth 10 cm, frame rate 0.67 Hz) was performed 2.5 h after symptom onset. ***b*** Contrast image with area of reduced contrast enhancement in the middle cerebral artery territory. Parametric images: ***c*** Pixelwise peak intensity image showing the area of reduced signal enhancement (dark) in the middle cerebral artery territory, ***d*** time to peak image showing the dark blue area of delayed perfusion, invalid data being displayed in gray, ***e*** area under the curve image, and ***f*** slope image.

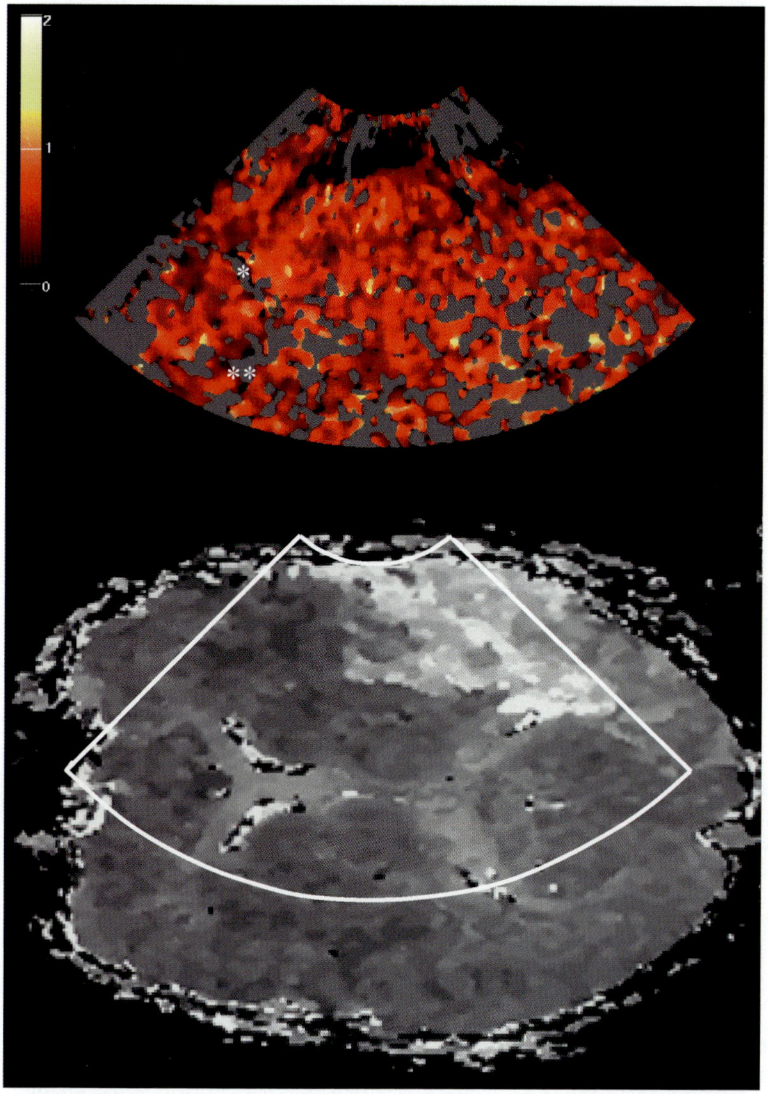

a

b

Fig. 4. Parametric image (***a***) of the perfusion coefficient of diminution imaging of a 67-year-old patient with acute MCA branch occlusion, 13.5 h after symptom onset (SonoVue infusion, 1.6 ml/min, 1.8/3.6 MHz, MI 1.6, frame rate 6.67 Hz). * = Anterior horn of ipsilateral ventricle; ** = anterior horn of contralateral ventricle. Note the dark area with a low perfusion coefficient, which corresponds to the area of delayed perfusion (white) in perfusion-weighted imaging (***b***), 10 h after symptom onset.

Besides the advantages of ultrasound perfusion imaging as a fast, semi-invasive bedside method, there are some disadvantages, such as the insonation artifacts, which occur in most of the studies (fig. 3), and potential side effects of the contrast agents, which restrict the employment of these substances in severe cardiac or pulmonary disease.

The major limitation of neurosonology is the ultrasound penetration through the skull. Even the temporal 'bone window' has an irregular thickness, which induces distortions in the ultrasound propagation. A significant rate of diagnostically insufficient acoustic windows has been encountered in clinical studies conducted so far (table 1). Because of these different insonation conditions, an interindividual comparison of intensity-based data remains problematic. A simple solution is the use of time-dependent parameters like TTP (bolus kinetics) of half-life (destruction kinetics). These parameters are depth independent [21] but, because of the low frame rate, the time resolution of TTP in high-MI imaging is not very high. One step towards minimizing insonation irregularities is the construction of ultrasound probes that are optimized for brain imaging. The ultrasound probes currently used were not specifically designed for transcranial sonography. Indeed, they are not optimized for the lower frequencies and higher MI imposed by the attenuation that is induced by the skull. Technical solutions to circumvent this problem are currently under investigation.

References

1 de Jong N: Mechanical Index. Eur J Echocardiogr 2002;3:73–74.

2 Burns PN: Harmonic imaging with ultrasound contrast agents. Clin Radiol 1996;51(suppl 1): 50–55.

3 Postema M, van Wamel A, Lancee CT, de Jong N: Ultrasound-induced encapsulated microbubble phenomena. Ultrasound Med Biol 2004;30:827–840.

4 Meyer K, Seidel G: Transcranial contrast diminution imaging of the human brain: A pilot study in healthy volunteers. Ultrasound Med Biol 2002;28:1433–1437.

5 Eyding J, Wilkening W, Reckhardt M, Schmid G, Meves S, Ermert H, Przuntek H, Postert T: Contrast burst depletion imaging (CODIM): A new imaging procedure and analysis method for semiquantitative ultrasonic perfusion imaging. Stroke 2003;34:77–83.

6 Federlein J, Postert T, Meves SH, Weber S, Przuntek H, Büttner T: Ultrasonic evaluation of pathological brain perfusion in acute stroke using second harmonic imaging. J Neurol Neurosurg Psychiatry 2000;69:616–622.

7 Seidel G, Albers T, Meyer K, Wiesmann M: Perfusion harmonic imaging in acute middle cerebral artery infarction. Ultrasound Med Biol 2003;29:1245–1251.

8 Seidel G, Meyer-Wiethe K, Berdien G, Hollstein D, Toth D, Aach T: Ultrasound perfusion imaging in acute middle cerebral artery infarction predicts outcome. Stroke 2004;35:1107–1111.

9 Shiogai T, Takayasu N, Mizuno T, Nakagawa M, Furuhata H: Comparison of transcranial brain tissue perfusion images between ultraharmonic, second harmonic, and power harmonic imaging. Stroke 2004;35:687–693.

10 Eyding J, Krogias C, Wilkening W, Postert T: Detection of cerebral perfusion abnormalities in acute stroke using phase inversion harmonic imaging (PIHI): Preliminary results. J Neurol Neurosurg Psychiatry 2004;75:926–929.
11 Bartels E, Bittermann HJ: Transcranial contrast imaging of cerebral perfusion in stroke patients following decompressive craniectomy. Ultraschall Med 2004;25:206–213.
12 Schlachetzki F, Hoelscher T, Dorenbeck U, Greiffenberg B, Marienhagen J, Ullrich OW, Bogdahn U: Sonographic parenchymal and brain perfusion imaging: Preliminary results in four patients following decompressive surgery for malignant middle cerebral artery infarct. Ultrasound Med Biol 2001;27:21–31.
13 Hynynen K, McDannold N, Sheikov NA, Jolesz FA, Vykhodtseva N: Local and reversible blood-brain barrier disruption by noninvasive focused ultrasound at frequencies suitable for trans-skull sonications. Neuroimage 2005;24:12–20.
14 Mychaskiw G 2nd, Badr AE, Tibbs R, Clower BR, Zhang JH: Optison (FS069) disrupts the blood-brain barrier in rats. Anesth Anal 2000;91:798–803.
15 Wiesmann M, Meyer K, Albers T, Seidel G: Parametric perfusion imaging with contrast-enhanced ultrasound in acute ischemic stroke. Stroke 2004;35:508–513.
16 Meairs S, Daffertshofer M, Neff W, Eschenfleder C, Hennerici M: Pulse-inversion contrast harmonic imaging: Ultrasonographic assessment of cerebral perfusion (letter). Lancet 2000;355:550–551.
17 Meyer K, Wiesmann M, Albers T, Seidel G: Harmonic imaging in acute stroke: Detection of a cerebral perfusion deficit with ultrasound and perfusion MRI. J Neuroimaging 2003;13:166–168.
18 Stolz E, Allendorfer J, Jauss M, Traupe H, Kaps M: Sonographic harmonic grey scale imaging of brain perfusion: Scope of a new method demonstrated in selected cases. Ultraschall Med 2002;23: 320–324.
19 Postert T, Federlein J, Weber S, Przuntek H, Büttner T: Second harmonic imaging in acute middle cerebral artery infarction: Preliminary results. Stroke 1999;30:1702–1706.
20 Kern R, Perren F, Schoeneberger K, Gass A, Hennerici M, Meairs S: Ultrasound microbubble destruction imaging in acute middle cerebral artery stroke. Stroke 2004;35:1665–1670.
21 Meves SH, Wilkening W, Thies T, Eyding J, Hölscher T, Finger M, Schmid G, Ermert H, Postert T: Comparison between echo contrast agent-specific imaging modes and perfusion-weighted magnetic resonance imaging for the assessment of brain perfusion. Stroke 2002;33:2433–2437.
22 Meyer-Wiethe K, Cangür H, Seidel G: Comparison of different mathematical models to analyse diminution kinetics of ultrasound contrast enhancement in a flow phantom. Ultrasound Med Biol 2005;31:93–98.

Prof. Dr. Günter Seidel
Neurologische Universitätsklinik
Ratzeburger Allee 160, DE–23538 Lübeck (Germany)
Tel. +49 451 500 3334, Fax +49 451 500 2489
E-Mail guenter.seidel@neuro.uni-luebeck.de

Baumgartner RW (ed): Handbook on Neurovascular Ultrasound.
Front Neurol Neurosci. Basel, Karger, 2006, vol 21, pp 140–149

Sonothrombolysis: Experimental Evidence

Michael Daffertshofer, Michael Hennerici

Department of Neurology, University of Heidelberg, University Hospital Mannheim, Mannheim, Germany

Abstract

Reopening of the occluded artery is the primary therapeutic goal in hyperacute ischemic stroke. Systemic treatment with tissue recombinant plasminogen activator (tPA) has been shown to be beneficial at least in a 3-hour door to needle window. Intra-arterial thrombolysis is favorable and opens the window of treatment up to at least 6 h but consequences invasive intra-arterial angiography in a high number of patients, of whom a significant number do not finally receive thrombolysis. The combination of ultrasound with thrombolytic agents may enhance the potential benefit by means of enzyme-mediated thrombolysis. When ultrasound is applied externally through skin or chest, attenuation will be very low. Attenuation, however, is significantly higher if penetration through the skull is required. Attenuation is frequency dependent, with ultrasound intensity being <10% of the output intensity for diagnostic frequencies (>1 MHz). This ratio nearly reverses in the kiloHertz range (<500 kHz). Ultrasound insonation is efficient for accelerating enzymatic thrombolysis within a wide range of intensities, from 0.5 W/cm^2 (MI ~0.3) to several watts per square centimeter, particularly in the nonfocused ultrasound field. Insonation with ultrasound increased tPA-mediated thrombolysis up to 20% in a static model, while it enhanced the recanalization rate from 30 to 90% in a flow model. Results from embolic rat models suggest that low-frequency ultrasound with 0.6 W/cm^2 significantly reduces infarct volume compared to pure tPA treatment. Safety of ultrasound exposure of the brain for therapeutic purposes has to address hemorrhage, heating, and direct tissue damage. Since animal studies suggested no increase of bleeding rate or harm to the blood-brain barrier, a clinical phase II study applying low-frequency ultrasound at ~300 kHz found a high number of secondary hemorrhages. Heating depends critically on the characteristics of the ultrasound. The most significant heating of the brain tissue itself is >1°C per hour using a 2 W/cm^2 probe; however, no significant heating could be found when using an emission protocol pulsing the ultrasound. The current experimental data helps to identify the optimal ultrasound characteristics for sonothrombolysis and supports the hypothesis combined treatment being a perspective in optimizing thrombolytic therapy in acute stroke.

More than two thirds of ischemic events are related to cerebral embolism. Clinical outcome depends on fast and efficient intracranial vessel recanalization [1]. Spontaneous recanalization of occluded intracerebral vessels occurs in 15–20% of patients within the first 24 h [2]. This rate may be increased to 34–47% by intravenous application and up to 90% by local intra-arterial application of thrombolytics. Beyond this breakthrough the reported low rate of recanalization after systemic application of tissue plasminogen activator tPA [3] may contribute to the still small rate of recovery and stimulated additional investigations to speed up clot lysis.

Experimental, as well as clinical studies, indicate that ultrasound can enhance tPA-mediated recanalization time after thrombotic coronary and peripheral artery occlusion with percutaneous [4] or endovascular application [5, 6], as well as thrombolysis after middle cerebral artery occlusion [7, 8].

In vitro Experimental Results

In vitro research has been conducted by a multitude of investigators on how ultrasound affects thrombolysis. There is evidence that ultrasound accelerates transport of tPA into a clot [9], affects binding of tPA to fibrin [10], causes a reversible disaggregation of fibrin fibers [11], and an increase of flow through the clot [12]. An enhancing effect of ultrasound on thrombolysis has been observed during continuous and intermittent ultrasound exposure over a wide range of frequencies (≤1 MHz) and intensities (≤16 W/cm^2) (table 1).

Although the potentially beneficial effect of external ultrasound on thrombolysis has been described much earlier, the feasibility of transcranial ultrasound for sonothrombolysis in stroke was first demonstrated at the end of the 1990s [17, 19]. Thrombolytic activity was significantly increased when applying low-frequency ultrasound during tPA treatment in a flow model positioned within a human skull. Another group also reported comparable results in an in vitro model and showed enhancement of thrombolysis with urokinase when additionally applying low-frequency ultrasound (211.5 kHz). Although attenuation of ultrasound in the cranial bone increases with frequency, a moderate acceleration of enzymatic thrombolysis can be found even at higher frequencies of 1 MHz or more (fig. 1) [22].

Ultrasound-Mediated Thrombolysis in vivo

Several animal studies [13, 23–25] showed increased thrombolytic activity when ultrasound was applied in combination with thrombolytic agents, with frequencies ranging from 27 to 200 kHz and intensities of 0.25 to >10 W/cm^2

Table 1. Characteristics of published reports of in vitro sonothrombolysis with ultrasound

Author	Year	Protocol	Frequency	Output intensity	Mode	Thrombolytic agent	Thrombolysis ratio*, %	Sonification time, min
Francis et al. [13]	1992	In vitro	1 MHz	1–8 W/cm^2	CW	tPA	140 (1 W/cm^2)	60
							150 (2 W/cm^2)	60
							178 (4 W/cm^2)	60
							458 (8 W/cm^2)	60
Lauer et al. [14]	1992	In vitro	1 MHz	1.75 W/cm^2	Interval	tPA	152	200
Luo et al. [6]	1993	In vitro	1 MHz	1–2.2 W/cm^2	CW	Streptokinase	55 (2.2 W/cm^2)	30
Harpaz et al. [15]	1994	In vitro	1 MHz	2.5 W/cm^2	CW	tPA	514.50	40
Kimura et al. [16]	1994	In vitro	300 kHz, 1 MHz	0.07, 0.4 W/cm^2	CW	tPA		
Francis et al. [9]	1995	In vitro	1 MHz	4 W/cm^2	PW	tPA	147 (tPA uptake)	60
							193 (tPA uptake)	240
Akiyama et al. [17]	1998	In vitro	211.5 kHz, 1.03 MHz	0.25 W/cm^2	CW	Urokinase	140	240
Suchkova et al. [18]	1998		40 kHz	0.25–1.5 W/cm^2	CW	tPA	175 (0.25 W/cm^2)	60
							290 (0.75 W/cm^2)	60
							375 (1 W/cm^2)	60
							385 (1.5 W/cm^2)	60
Behrens et al. [19]	1999	In vitro	33.3 kHz, 71.4 kHz	0.5–3.4 W/cm^2	CW	tPA	130 (33 kHz)	60
							152 (33 kHz)	180
							143 (71 kHz)	60
							171 (71 kHz)	180
Pfaffenberger et al. [20]	2005	In vitro	1.8 MHz	105 mW/cm^2	PW	tPA	21.8 (control)	60
							23.0 (1.8 MHz); ns	
Nedelmann et al. [21]	2005	In vitro	20 kHz	0.2 W/cm^2	CW	ø	52.4 (20 kHz)	10
			40 kHz				49.4 (40 kHz)	10
			60 kHz				21.4 (60 kHz)	10

CW = Continuous wave; PW = pulsed wave; and interval, intermittent insonation.
* Compared with control results.

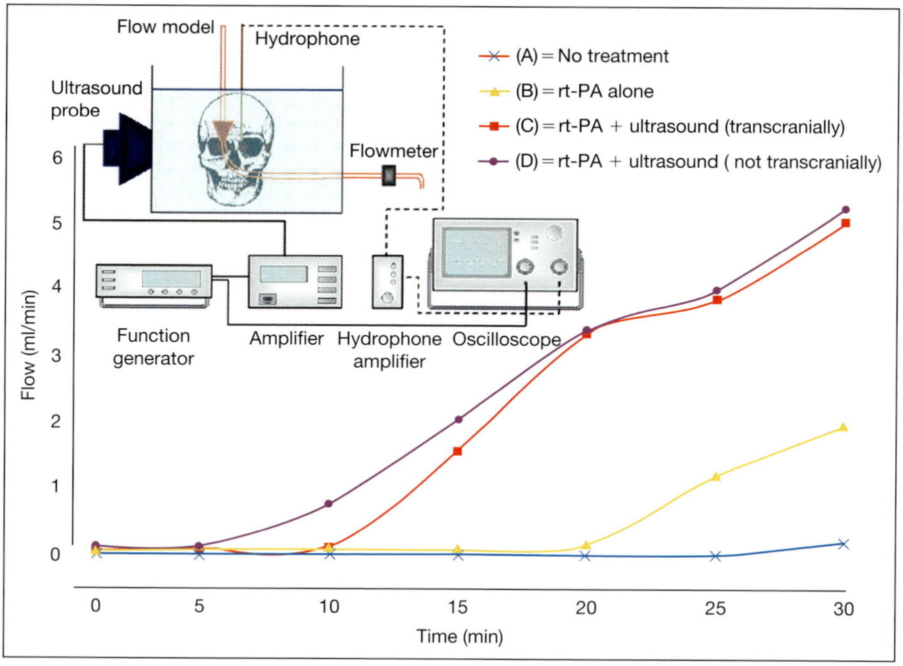

Fig. 1. Flow rate over time in a tube model [19]. Measurement of recanalization after complete occlusion from a fibrin clot in different treatment groups: spontaneously (A), when treating with rt-PA only (B), when treating with rt-PA and ultrasound (1 MHz pulsed wave) (D), and (C) when treating with rt-PA and ultrasound (1 MHz pulsed wave) transcranially (cadaver skull bone). The addition of ultrasound to tPA treatment showed a further decrease of recanalization time.

(table 2). The degree of thrombolysis enhancement varied with ultrasound characteristics, dosage of the thrombolytic agent and is also depended on various biological parameters, e.g., the clot characteristics [31]. Most studies demonstrated the potential usefulness of ultrasound for the treatment of arterial or venous thrombosis. Ultrasound may also have pro-thrombic effects. High-intensity ultrasound [e.g., 6.3 W/cm^2] initially resulted in rapid recanalization of occluded femoral arteries in rabbits, but a higher rate of vessel reocclusion was observed [26]. This may be explained by platelet activation [32] or by an increased inflammatory response due to augmentation of the adhesion of leukocytes to the endothelium [33] caused by high-intensity ultrasound.

The promising results obtained with low-intensity ultrasound in peripheral vessels were expanded to include stroke in an animal model. In an embolic rat model with occlusion of the middle cerebral artery by an autologous arterial clot [34, 35], thrombolysis with tPA reduced infarct volume compared to a control group (26 vs. 44% infarction of the entire hemisphere), and insonation with

Table 2. Characteristics of published reports of in vivo (animal experiments) sonothrombolysis with ultrasound

Author	Year	Protocol	Model	Frequency	Output intensity, W/cm^2	Mode	Thrombolytic agent	Reflow ratio or % flow ratio*	Sonification time, min
Lauer et al. [14]	1992	In vivo	Rabbit jugular vein	1 MHz	1.75	Interval	tPA	916	180
Kornowski et al. [26]	1994	In vivo	Rabbit femoral artery	1 MHz	6.3	Interval	tPA		120
Luo et al. [27]	1996	In vivo	Rabbit femoral artery	26 kHz	16		Streptokinase	983	30
Riggs et al. [28]	1997	In vivo	Rabbit femoral artery	1 MHz	2	Interval	Streptokinase	410	120
Luo et al. [29]	1998	In vivo	Rabbit femoral artery	37 kHz	160	PW	Streptokinase	1,492	60
Suchkova et al. [30]	2000	In vivo	Rabbit femoral artery	40 kHz	0.75	CW	Streptokinase	1,185	120
Daffertshofer et al. [8]	2004	In vivo	Rat embolic MCA	27 KHz	0.6	PW	tPA	34 (tPA only)** 68 (US + tPA)*	60

CW = Continuous wave; PW = pulsed wave; and interval, intermittent insonation.
*Compared with control results; ** Reduction of infarct volume compared to control results.

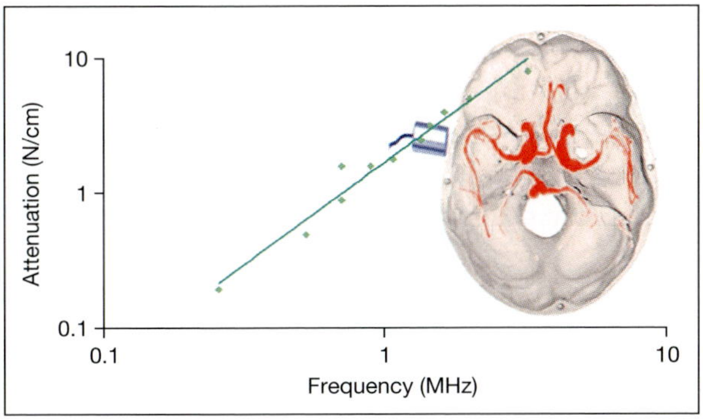

Fig. 2. The diagram demonstrates the attenuation of ultrasound through the skull dependent on the used frequency, showing the strong reversed correlation between decrease of intensity and increase of frequency.

ultrasound (27.5 kHz, 0.6 W/cm^2 20% duty cycle) caused a significant additional reduction of infarct size (11% infarction of the entire hemisphere). Feasibility of ultrasound exposure through the skull was confirmed [36] using a model of a rabbit femoral artery. The authors administered monteplase (mt-PA) intravenously and applied ultrasound (490 kHz, 0.13 W/cm^2) through an external piece of temporal bone. The recanalization rate was 16.7% in the mt-PA group and 66.7% in the mt-PA plus ultrasound group. Despite several clinical human studies using ultrasound devices approved for diagnostic use [7, 37], in vivo studies on animal stroke models using diagnostic frequency (>1 MHz), intensity (0.5–1.0 W/cm^2), or both are still almost completely lacking.

Application of Ultrasound through the Skull

Focused pulsed-wave ultrasound with frequencies above 1 MHz might be transmitted with weak and tolerable attenuation through the skull [28, 38] and is established for diagnostic transcranial routine application [29, 39].

Within 0.25- and 6.0-MHz ultrasound frequencies, the increase of insertion loss (fig. 2) through the skull is not only roughly proportionally related to an increased intensity, but also directly linked to the thickness of the diploë and the skull bone [40]. Pfaffenberger et al. [20], measured the ultrasound attenuation of 2-MHz standard diagnostic transducers and found decreases of output intensity of 86.8% (8.8 dB) to 99.2% (21.2 dB), depending on temporal bone thickness (1.91–5.01 mm). These data indicate to use ultrasound at low to mid-kiloHertz frequencies and suggest that only those frequencies may reach the brain and intracranial vessels with thermally acceptable levels. We investigated these effects within the range of 20–100 kHz and demonstrated low ultrasound attenuation through a sample of different postmortem skulls by transtemporal and -occipital insonation [19]. The average attenuation through the skull was 0.1 ± 0.9 dB for transtemporal, 1.5 ± 0.6 dB for transoccipital, and 6.0 ± 0.8 dB for transorbital insonation with 33.3 kHz and an intensity of 0.5 W/cm^2. At 71.4 kHz with an intensity of 3.4 W/cm^2, the average attenuation was 5.2 ± 1.3 dB, 7.5 ± 1.5 dB, and 8.9 ± 1.0 dB for transtemporal, -occipital, and -orbital application, respectively. Different data show that the brain may be accessible for noninvasive transcranial treatment with ultrasound, indicating that a frequency of 300–500 kHz allows an attenuation of only 0.2 N/cm when transmitted through the skull.

Endovascular Application of Ultrasound

Miniaturized transducers have also been attached to catheters for direct endovascular use, offering the potential of localized ultrasound thrombolysis, while avoiding attenuation of intensity through the skull and reducing insonation of the surrounding tissue. Tachibana and Koga [41] demonstrated enhanced clot lysis in vitro using a microtransducer operating at 225 kHz and similar in vitro results were demonstrated for combined application of ultrasound (170 kHz, 0.5 W/cm^2) and urokinase [41]. These catheter-mounted transducers showed similar qualitative results to those with larger transducers, but the potential endovascular use of microcatheters for acute stroke treatment is limited to specialized centers and a broader applicability seems unrealistic.

Limitations of Therapeutic Ultrasound

Safety is of primary concern in the clinical application of therapeutic ultrasound in potential stroke treatment. Within the low range of up to 2 W/cm^2, it is likely that ultrasound can be delivered safely during fibrinolytic therapy without causing acute side effects; however, continuous wave ultrasound at 1 MHz with an intensity of 1.6 W/cm^2 is known to potentiate the inflammatory response by augmenting the adhesion of leukocytes to the endothelium, but without irreversible damage of the endothelial cells [33]. Also, nonthermal effects of therapeutic ultrasound exposure may lead to an increase of intracellular calcium by a perturbation of the membrane, and therefore cause toxic in-cell activation [42]. Toxicity from ultrasound heating is primarily related to the absolute increase of temperature and demonstrated negligible effects below 40°C [43]. Investigations performed by us in rats showed that continuous exposure of 185-kHz ultrasound with 2-W/cm^2 spatial average intensity may elevate temperatures by 6–8°C above normal values of 37°C on the surface of the transducer after 90 min of exposure time. However, the systemic body temperature was not increased (±0.2°C), and the blood-brain barrier not disrupted. In general, optimal coupling of the ultrasound transducer to the skin may help to minimize heating effects.

Other bioeffects of ultrasound are related to acoustic cavitation, which refers to the expansion and collapse of gas bubbles, resulting from sudden pressure changes in a liquid medium during the passage of the sound wave [44]. This transient cavitation can produce additional local heating and liberation of free radicals and shock waves which may cause tissue and endothelial damage [45], but is a more common phenomenon in high-intensity ultrasound fields and its significance and occurrence in low-intensity fields is still debatable.

Future Aspects

Clinical trials (observational and phase II) utilizing standard diagnostic ultrasound devices already suggest a small thrombolytic effect on recanalization, but currently without significant clinical benefit. Experimental data indicate lower frequency ultrasound being more suitable for transcranial sonothrombolysis. A small clinical trial with a low-frequency insonator (300 kHz), however, was stopped because of a high number of bleedings [46]. The optimal ultrasound intensity, frequency, and insonation characteristics still have to be determined [47]. Therapeutic ultrasound probably has various effects on vascular/brain tissue that are hard to control and may depend on the insonation characteristics. There is some evidence that ultrasound can increase cerebral perfusion [48], open the blood-brain barrier, or even cause cellular membranes to be more permeable (sonoporation), etc. However one major future aspect of sonothrombolysis may be to reduce the main side effect of enzymatic thrombolysis – intracranial bleeding – by reducing tPA. Some pilot studies indicated that microbubbles can facilitate sonothrombolysis [49].

Transcranial sonothrombolysis with ultrasound alone would mean to apply ultrasound intensities that per se could cause serious tissue damage. A clinically applicable scenario of transcranial sonothrombolysis needs the combination of ultrasound with a thrombolytic agent or with microbubbles [21, 50] or with platelet-inhibitor-connected microbubbles [49], thus using a therapeutic system that combines several experimental aspects. Therefore, it is important to provide proven experimental data before applying such a therapy in clinical practice.

References

1 Bozzao L, Fantozzi LM, et al: Early collateral blood supply and late parenchymal brain damage in patients with middle cerebral artery occlusion. Stroke 1989;20:735–740.

2 Mori E, Yoneda Y, et al: Intravenous recombinant tissue plasminogen activator in acute carotid artery territory stroke. Neurology 1992;42:976–982.
3 The National Institute of Neurological Disorders and Stroke rt-PA Stroke Study Group: Tissue plasminogen activator for acute ischemic stroke. N Engl J Med 1995;333:1581–1587.
4 Siegel RJ, Cumberland DC, et al: Percutaneous peripheral ultrasonic angioplasty. Herz 1990;15:329–334.
5 Siegel RJ, Cumberland DC, et al: Ultrasound recanalization of diseased arteries. From experimental studies to clinical application. Surg Clin North Am 1992;72:879–897.
6 Luo H, Steffen W, et al: Enhancement of thrombolysis by external ultrasound. Am Heart J 1993;125:1564–1569.
7 Alexandrov AV, Molina CA, et al: Ultrasound-enhanced systemic thrombolysis for acute ischemic stroke. N Engl J Med 2004;351:2170–2178.
8 Daffertshofer M, Huang Z, et al: Efficacy of sonothrombolysis in a rat model of embolic ischemic stroke. Neurosci Lett 2004;361:115–119.
9 Francis CW, Blinc A, et al: Ultrasound accelerates transport of recombinant tissue plasminogen activator into clots. Ultrasound Med Biol 1995;21:419–424.
10 Siddiqi F, Odrljin TM, et al: Binding of tissue-plasminogen activator to fibrin: Effect of ultrasound. Blood 1998;91:2019–2025.
11 Braaten JV, Goss RA, et al: Ultrasound reversibly disaggregates fibrin fibers. Thromb Haemost 1997;78:1063–1068.
12 Siddiqi F, Blinc A, et al: Ultrasound increases flow through fibrin gels. Thromb Haemost 1995;73:495–498.
13 Francis CW, Onundarson PT, et al: Enhancement of fibrinolysis in vitro by ultrasound. J Clin Invest 1992;90:2063–2068.
14 Lauer CG, Burge R, et al: Effect of ultrasound on tissue-type plasminogen activator-induced thrombolysis. Circulation 1992;86:1257–1264.
15 Harpaz D, Chen X, et al: Ultrasound accelerates urokinase-induced thrombolysis and reperfusion. Am Heart J 1994;127:1211–1219.
16 Kimura M, Iijima S, et al: Evaluation of the thrombolytic effect of tissue-type plasminogen activator with ultrasonic irradiation: In vitro experiment involving assay of the fibrin degradation products from the clot. Biol Pharm Bull 1994;17:126–130.
17 Akiyama M, Ishibashi T, et al: Low-frequency ultrasound penetrates the cranium and enhances thrombolysis in vitro. Neurosurgery 1998;43:828–832.
18 Suchkova V, Siddiqi FN, et al: Enhancement of fibrinolysis with 40-kHz ultrasound. Circulation 1998;98:1030–1035.
19 Behrens S, Daffertshofer M, et al: Low-frequency, low-intensity ultrasound accelerates thrombolysis through the skull. Ultrasound Med Biol 1999;25:269–273.
20 Pfaffenberger S, Devcic-Kuhar B, et al: Can a commercial diagnostic ultrasound device accelerate thrombolysis?: An in vitro skull model. Stroke 2005;36:124–128.
21 Nedelmann M, Brandt C, et al: Ultrasound-induced blood clot dissolution without a thrombolytic drug is more effective with lower frequencies. Cerebrovasc Dis 2005;20:18–22.
22 Spengos K, Behrens S, et al: Acceleration of thrombolysis with ultrasound through the cranium in a flow model. Ultrasound Med Biol 2000;26:889–895.
23 Hamano K: Thrombolysis enhanced by transcutaneous ultrasonic irradiation. Jikeikai Med J 1991;106:533–542.
24 Goyen M, Kroger K, et al: Intravascular ultrasound angioplasty in peripheral arterial occlusion. Preliminary experience. Acta Radiol 2000;41:122–124.
25 Teal P, Hill MD, et al: Intra-arterial ultrasound catheter (EKOS) facilitated thrombolysis. 7th International Symposium on Thrombolysis and Acute Stroke Therapy, 2002. http://www.thrombolysis-acute-stroke.org/lyon/
26 Kornowski R, Meltzer RS, et al: Does external ultrasound accelerate thrombolysis? Results from a rabbit model. Circulation 1994;89:339–344.
27 Luo H, Nishioka T, et al: Transcutaneous ultrasound augments lysis of arterial thrombi in vivo. Circulation 1996;94:775–778.
28 Riggs PN, Francis CW, et al: Ultrasound enhancement of rabbit femoral artery thrombolysis. Cardiovasc Surg 1997;5:201–207.

29 Luo H, Birnbaum Y, et al: Enhancement of thrombolysis in vivo without skin and soft tissue damage by transcutaneous ultrasound. Thromb Res 1998;89:171–177.
30 Suchkova VN, Baggs RB, et al: Effect of 40-kHz ultrasound on acute thrombotic ischemia in a rabbit femoral artery thrombosis model: Enhancement of thrombolysis and improvement in capillary muscle perfusion. Circulation 2000;101:2296–2301.
31 Nedelmann M, Eicke BM, et al: Low-frequency ultrasound induces nonenzymatic thrombolysis in vitro. J Ultrasound Med 2002;21:649–656.
32 Williams AR, Chater BV, et al: Release of beta-thromboglobulin from human platelets by therapeutic intensities of ultrasound. Br J Haematol 1978;40:133–142.
33 Maxwell L, Collecutt T, et al: The augmentation of leucocyte adhesion to endothelium by therapeutic ultrasound. Ultrasound Med Biol 1994;20:383–390.
34 Busch E, Kruger K, et al: Improved model of thromboembolic stroke and rt-PA induced reperfusion in the rat. Brain Res 1997;778:16–24.
35 Zhang RL, Chopp M, et al: A rat model of focal embolic cerebral ischemia. Brain Res 1997;766: 83–92.
36 Ishibashi T, Akiyama M, et al: Can transcranial ultrasonication increase recanalization flow with tissue plasminogen activator? Stroke 2002;33:1399–1404.
37 Alexandrov AV: Ultrasound-enhanced thrombolysis for stroke: Clinical significance. Eur J Ultrasound 2002;16:131–140.
38 Fry FJ, Goss SA, et al: Transkull focal lesions in cat brain produced by ultrasound. J Neurosurg 1981;54:659–663.
39 Aaslid R, Markwalder TM, et al: Noninvasive transcranial Doppler ultrasound recording of flow velocity in basal cerebral arteries. J Neurosurg 1982;57:769–774.
40 Fry FJ, Barger JE: Acoustical properties of the human skull. J Acoust Soc Am 1978;63: 1576–1590.
41 Tachibana S, Koga E: Ultrasonic vibration for boosting fibrinolytic effect of urokinase. Blood and Vessel 1981;12:450–453.
42 Mortimer AJ, Dyson M: The effect of therapeutic ultrasound on calcium uptake in fibroblasts. Ultrasound Med Biol 1988;14:499–506.
43 National Council on Radiation Protection and Measurement: Exposure criteria for medical diagnostic ultrasound. I. Criteria based on thermal mechanisms. NCRP Report No. 113, Bethesda, MD, 1992.
44 Apfel RE: Acoustic cavitation: A possible consequence of biomedical uses of ultrasound. Br J Cancer Suppl 1982;45:140–146.
45 Dalecki D, Raeman CH, et al: Hemolysis in vivo from exposure to pulsed ultrasound. Ultrasound Med Biol 1997;23:307–313.
46 Daffertshofer M, Gass A, et al: Transcranial low-frequency ultrasound-mediated thrombolysis in brain ischemia: Increased risk of hemorrhage with combined ultrasound and tissue plasminogen activator: Results of a phase II clinical trial. Stroke 2005;36:1441–1446.
47 Dijkmans PA, Juffermans LJ, et al: Microbubbles and ultrasound: From diagnosis to therapy. Eur J Echocardiogr 2004;5:245–256.
48 Sedlaczek O, Gunther M, et al: Bio-effects of transcranial Doppler visualised by serial MR-arterial spin labeling. Cerebrovasc Dis 2005;19(suppl 2):8.
49 Wu Y, Unger EC, et al: Binding and lysing of blood clots using MRX-408. Invest Radiol 1998;33: 880–885.
50 Cintas P, Le Traon AP, et al: High rate of recanalization of middle cerebral artery occlusion during 2-MHz transcranial color-coded doppler continuous monitoring without thrombolytic drug. Stroke 2002;33:626–628.

Dr. M. Daffertshofer
Department of Neurology, Klinikum Mittelbaden
Balgerstrasse 50
DE–76532 Baden-Baden (Germany)
Tel. +49 7221 91 2730, Fax +49 7221 91 2440
E-Mail m.daffertshofer@klinikum-mittelbaden.de

Baumgartner RW (ed): Handbook on Neurovascular Ultrasound.
Front Neurol Neurosci. Basel, Karger, 2006, vol 21, pp 150–161

Acute Stroke: Therapeutic Transcranial Doppler Sonography

R. Mikulik, A.V. Alexandrov

Department of Neurology, University of Texas Health Science Center at Houston, Houston, Tex., USA

Abstract

Ultrasound (US) has emerged as a new tool to treat ischemic stroke. The potential advantage of US is decreased risk of systemic bleeding complications due to its site-specific effect. Moreover, external application is noninvasive and is readily available. Experimental studies showed that low intensity ($\leq$2 W/cm^2) US safely enhanced thrombolytic drug activity within a wide range of frequencies (0.04–3.4 MHz). In humans, transcranial sonothrombolysis with mid-kHz frequencies showed an unacceptably high rate of intracranial bleeding, while the use of 2 MHz yielded promising results in The Combined Lysis of Thrombus in Brain Ischemia Using Transcranial Ultrasound and Systemic TPA (CLOTBUST) study. This study was a phase II randomized clinical trial that included patients with middle cerebral artery (MCA) occlusion within 3 h of stroke onset, who were treated with standard dose of tissue plasminogen activator (t-PA). Residual flow in MCA was monitored with 2 MHz US in one group, and the rate of complete recanalization and dramatic clinical recovery significantly increased as compared to t-PA alone. This chapter further discusses diagnosis of an acute occlusion and recanalization using the thrombolysis in brain ischemia (TIBI) waveform flow grading scale, application of fast track insonation protocol, and administration of US. Also, the potential enhancement of sonothrombolysis with microbubbles is discussed.

This chapter will cover the general application of therapeutic ultrasound (US) in acute stroke patients. Up to 60% of stroke patients with middle cerebral artery (MCA) occlusions fail to achieve early complete recanalization [1]. US has emerged as a new tool to increase recanalization when used with thrombolytics or alone. The advantage of US is decreased risk of systemic bleeding complications due to its site-specific effect. Moreover, external application is noninvasive and is readily available.

Background

Two approaches with different mechanism of action can be used. The first approach uses intraarterial delivery of high-intensity (tens of W/cm^2) and low-frequency (20–25 kHz) US to mechanically disrupt the clot or atherosclerotic plague. The second uses either externally or intraarterially applied low-intensity US (0.25–8 W/cm^2) within a whole range of frequencies (tens of Hz up to several MHz), to enhance enzymatic effect of thrombolytics. This effect was confirmed by numerous in vitro and in vivo studies, which also showed that the effect of US could be explained by an alteration of fibrin structure with improved transport and increased binding of thrombolytics.

This chapter will focus on transcranial application of low-intensity US. Experimental data, therapeutic use of transcranial color duplex sonography, and intraarterial application of low-intensity US will be covered elsewhere.

Human Studies

The therapeutic effect of US has been tested in human studies with two different modalities: (1) one approach was to use kHz frequencies that offer less attenuation with propagation through the bone. Special devices had to be developed for this purpose. (2) In contrast, the other approach relies on readily available, inexpensive, and approved TCD technology based on low MHz frequencies, which are routinely used for diagnostic purposes. In fact, the first promising results using 2 MHz probe have been shown in phase I and II CLOTBUST studies (Combined Lysis of Thrombus in Brain Ischemia Using Transcranial Ultrasound and Systemic TPA). Results of smaller studies with transcranial color duplex sonography have also been reported and will be discussed in another chapter.

Studies using kHz Frequencies

The first devices operating on low-kHz frequencies for use in humans were developed by Walnut Technologies (Boston, Mass., USA). These frequencies were, however, intolerable for stroke patients, causing tinnitus. Using mid-kHz range, another device was developed and later tested in Germany in a multicenter trial (Transcranial Low-Frequency Ultrasound-Mediated Thrombolysis in Brain Ischemia, TRUMBI) [2]. This prospective, randomized study aimed to show safety and effectiveness of US as an accelerator of enzymatic t-PA-mediated thrombolysis. A standard 0.9 mg/kg t-PA dose was given to acute stroke patients within the 0- to 6-hour window, alone or in combination with 90 min of transcranial insonation with 300 kHz, 700 mW/cm^2 pulse-wave US device.

US exposure and t-PA led to intracranial bleeding diagnosed on MRI in 13 out of 14 patients, as compared to 5 out of 12 with t-PA alone. Interestingly, there was no difference in early recanalization rate. The trial was terminated for safety concerns.

One speculative explanation for such bleedings is potential injury to the endothelium and blood-brain barrier caused by the mechanical stretching and creation of standing waves due to long spatial pulse duration [3].

CLOTBUST Studies

Three factors position the CLOTBUST studies as an alternative and promising method for performing sonothrombolysis with frequency and power ranges of diagnostic US.

(1) The diagnostic US has been used for prolonged monitoring and emboli detection, with no harmful effect reported.

(2) Low-MHz frequencies enhanced sonothrombolysis in in vivo and in vitro studies.

(3) Delivery of US energy through the skull is probably sufficient. The following section will outline the results of CLOTBUST trials and then give more detailed instructions on how to perform its technique.

Preliminary data that led to CLOTBUST studies originated in 2000 through the work of Alexandrov et al. [4], who reported a high rate of recanalization and dramatic recovery during t-PA infusion in 40 acute stroke patients with intracranial artery occlusions when continuously monitored with 2-MHz TCD probe. Recanalization on TCD was complete in 30% and partial in 40% of patients, which was higher than previously reported [1]. Also, the response rate to t-PA therapy at 24 hours was higher than in the NINDS rt-PA Stroke Study (40 vs. 27% improvement by 10+ points in NIHSS at 24 h). This study also showed that an US beam can be steadily focused at presumed intracranial thrombus location using a headframe, and arterial recanalization can be monitored in real time. The number of patients in the original cohort was extended to obtain data regarding safety, rates of early recanalization, and clinical dramatic recovery, reported as phase I data of the CLOTBUST trial.

CLOTBUST I included stroke patients with intracranial arterial occlusion who received intravenous standard dose of 0.9 mg/kg t-PA within 3 h of stroke onset and underwent monitoring with portable diagnostic TCD. Complete recanalization was defined as thrombolysis in brain ischemia (TIBI) flow grades 4–5. Fifty-five patients had a median NIHSS 18. Complete recanalization on TCD within 2 h after bolus was found in 36% of patients. Dramatic recovery (NIHSS score ≤ 3) occurred in 20% at 2 h and in 24% at 24 h. Improvement was significantly associated with recanalization during, or shortly after, t-PA infusion.

Based on the results of CLOTBUST I, a phase II trial was designed [5]. Efficacy was determined by a combined primary endpoint of complete recanalization within 2 h after t-PA bolus demonstrated by TCD, or early clinical recovery by ≥10 NIHSS points, or total NIHSS score ≤3 within 2 h after t-PA bolus. The clinical endpoints were both chosen as a better way of describing dramatic clinical recovery after early recanalization [6]. The primary safety endpoint was defined as intracerebral hemorrhage with clinical worsening (indicated by an NIHSS score of ≥4) within 72 h of the onset of stroke.

CLOTBUST Phase II study was a multicenter, randomized clinical trial with blinded clinical endpoints. Patients received standard intravenous t-PA therapy (i.e., 0.9 mg/kg body weight). Therapy was initiated within 3 h of the onset of symptoms of stroke, either with 2 h of continuous monitoring with the use of TCD (the target group), or with placebo monitoring (the control group). A total of 126 patients were included with median NIHSS of 16. Symptomatic intracerebral hemorrhage occurred in 3 patients in both groups. Complete recanalization or dramatic clinical recovery within 2 h after the administration of a t-PA bolus occurred in 49% in the target group, as compared to 30% ($p = 0.03$) in the control group. Complete recanalization occurred within 2 h after the t-PA bolus in 46% of patients in the target group and 18% in the control group ($p < 0.001$). At 3 months, 42% of patients in the target group and 29% of patients in the control group had favorable outcomes, as indicated by a score of 0–1 on the modified Rankin scale ($p = 0.20$).

General Instructions for Diagnosis and Performing TCD

The following section outlines the diagnosis of an acute arterial occlusion, diagnostic protocol, administration of US and monitoring of recanalization process in CLOTBUST studies. In order to perform these procedures, a good window of insonation is the most critical prerequisite.

Diagnosis of an Acute Arterial Occlusion

Acute occlusion of intracranial artery produces both changes in residual flow throughout an artery occluded by a fresh clot and frequent development of collateral channels to compensate for a lesion [7]. Clot dissolution can be associated with the presence of microembolic signals [8]. To achieve the maximum benefit from TCD, it is thus important that the examiners pay attention not only to velocity measurements, but also to flow waveforms, presence of flow diversion, or microembolic signals [9]. The following section will discuss the

Table 1. Diagnostic criteria for acute intracranial occlusion

Site of occlusion	Depth of occlusion and abnormal waveform (TIBI 0–3), window of insonation	Additional signs of acute intracranial occlusion
ICA	62–70 mm for distal ICA occlusion, transorbital window	Blunted MCA signal, reversed OA for occlusions below the origin of OA, reversed ipsilateral A1 ACA and increased contralateral ICA and A1 ACA, high-velocity flow ('stenotic like signal') in the ACoA-cross-filling (70–80 mm) and PCoA (60–75 mm) towards the probe. For T-type of distal ICA occlusion, no flow in ACA + MCA, with good flow in PCA. Possible embolic signals in MCA
M1 MCA	45–65 mm, transtemporal window	ACA or PCA > MCA by ≥10%, possible embolic signals in distal MCA
M2 MCA	30–45 mm, transtemporal window	ACA or PCA > MCA by ≥10%, M2 > M1
BA proximal	80–90 mm, suboccipital window	PICA > VA, reversed flow in distal BA (stenotic or low resistance), increased flow in PCoA away from the probe, abnormal flow in one or both VA
BA distal	90–100 mm, suboccipital window	AICA > BA, increased flow in PCoA away from the probe, decreased velocity in distal BA

ACA, MCA and PCA = Anterior, middle, and posterior cerebral arteries; OA = ophthalmic artery; ACoA and PCoA = anterior and posterior communicating artery; AICA and PICA = anterior and posterior inferior cerebellar artery; VA = vertebral artery; BA = basilar artery.

description of residual flow patterns in an artery occluded by a clot and then supportive findings that help to establish diagnosis (table 1). The TCD diagnostic criteria discussed here have been validated in several studies and can identify thrombus location with accuracy >90% for MCA and ICA [10–12].

TCD Grading System to Measure Residual Flow

An acute arterial occlusion is different from chronic occlusion for two reasons: it is often partial and incomplete creating several patterns of residual flow [12] and it is a dynamic process of thrombus dissolution, propagation, and reocclusion [13], leading to frequent changes in flow pattern. Waveform morphology rather than velocity itself discloses more information about clot

Grade	Definition	Waveform
Grade 0 Absent	Absent flow signals are defined by the lack of regular pulsatile flow signals despite varying degrees of background noise	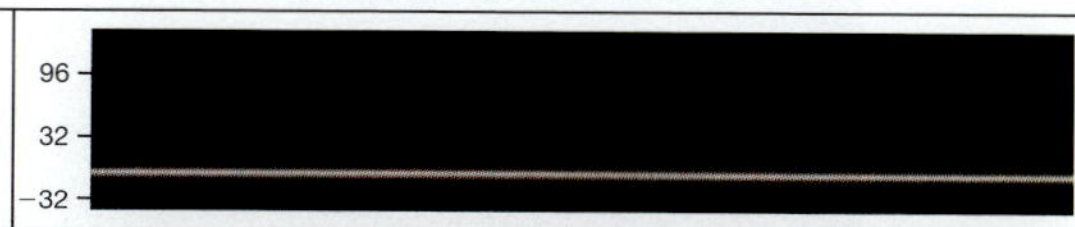
Grade 1 Minimal	Systolic spikes of variable velocity and duration Absent diastolic flow during all cardiac cycles based on visual interpretation of periods of no flow during end-diastole. Reverberating flow is a type of minimal flow	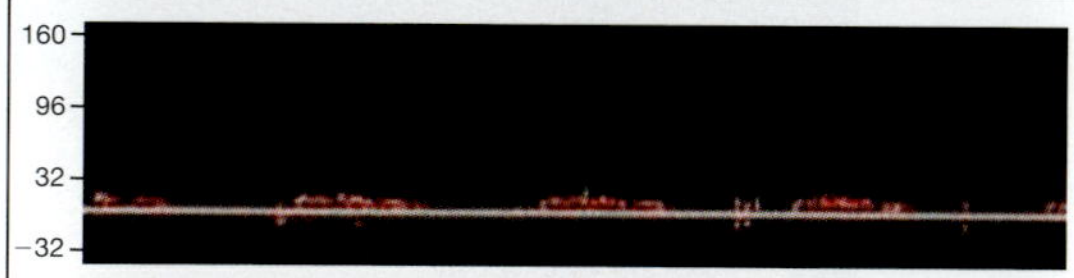
Grade 2 Blunted	Flattened systolic flow acceleration of variable duration compared to control Positive end-diastolic velocity and pulsatility index <1.2	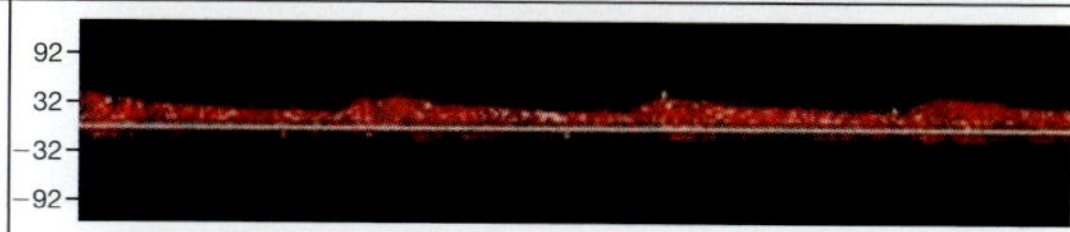
Grade 3 Dampened	Normal systolic flow acceleration Positive end-diastolic velocity Decreased mean flow velocity (MFV) by ≥30% compared to control	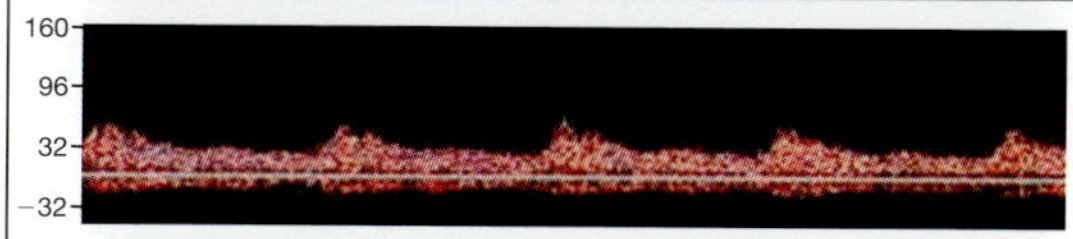
Grade 4 Stenotic	MFV of ≥80 cm/s *and* velocity difference of ≥30% compared to control side; if velocity difference is <30%, additional sign of stenosis, i.e. turbulence, spectral narrowing OR If both affected and comparison sides have MFV < 80 cm/s due to low end-diastolic velocities, MFV >30% compared to the control side *and* signs of turbulence	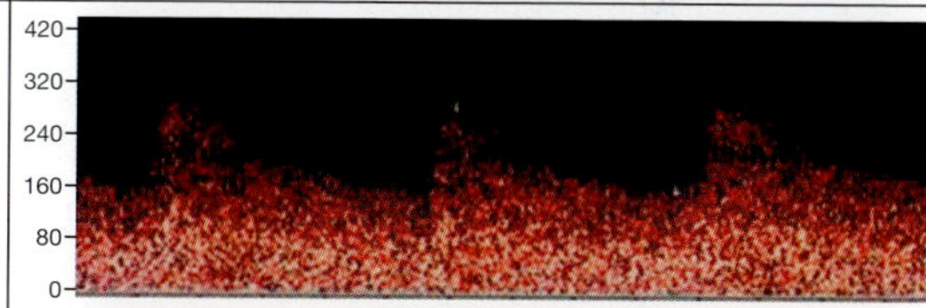
Grade 5 Normal	<30% mean velocity difference compared to control Similar waveform shapes compared to control	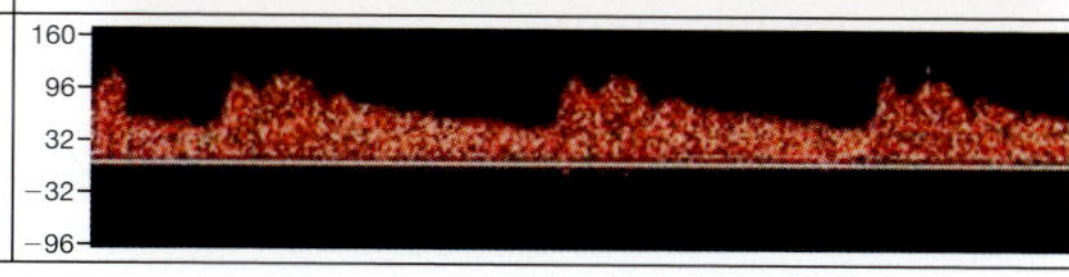

Fig. 1. TIBI flow grading system. Modified from [12].

location, hemodynamic significance of obstruction, and resistance in the distal vasculature [9].

To describe waveform morphology on TCD, TIBI residual flow grading system was developed, which was derived from angiographic classification of residual flow called thrombolysis in myocardial infarction (TIMI) [12]. TIBI grades range from 0 to 5: absent, minimal, blunted, dampened, stenotic, and normal flow, respectively, (for definitions, see fig. 1). To diagnose acute arterial occlusion, the primary finding is the presence of TIBI flow grades 0–3 [12] (absent, minimal, blunted, or dampened) in the vessel supplying a territory affected by ischemia (fig. 2). For specific occlusions and depth of abnormal TIBI flow, see table 1. TIBI flow grades correlate with baseline and 24-hour NIHSS, as well as recanalization and in-hospital mortality (lower TIBI

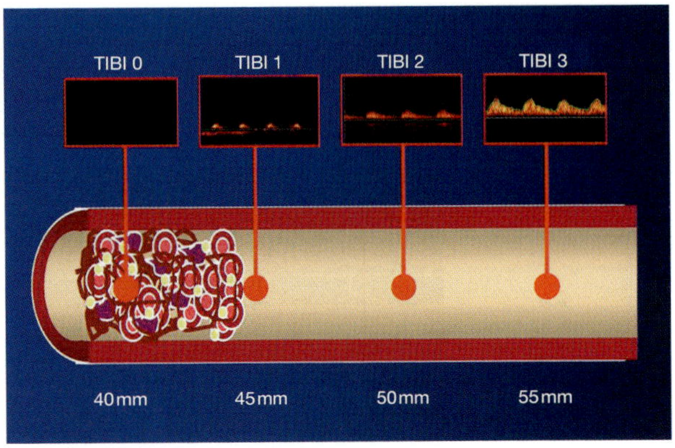

Fig. 2. Examples of TIBI flow grades at different depths in acute middle cerebral artery occlusion. Modified figure courtesy of Carlos Molina, MD.

predicts less recanalization and higher NIHSS and mortality) [12]. In CLOTBUST studies, all sonographers successfully passed a computerized tutorial and multiple-choice examination in TIBI waveform interpretation (TIBI Tutorial and Examination, ©Health Outcomes Institute, Inc., www.health-outcomes-institute.com).

Secondary Supportive Findings

Secondary supportive findings include evidence of collateralization (flow 'diversion'), presence of microembolic signals, stenotic signals, or flow pulsatility changes. Collateralization or flow 'diversion' refers to the increased and/or reversed blood flow to compensate for hemodynamically significant lesions in intra- or extracerebral circulation. Anatomically, it is enabled by connections either through Circle of Willis or leptomeningeal collaterals.

Table 1 elaborates collateral pathways, as well as other supportive findings, in the case of certain occlusions.

Diagnostic Protocol

Because no delay in treatment is justified in acute stroke patients [14], TCD should usually take place simultaneously with other procedures performed in the emergency room. In addition, knowledge of artery status before treatment initiation is useful in many circumstances. For rapid diagnosis and clot location, fast-track (<15 min) insonation protocol was developed [15]

Table 2. Fast-track TCD insonation protocol

Clinical diagnosis of cerebral ischemia in the anterior circulation

1. If time permits, begin insonation on the nonaffected side to establish the transtemporal window, normal MCA waveform (M1 depth 45–65 mm, M2 30–45 mm), and velocity for comparison to the affected side.
2. If short on time, start on the affected side: first assess MCA at 50 mm. If no signal is detected, increase the depth to 62 mm. If an antegrade flow signal is found, reduce the depth to trace the MCA stem or identify the worst residual flow signal. Search for possible flow diversion to the ACA, PCA, or M2 MCA. Evaluate and compare waveform shapes and systolic flow acceleration.
3. Continue on the affected side (transorbital window). Check flow direction and pulsatility in the OA at depths 40–50 mm followed by ICA siphon at depths 55–65 mm.
4. If time permits, or in patients with pure motor or sensory deficits, evaluate BA (depth 80–100 mm) and terminal VA (40–80 mm).

Clinical diagnosis of cerebral ischemia in the posterior circulation

1. Start suboccipital insonation at 75 mm (VA junction) and identify BA flow at 80–100 mm.
2. If abnormal signals are present at 75–100 mm, find the terminal VA (40–80 mm) on the nonaffected side for comparison and evaluate the terminal VA on the affected side at similar depths.
3. Continue with transtemporal examination to identify PCA (55–75 mm) and possible collateral flow through the posterior communicating artery (check both sides).
4. If time permits, evaluate both MCAs and ACAs (60–75 mm) for possible compensatory velocity increase as an indirect sign of BA obstruction.

ACA, MCA and PCA = Anterior, middle, and posterior cerebral arteries; OA = ophthalmic artery; VA = vertebral artery; BA = basilar artery; ICA = internal carotid artery.

(table 2). This protocol is tailored for different clinical situations based on presumed artery clot location.

Administration of US and Monitoring of an Acute Arterial Occlusion and Recanalization

After the occlusion is diagnosed by handheld examination, a head frame is used for monitoring purposes. In CLOTBUST studies, the headframe (Marc series, Spencer Technologies, Va., USA) allowed for steady positioning of transducer over the temporal bone at a constant angle. If the basilar artery was occluded, handheld monitoring was performed via the suboccipital window.

The reason for monitoring is two-fold: (1) to deliver ultrasonic energy to the clot to enhance the effect of thrombolytics [6, 16] and (2) to monitor beginning, timing, and amount of recanalization process induced by therapy in real time [17]. These are discussed below:

(1) Since more than one abnormal TIBI flow grades can be present in the same patient (fig. 2), the depth with the worst residual flow signal has to be selected for monitoring. This is the site in the course of occluded artery with any detectable flow closest to the thrombus location. This ensures that the clot receives maximum US energy. The sample volumes are set at 3–6 mm for power-motion Doppler [18] units and 10–15 mm for all other single-channel TCD units. Emitted-power output is set at the maximal achievable level with selected insonation depths under the FDA-allowed threshold of 750 mW.

(2) Monitoring allows following the processes of recanalization and reocclusion in real time. In CLOTBUST studies, recanalization was graded as complete, partial, or absent using previously validated classification predictive of the TIMI flow grades [11]. Complete recanalization was diagnosed when a normal waveform (TIBI 5), or a low resistance stenotic signal (TIBI 4), appeared at the selected depth of insonation, suggesting low resistance in the distal circulatory bed. This correlates with unobstructed passage of contrast (TIMI grade 3 flow). In patients with concomitant severe stenosis or occlusion of the proximal internal carotid artery, complete recanalization of the MCA was considered to have been achieved if a blunted and low-resistance waveform was seen over both M1 and M2 segments on TCD [11], with an improvement in mean flow velocity to more than 20 cm/s. These TCD criteria predict TIMI grade 3 flow in the MCA with a rate of accuracy >90% [11]. Recanalization process can also be indicated by flow velocity improvement by ≥30% at a constant angle of insonation or appearance of embolic signals [8, 9].

Partial recanalization was diagnosed if flow improved by one or more grades from the baseline, but not to the level of grade 5 on the TIBI scale [16]. Lack of change in the abnormal flow signals indicated that no recanalization had occurred.

Reocclusion was diagnosed if flow worsened by at least one TIBI grade [19] in the absence of circulatory conditions that could explain this change, i.e. blood pressure drop.

Conclusions on CLOTBUST Findings

The CLOTBUST II results indicate a biological effect of US that could enhance intravenous thrombolysis in patients with acute ischemic stroke. The main limitation in the CLOTBUST II study is that the recanalization endpoint could not be assessed on a blinded principle and was unconfirmed by angiographic techniques. The 'blinded' clinical endpoint, however, also favored the target US group. Thus, it is likely that the observed difference in recanalization frequencies existed.

Strong operator dependency is the general limitation in the administration of US; experienced sonographers need to be available. To prove the efficacy of sonothrombolysis in phase III trials, it will be necessary either to train more operators or to develop an operator-independent US machine. In the meantime, a new approach to increase the effectiveness of sonothrombolysis with the use of echocontrast agents is under way.

Use of Echocontrast Agents (Microbubbles)

Microbubbles are 1- to 5-μm gas cavities stabilized by a coating with either lipids or human albumin. They have been used for diagnostic purposes in US imaging due to good reflection of US waves.

Several in vitro and in vivo studies showed that the presence of microbubbles could further enhance the effect of US on thrombolysis [20, 21]. Other such studies noted that even without the presence of thrombolytics, the combination of US and microbubbles could dissolve the clot [22, 23].

Molina et al. [24] provided the first data on human stroke. In patients with MCA occlusion treated within the first 3 h, the recanalization rate achieved through a combination of t-PA plus microbubbles plus US (2-MHz diagnostic probe) was significantly higher (54.5%), when compared to those given t-PA plus US (23.9%) or t-PA alone (23.9%). The mechanism by which microbubbles exert a positive effect is probably related to transient cavitation and increased permeation of exo- or endogenous t-PA [25].

The use of microbubbles holds potential for the future. Microbubbles targeted to the GPIIb/IIIa receptor have already shown promise in in vitro and in vivo studies [23]. Theoretically, microbubbles can be used to carry thrombolytic drugs directly to the thrombus.

References

1 del Zoppo GJ, Poeck K, Pessin MS, Wolpert SM, Furlan AJ, Ferbert A, Alberts MJ, Zivin JA, Wechsler L, Busse O, et al: Recombinant tissue plasminogen activator in acute thrombotic and embolic stroke. Ann Neurol 1992;32:78–86.

2 Daffertshofer M, Gass A, Ringleb P, Sitzer M, Sliwka U, Els T, Sedlaczek O, Koroshetz WJ, Hennerici MG: Transcranial low-frequency ultrasound-mediated thrombolysis in brain ischemia: increased risk of hemorrhage with combined ultrasound and tissue plasminogen activator: results of a phase II clinical trial. Stroke 2005;36:1441–1446.

3 Culp WC, McCowan TC: Ultrasound augmented thrombolysis. Current Medical Imaging Reviews 2005;1:5–12.

4 Alexandrov AV, Demchuk AM, Felberg RA, Christou I, Barber PA, Burgin WS, Malkoff M, Wojner AW, Grotta JC: High rate of complete recanalization and dramatic clinical recovery during t-PA infusion when continuously monitored with 2-MHz transcranial doppler monitoring. Stroke 2000;31:610–614.

5 Alexandrov AV, Wojner AW, Grotta JC: CLOTBUST: Design of a randomized trial of ultrasound-enhanced thrombolysis for acute ischemic stroke. J Neuroimaging 2004;14:108–112.

6 Alexandrov AV, Demchuk AM, Burgin WS, Robinson DJ, Grotta JC: Ultrasound-enhanced thrombolysis for acute ischemic stroke. I. Findings of the CLOTBUST trial. J Neuroimaging 2004;14:113–117.

7 Demchuk AM, Christou I, Wein TH, Felberg RA, Malkoff M, Grotta JC, Alexandrov AV: Specific transcranial doppler flow findings related to the presence and site of arterial occlusion. Stroke 2000;31:140–146.

8 Alexandrov AV, Demchuk AM, Felberg RA, Grotta JC, Krieger DW: Intracranial clot dissolution is associated with embolic signals on transcranial Doppler. J Neuroimaging 2000;10: 27–32.

9 Alexandrov AV: Cerebrovascular Ultrasound in Stroke Prevention and Treatment. New York, Blackwell Publishing, 2004, pp 99–102, 242.

10 Demchuk AM, Christou I, Wein TH, Felberg RA, Malkoff M, Grotta JC, Alexandrov AV: Accuracy and criteria for localizing arterial occlusion with transcranial Doppler. J Neuroimaging 2000;10:1–12.

11 Burgin WS, Malkoff M, Felberg RA, Demchuk AM, Christou I, Grotta JC, Alexandrov AV: Transcranial Doppler ultrasound criteria for recanalization after thrombolysis for middle cerebral artery stroke. Stroke 2000;31:1128–1132.

12 Demchuk AM, Burgin WS, Christou I, Felberg RA, Barber PA, Hill MD, Alexandrov AV: Thrombolysis in brain ischemia (TIBI) transcranial Doppler flow grades predict clinical severity, early recovery, and mortality in patients treated with intravenous tissue plasminogen activator. Stroke 2001;32:89–93.

13 Alexandrov AV: Ultrasound identification and lysis of clots. Stroke 2004;35:2722–2725.

14 Hacke W, Donnan G, Fieschi C, Kaste M, von Kummer R, Broderick JP, Brott T, Frankel M, Grotta JC, Haley EC Jr, Kwiatkowski T, Levine SR, Lewandowski C, Lu M, Lyden P, Marler JR, Patel S, Tilley BC, Albers G, Bluhmki E, Wilhelm M, Hamilton S: Association of outcome with early stroke treatment: Pooled analysis of ATLANTIS, ECASS, and NINDS rt-PA stroke trials. Lancet 2004;363:768–774.

15 Alexandrov AV, Demchuk AM, Wein TH, Grotta JC: Yield of transcranial Doppler in acute cerebral ischemia. Stroke 1999;30:1604–1609.

16 Alexandrov AV, Molina CA, Grotta JC, Garami Z, Ford SR, Alvarez-Sabin J, Montaner J, Saqqur M, Demchuk AM, Moye LA, Hill MD, Wojner AW: Ultrasound-enhanced systemic thrombolysis for acute ischemic stroke. N Engl J Med 2004;351:2170–2178.

17 Alexandrov AV, Burgin WS, Demchuk AM, El-Mitwalli A, Grotta JC: Speed of intracranial clot lysis with intravenous tissue plasminogen activator therapy: Sonographic classification and short-term improvement. Circulation 2001;103:2897–2902.

18 Moehring MA, Spencer MP: Power M-mode Doppler (PMD) for observing cerebral blood flow and tracking emboli. Ultrasound Med Biol 2002;28:49–57.

19 Alexandrov AV, Grotta JC: Arterial reocclusion in stroke patients treated with intravenous tissue plasminogen activator. Neurology 2002;59:862–867.

20 Tachibana K, Tachibana S: Albumin microbubble echo-contrast material as an enhancer for ultrasound accelerated thrombolysis. Circulation 1995;92:1148–1150.

21 Porter TR, LeVeen RF, Fox R, Kricsfeld A, Xie F: Thrombolytic enhancement with perfluorocarbon-exposed sonicated dextrose albumin microbubbles. Am Heart J 1996;132:964–968.

22 Birnbaum Y, Luo H, Nagai T, Fishbein MC, Peterson TM, Li S, Kricsfeld D, Porter TR, Siegel RJ: Noninvasive in vivo clot dissolution without a thrombolytic drug: Recanalization of thrombosed iliofemoral arteries by transcutaneous ultrasound combined with intravenous infusion of microbubbles. Circulation 1998;97:130–134.

23 Culp WC, Porter TR, Lowery J, Xie F, Roberson PK, Marky L: Intracranial clot lysis with intravenous microbubbles and transcranial ultrasound in swine. Stroke 2004;35:2407–2411.

24 Molina CA, Ribó M, Arenillas JF, Rubiera M, Montaner J, Santamarina E, Huertas R, Dealgado P, Purroy F, Alvarez-Sabín J: Microbubbles administration accelerates clot lysis during continuous 2 MHz ultrasound monitoring in stroke patients treated with intravenous tpa. International Stroke Conference, New Orleans, Luisiana, Feb 2–4, 2005.
25 Unger EC, Porter T, Culp W, Labell R, Matsunaga T, Zutshi R: Therapeutic applications of lipid-coated microbubbles. Adv Drug Deliv Rev 2004;56:1291–1314.

Robert Mikulik, MD
Department of Neurology, University of Texas
Health Science Center at Houston
6431 Fannin, MSB 7.124
Houston, TX 77030 (USA)
Tel. +1 281 380 1930, Fax +1 713 500 0660
E-Mail mikulik@hotmail.com

Baumgartner RW (ed): Handbook on Neurovascular Ultrasound.
Front Neurol Neurosci. Basel, Karger, 2006, vol 21, pp 162–170

Acute Stroke: Therapeutic Transcranial Color Duplex Sonography

Jürgen Eggers

Neurology, Segeberger Kliniken, Bad Segeberg, Germany

Abstract

The enhancement of thrombolysis by ultrasound energy (sonothrombolysis) is an emerging field of interest in the treatment of acute ischemic stroke. Recent in vitro and clinical studies have investigated the effects of using transcranially applied 'diagnostic' ultrasound for this purpose. Using transcranial color duplex sonography (TCDS) allows an examiner to identify the site of occlusion and focus the ultrasound beam on it. Clinical studies using TCDS to enhance thrombolysis in acute middle cerebral artery occlusions have revealed an accelerating effect on recanalization, as well as a tendency for a better outcome. Data from small sample studies suggest that this effect on recanalization is present not only in combination with recombinant tissue plasminogen activator (rt-PA), but also with any thrombolytic drug. However, when TCDS was used in combination with rt-PA, an increase in the rate of asymptomatic and symptomatic intracerebral hemorrhages tended to occur compared to patients treated with thrombolysis alone. Larger sample-sized clinical studies should be conducted in the future to evaluate the safety and efficacy of using TCDS for sonothrombolysis. This method should also be further developed to determine its effect when used in combination with other types of ultrasound and thrombolytic drugs.

The thrombolytic effect of ultrasound (US) has been known for many decades [1]. The first time it was shown that this method works, even after application through a human skull, was in 1999 when Akiyama et al. [2] found that combining US and urokinase caused a reduction of thrombus weight in vitro. The low-frequency US used in this study penetrated the skull much better than the high-frequency, low-energy US used for diagnostic purposes in transcranial examinations, where the attenuation of the skull was shown to be about 90% [3]. However, using a diagnostic 1-MHz US Doppler probe was also shown to have an effect on thrombus dissolution in vitro after application through a human temporal bone [4].

The clinical use of transcranial 'diagnostic' Doppler US for sonothrombolysis started when physicians, who extensively used this method during their examination of stroke patients with acute intracranial vessel occlusions, observed, independently from each other, an unexpected increase in the rate of recanalization. The first description of a possible impact on the clinical course of patients with acute ischemic stroke was made by Alexandrov et al. [5] from Houston, Texas, when performing continuous transcranial Doppler sonography monitoring in acute ischemic stroke patients. Using transcranial color duplex sonography (TCDS) in the examination of acute middle cerebral artery (MCA) occlusions also produced an unexpected rise in the frequency of recanalization. This happened shortly after, and even before, the start of recombined tissue-type plasminogen activator (rt-PA) infusion. After this phenomenon was observed in Lübeck a randomized study on this observation was initiated there [6, 7].

TCDS for Sonothrombolysis

TCDS has been shown to be a reliable tool in the diagnosis of intracranial vascular disease [8–10]. Compared with TCD, which simply provides the Doppler signal from a defined insonation depth, TCDS is a more advanced tool. When given a sufficient acoustic bone window, TCDS provides mainly three types of information: (1) the B-mode gray-scale two-dimensional picture of parenchymal and other structures of the brain, (2) the color-coded flow signal of intracranial vessels, and (3) the Doppler spectra detected within the vessel. The main segments of the basal brain arteries can be easily identified based on these three pieces of information. To give an example, the MCA-M1, which runs in the lateral fissure, is displayed as a structure of higher intensity compared with the surrounding brain parenchyma. An intracranial vessel occlusion can be diagnosed if the color-coded signal, as well the Doppler signal, is missing at the typical site of the vessel (fig. 1). During sonothrombolysis, the Doppler sample volume is placed on the site of occlusion to focus the pulsed-wave US beam on it. Because acute stroke patients can be very uncooperative and agitated during this procedure, frequent supervision of the correct placement of the US beam on its target is required. To minimize the deviation of the US beam, the US device's combined B-mode and color-coded mode should be intermittently activated (e.g., every 10 s), a technique which is referred to as 'refreshing'. Because continuous readjustment of the US beam is required throughout the insonation, the probe should be held by hand. In all of the studies that made use of TCDS, the duration of insonation was 1 h. However, even a shorter insonation time might lead to an acceleration of recanalization (see next page).

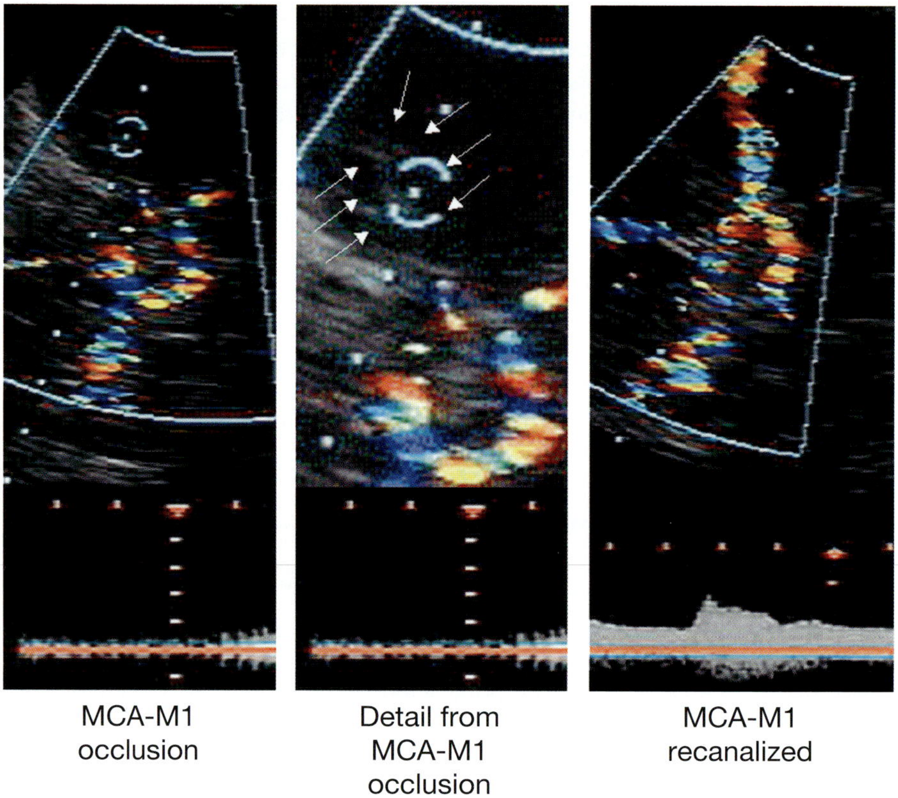

Fig. 1. TCDS of the circle of Willis, showing an occlusion of the MCA-M1 (left). Please note the missing Doppler spectra and the lateral fissure displayed as an echogenic structure marked by the arrows in the detail of the picture showing the occlusion (middle). Reconstituted flow after recanalization with normalized Doppler spectra (right).

Clinical Studies

Only patients with an acute occlusion of the main stem of the MCA (MCA-M1) were included in these clinical studies that used TCDS for sonothrombolysis. This restriction was mainly done for two reasons. From a practical point of view, MCA-M1 can be easily identified, even in the case of occlusion. The aforementioned restriction led also to a very homogeneous sample of (severely affected) patients. In all of these clinical studies, patients with an insufficient acoustic window (about 10%) were excluded.

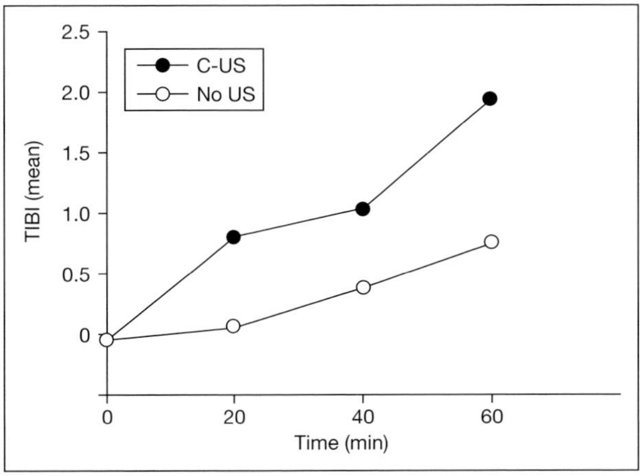

Fig. 2. Recanalization during insonation. Data from 37 patients with acute MCA-M1 occlusion who were treated with continuous ultrasound (C-US) plus rt-PA treatment or no US with rt-PA alone. Continuous insonation was started at the time of rt-PA bolus injection. Thrombolysis in brain ischemia (TIBI) Doppler flow [21] was graded as follows: 0 = absent; 1 = minimal; 2 = blunted; 3 = dampened; 4 = stenotic; and 5 = normal. Improved TIBI grades of the C-US group compared to the no US group was observed after 20, 40 and 60 min (exploratory two-sided p values <0.05, Wilcoxon test).

TCDS in Combination with rt-PA

Results of a randomized clinical study of 37 patients with TCDS-proven MCA-M1 occlusion, who underwent standard rt-PA intravenous treatment, revealed a faster rate of recanalization if the occlusion site was continuously insonated for one hour by TCDS-guided pulsed-wave US (rt-PA plus US). The continuous insonation was started at the time of the rt-PA bolus injection. Interestingly, recanalization in the rt-PA-plus-US-treated group was already higher after 20 min in comparison to the control group treated with rt-PA alone (fig. 2). This finding might contribute to the discussion of how long the US should be administered to have a measurable effect on thrombolysis. The patients from the rt-PA plus US group had a more favorable short-term clinical course during the first 4 days as measured on the National Institutes of Health Stroke Scale (NIHSS). When compared with the NIHSS score at baseline, the patients from the rt-PA plus US group showed a better improvement than the patients treated with rt-PA alone (fig. 3). A favorable outcome (modified Rankin Score ≤ 1) after 3 months was rare in these severely affected patients and present only in patients of the rt-PA plus US group (4/19, 21.1%). The frequency of symptomatic (3/19, 15.8% vs. 1/18, 5.6%) as well as asymptomatic intracerebral

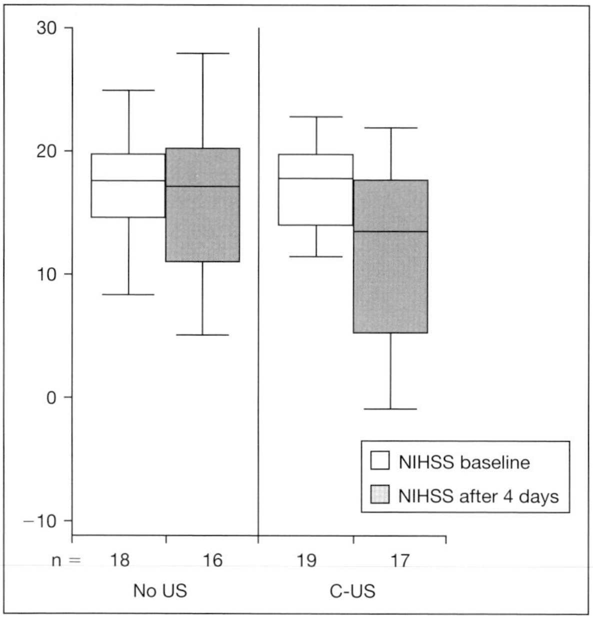

Fig. 3. The National Institutes of Health Stroke Scale (NIHSS) at baseline and after 4 days. The values are displayed as box plots with the middle line indicating the median, the boxes on both sides of it the interquartile range, and the lines that extend from the box to the highest and lowest values, excluding outliers, which were not present in these data. The mean NIHSS improvement was 5.65 ± 6.27 in the C-US group (n = 17) vs. 1.25 ± 4.78 in the no US group (n = 16) (two-sided exploratory p = 0.025, Mann-Whitney U test). All missing subjects (2 from each group) had died or could not be evaluated because of artificial respiration.

hemorrhages tended to be higher in the rt-PA plus US group, thus suggesting a possible side effect of using US. The type of hemorrhage was also retrospectively analyzed on the basis of the morphology displayed by cranial computed tomography, graded as hemorrhagic infarction type 1 or 2 and parenchymal hematoma type 1 or 2 [11]. The results confirmed the tendency of an increased rate of intracranial hemorrhages in the rt-PA plus US group in comparison to the group treated with rt-PA alone. However, the differences were not statistically significant, and overall, the increased rate of intracranial hemorrhages did not result in a worse clinical course; in fact, the patients from the rt-PA plus US group tended to have a more favorable clinical course. The intracranial hemorrhages might be caused by a direct US effect and also as a result of a reperfusion trauma after a faster rate of recanalization in the patients treated with rt-PA plus US [12]. Deaths after 3 months were equally distributed in both groups (3/19, 15.8% of the rt-PA plus US group vs. 2/18, 11.8% of the rt-PA group).

Using TCDS without Thrombolytic Drugs

Presently, intravenous rt-PA is still the only treatment option for patients with acute ischemic stroke. Many patients have to be excluded from this therapy because of the restrictive clinical indications of this potentially harmful treatment. Sonothrombolysis could offer an alternative method of accelerating recanalization in patients with an acute intracranial arterial occlusion who also have contraindications for rt-PA. Results from a randomized clinical study on a small sample of 15 patients with acute MCA-M1 occlusion, but with contraindications for rt-PA treatment and included within a time window of 6 instead of 3 h, showed significantly better (incomplete) recanalization. As in the study involving the treatment of patients with a combination of rt-PA and US, the early clinical course was more favorable in those patients treated with US. No intracranial hemorrhages occurred in the US-treated group. No major differences were present in terms of the outcome after 3 months. The results regarding recanalization were consistent with the findings from a series of 6 patients, also with MCA-M1 occlusion, who were similarly treated with TCDS-guided pulsed-wave US as those in the randomized study [13].

Both methods, TCDS-guided sonothrombolysis with and without rt-PA, need to be tested in larger samples of patients to determine their safety and efficacy. At present, recanalization does indeed seem to be accelerated by insonation with transcranial 'diagnostic' US, but the sample sizes are too small to prove an effect on the outcome after 3 months. The initiation of recanalization was detected in most patients after a continuous insonation time of 20 min in all studies utilizing TCDS, with or without rt-PA. Therefore, it can be speculated that an insonation time shorter than one hour may be sufficient to induce recanalization. If a shorter insonation time is eventually found to be sufficient to induce recanalization, it is possible that the occurrence of intracranial hemorrhages, which appeared in patients treated with US in combination with rt-PA, may be prevented.

Originally designed as a diagnostic tool, TCDS can be used to identify only the major brain vessels; the more distal branches of these arteries cannot be displayed or insonated using this method. As a result, this characteristic of TCDS may limit its ability to be used for sonothrombolysis. The energy transmitted through the skull is very low; nevertheless, it obviously has an effect on recanalization and may even cause an increase in the rate of intracranial hemorrhages. The impact on thrombolysis of US emitted by a commercial probe, as similarly used in the clinical studies described above, in combination with rt-PA was tested in an in vitro setting [14]. Compared with the duplex-Doppler and the continuous wave Doppler, the pulsed-wave Doppler mode was most operant on thrombus weight reduction. A reduction of thrombus weight was present only if the experiment was performed without a human temporal bone placed between the US probe and the thrombus. Measurements indicated that the US energy was reduced by about 90% when passed through the skull. However, this in vitro model might not accurately reproduce the complex situation that occurs in the human brain during acute stroke. In addition, data from other in vitro studies have determined that transcranial-applied US has an effect on thrombolysis, but the mechanism of action is still unknown. Data from in vitro studies investigating the effect of US that is of a lower frequency and higher energy than used in the clinical setting suggest that the penetration of rt-PA into the thrombus may be enhanced under these conditions [15]. It is also known that US enhances the binding of rt-PA to fibrin; interestingly, this effect is reversible [16]. Because it could explain the improved short-time outcome of the investigated patients, it is important to note that both the thrombus and endothelium show changes after insonation, because both may contribute to the improved patient outcome after US treatment [17].

Further Developments

Because TCDS-guided sonothrombolysis used in combination with rt-PA appears to increase the rate of intracranial hemorrhages, this finding raises the question of whether the US should be modified to substitute rt-PA or if the US should be used in combination with other thrombus-dissolving drugs. It has been recently shown that 2-MHz pulsed-wave US used in combination with the glycoprotein IIb/IIIa inhibitor abciximab can enhance the dissolution of a thrombus [18]. As shown in vitro by Larrue and coworkers [19], using TCDS in combination with an US contrast enhancer (Levovist™) may also represent another method of amplifying the power of sonothrombolysis. A randomized, multicenter clinical trial (Microbubbles and Ultrasound in Stroke Trial, MUST) was recently launched to test the effect of using microbubbles, rt-PA, and US in combination on recanalization and patient outcome. Specific transcranial US devices operating at 1-MHz are also currently being developed [20].

TCDS is a widely available diagnostic tool that is used not only to visualize the site of an intracranial vessel occlusion but can also be used to treat this occlusion by focusing an US beam on it. Presently, rt-PA is the only established therapy used in the treatment of acute ischemic stroke. However, based on recent research findings, sonothrombolysis has the potential of becoming another treatment option.

References

1 Trübestein G, Engel C, Etzel F, Sobbe A, Cremer H, Stumpff U: Thrombolysis by ultrasound. Clin Sci Mol Med Suppl 1976;3:s697–s698.

2 Akiyama M, Ishibashi T, Yamada T, Furuhata H: Low-frequency ultrasound penetrates the cranium and enhances thrombolysis in vitro. Neurosurgery 1998;43:828–832.

3 Grolimund P: Transmission of ultrasound through the temporal bone; in Aaslid R (ed.): Transcranial Doppler sonography. Wien, New York, Springer-Verlag, 1986, pp 10–21.

4 Behrens S, Spengos K, Daffertshofer M, Schroeck H, Dempfle CE, Hennerici M: Transcranial ultrasound-improved thrombolysis: Diagnostic vs. therapeutic ultrasound. Ultrasound Med Biol 2001;27:1683–1689.

5 Alexandrov AV, Demchuk AM, Felberg RA, Christou I, Barber PA, Burgin WS, Malkoff M, Wojner AW, Grotta JC: High rate of complete recanalization and dramatic clinical recovery during tPA infusion when continuously monitored with 2-MHz transcranial Doppler monitoring. Stroke 2000;31:610–614.

6 Eggers J, Koch B, Meyer K, Konig I, Seidel G: Effect of ultrasound on thrombolysis of middle cerebral artery occlusion. Ann Neurol 2003;53:797–800.

7 Eggers J, Seidel G, Koch B, Konig IR: Sonothrombolysis in acute ischemic stroke for patients ineligible for rt-PA. Neurology 2005;64:1052–1054.

8 Gerriets T, Goertler M, Stolz E, Postert T, Sliwka U, Schlachetzki F, Seidel G, Weber S, Kaps M: Feasibility and validity of transcranial duplex sonography in patients with acute stroke. J Neurol Neurosurg Psychiatry 2002;73:17–20.

9 Gerriets T, Postert T, Goertler M, Stolz E, Schlachetzki F, Sliwka U, Seidel G, Weber S, Kaps M: DIAS I: Duplex-sonographic assessment of the cerebrovascular status in acute stroke: A useful tool for future stroke trials. Stroke 2000;31:2342–2345.

10 Kenton AR, Martin PJ, Abbott RJ, Moody AR: Comparison of transcranial color-coded sonography and magnetic resonance angiography in acute stroke. Stroke 1997;28:1601–1606.

11 Berger C, Fiorelli M, Steiner T, Schabitz WR, Bozzao L, Bluhmki E, Hacke W, von Kummer R: Hemorrhagic transformation of ischemic brain tissue: Asymptomatic or symptomatic? Stroke 2001;32:1330–1335.

12 Molina CA, Alvarez-Sabin J, Montaner J, Abilleira S, Arenillas JF, Coscojuela P, Romero F, Codina A: Thrombolysis-related hemorrhagic infarction: A marker of early reperfusion, reduced infarct size, and improved outcome in patients with proximal middle cerebral artery occlusion. Stroke 2002;33:1551–1556.

13 Cintas P, Le Traon AP, Larrue V: High rate of recanalization of middle cerebral artery occlusion during 2-MHz transcranial color-coded Doppler continuous monitoring without thrombolytic drug. Stroke 2002;33:626–628.

14 Pfaffenberger S, Devcic-Kuhar B, Kollmann C, Kastl SP, Kaun C, Speidl WS, Weiss TW, Demyanets S, Ullrich R, Sochor H, Wober C, Zeitlhofer J, Huber K, Groschl M, Benes E, Maurer G, Wojta J, Gottsauner-Wolf M: Can a commercial diagnostic ultrasound device accelerate thrombolysis? An in vitro skull model. Stroke 2005;36:124–128.

15 Francis CW, Blinc A, Lee S, Cox C: Ultrasound accelerates transport of recombinant tissue plasminogen activator into clots. Ultrasound Med Biol 1995;21:419–424.

16 Siddiqi F, Odrljin TM, Fay PJ, Cox C, Francis CW: Binding of tissue-plasminogen activator to fibrin: Effect of ultrasound. Blood 1998;91:2019–2025.

17 Suchkova VN, Baggs RB, Francis CW: Effect of 40-kHz ultrasound on acute thrombotic ischemia in a rabbit femoral artery thrombosis model: Enhancement of thrombolysis and improvement in capillary muscle perfusion. Circulation 2000;101:2296–2301.

18 Eggers J, Ossadnik S, Seidel G: Ultrasound-enhanced thrombolysis: Effect of combination of 2-MHz ultrasound and abciximab in vitro. Cerebrovasc Dis 2005;19(suppl 2):11.

19 Cintas P, Nguyen F, Boneu B, Larrue V: Enhancement of enzymatic fibrinolysis with 2-MHz ultrasound and microbubbles. J Thromb Haemost 2004;2:1163–1166.

20 Culp WC, McCowan TC: Ultrasound augmented thrombolysis. Current Medical Imaging Review; 2005;1:5–12.

21 Demchuk AM, Burgin WS, Christou I, Felberg RA, Barber PA, Hill MD, Alexandrov AV: Thrombolysis in brain ischemia (TIBI) transcranial Doppler flow grades predict clinical severity, early recovery, and mortality in patients treated with intravenous tissue plasminogen activator. Stroke 2001;32:89–93.

Jürgen Eggers, MD
Neurology, Segeberger Kliniken
Hamdorfer Weg 3
DE–23795 Bad Segeberg (Germany)
Tel. +49 4551 802 6854, Fax +41 4551 802 5905
E-Mail juergen.eggers@segebergerkliniken.de

Baumgartner RW (ed): Handbook on Neurovascular Ultrasound.
Front Neurol Neurosci. Basel, Karger, 2006, vol 21, pp 171–181

Cerebral Aneurysms and Arteriovenous Malformations

Christof Klötzsch[a], Judith U. Harrer[b]

[a]Department of Neurology, Kliniken Schmieder, Allensbach, and Hegau-Hospital Singen, and [b]Department of Neurology, University Hospital Aachen, Aachen, Germany

Abstract

Cerebral aneurysms and arteriovenous malformations (AVMs), including arteriovenous fistulae, are rather seldom investigated by means of transcranial color-coded duplex sonography (TCCS). Nevertheless, the continuous improvements in high-quality scanners, ultrasound contrast enhancers, and special software, such as three-dimensional reconstruction tools, make these lesions assessable in a high number of patients. In particular, the possibility of investigating hemodynamics and hemodynamic changes in a noninvasive manner is a unique feature of TCCS, which is therefore particularly valuable for monitoring stepwise transcatheter treatment of these lesions. Limitations of the technique, mainly caused by restrictions of the insonated bone windows, render this method inadequate as a screening tool. However, TCCS has proven to be a highly useful technique for follow-up investigations of treated and untreated cerebral aneurysms and AVMs. This chapter explains the investigation of these lesions and gives an insight into the most important up-to-date literature.

Cerebral Aneurysms

Several investigators have reported on the detection of intracranial aneurysms using transcranial color-coded duplex sonography (TCCS) [1–12]. The prime criterion for the diagnosis of an aneurysm is a color-coded appendix (fig. 1, 2) connected with a vessel; additional criteria are (1) a red and a blue zone within the lumen of the aneurysm due to bidirectional flow within larger aneurysms and (2) a circular echogenic structure in B-mode imaging, demonstrated by fast switching from color-coded mode to B-mode [4]. Aneurysms with thrombosed components (fig. 3) appear as an echogenic, often calcified

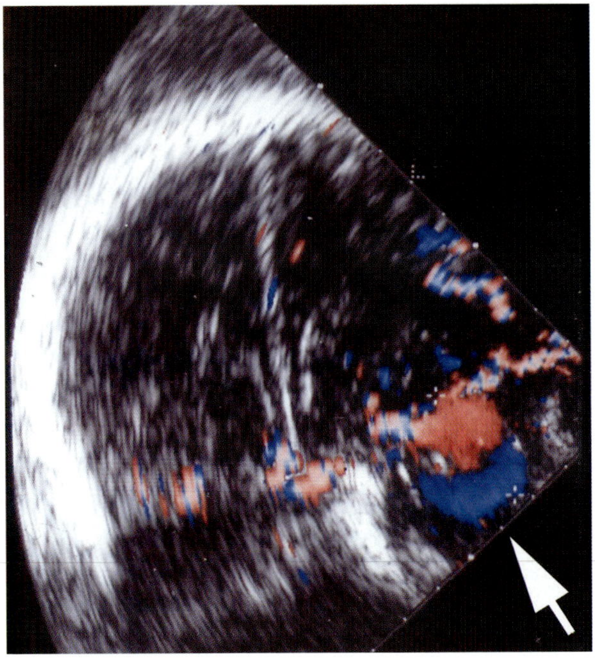

Fig. 1. Middle cerebral artery aneurysm. Coronal plane section, insonation through the temporal bone window: the arrow indicates a large aneurysm of the middle cerebral artery with a bicolored zone, which results from simultaneous inflow and outflow within the aneurysmal lumen. The echo-intense small structure in the midline is caused by the cerebral falx.

shell, which surrounds the less echogenic thrombosed portions. The maximum diameter of the color-coded lumen of the aneurysm should be measured in two planes. In a study conducted by Percival et al. [9] in 39 aneurysms, the maximum (systolic) and minimum (end-diastolic) area of each aneurysm was measured by two observers without significant differences. Thus, the aneurysm size may be measured in either part of the heart cycle; although, the authors suggest maintaining any of the sizing method in repeated measurements of individual patients to minimize errors. Several typical Doppler signals may be measured in cerebral aneurysms. Klötzsch et al. [4] observed a pathological pulse-wave Doppler spectrum with low-frequency signals in the lumen, caused by turbulent flow in 44% of the investigated aneurysms. In large saccular aneurysms with a small neck and a diameter >10 mm, a bidirectional pulse-wave Doppler signal along with the above-mentioned red and blue areas within the lumen can be detected in color-coded duplex mode. In small aneurysms with a diameter of <6 mm, the sample volume is too large to obtain any Doppler signal, which is

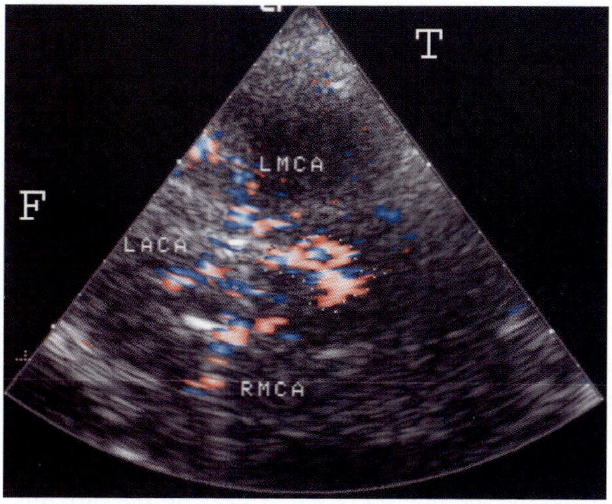

Fig. 2. Basilar artery aneurysm. Transversal insonation plane, insonation through the temporal bone window: this figure demonstrates the circle of Willis with a giant aneurysm (surrounded by dotted line) at the top of the basilar artery compressing the brain stem. LMCA = Left middle cerebral artery; LACA = left anterior cerebral artery; RMCA = right middle cerebral artery; F = frontal; T = temporal.

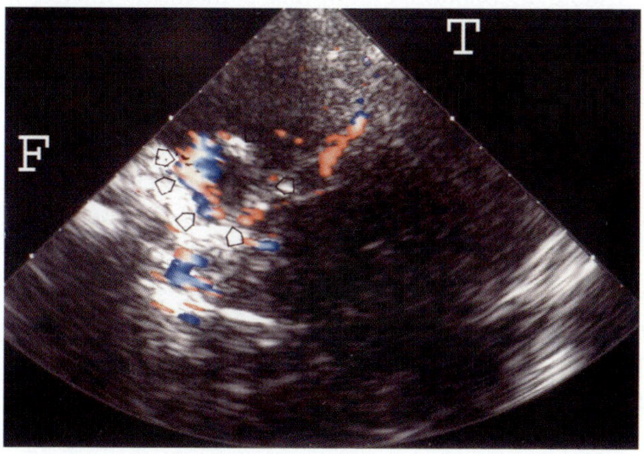

Fig. 3. Thrombosed aneurysm. Transversal insonation plane, insonation through the temporal bone window: this figure shows a particularly thrombosed large aneurysm (arrows) of the distal segment of the internal carotid artery. Half of the aneurysm is occluded by thrombosed (black signal) and calcified material (bright signal), while blood flow is detectable in the other half of the lesion. The bright signal in frontomedial position to the aneurysm is the base of the skull (os sphenoidale). F = Frontal, T = temporal.

not contaminated by flow signals from the parent artery. Low-flow options allow detection of velocities as low as 1 cm/s within the aneurysms.

Sensitivity of aneurysm detection depends on aneurysm size and location. White et al. [11] investigated 171 patients with suspected intracranial aneurysm. Sensitivity per patient was 78% for any aneurysm, but ranged from 35% for aneurysms ≤5 mm to 81% for aneurysms >5 mm. Accuracy was lower for detecting aneurysms of the cavernous and terminal segments of the internal carotid artery (ICA), including posterior communicating artery origin (71%), than for those of the anterior (82%) or the middle cerebral arteries (79%). Small ICA aneurysms with a diameter of <6 mm near the origin of the ophthalmic artery (infra- and supraclinoid), where the ICA performs a 180° turn, are often not demonstrable, because the C3 and C4 segment of the ICA lie too close together. Another anatomically difficult region is the intracranial vertebral artery and its branch, the posterior inferior cerebellar artery. Although it is possible to show the y-shape of the intracranial vertebral artery and the proximal part of the basilar artery, the image quality is not comparable with that obtained from the anterior circulation, because the insonation depth varies from 50 to 110 mm between individuals. Aneurysms in this location often cannot be differentiated reliably due to the frequent tortuosity of these vessels.

Multiple two-dimensional-TCCS images must be integrated in the sonographer's mind to develop a three-dimensional (3D) impression of the intracranial vessel anatomy. The restriction to only a few insonation windows (temporal, nuchal, transorbital) with variable insonation conditions sometimes makes it impossible to obtain optimal image planes for diagnosis of vascular changes. In the past few years computerized technology has advanced sufficiently to allow the development of visualization techniques capable for 3D-TCCS. Power-based TCCS is better suited than mean-frequency-based TCCS for 3D reconstruction, because it allows a more sensitive detection of low flow near the vessel wall and is less degraded by noise and clutter [3]. Administration of an echo contrast enhancer enables 3D reconstruction even of small vascular alterations, avoids vessel discontinuity, and significantly improves the differentiation from disturbing background signals. To achieve a stable contrast enhancement of 15–20 dB for 8–10 min without blooming artifacts, a contrast enhancer should be applied with an infusion pump rather than as a single intravenous bolus injection [10]. For precise demonstration of vessel dimensions, it is important to extremely reduce color persistence and color Doppler gain to avoid blooming artifacts. Filter settings should be adjusted individually. By means of 3D-TCCS, Klötzsch et al. [10] detected 29 of 30 angiographically proven intracranial aneurysms (97%). A comparison of the aneurysmal size in the three main diameters of each aneurysm revealed a correlation coefficient of 0.95 between digital subtraction angiography and 3D-TCCS, even though the aneurysmal diameter estimated by digital subtraction angiography ranged from as little as 3–16 mm. The high interobserver correlation (o = 0.96) of 3D-determined aneurysmal size reflects the high reliability of the technique. Compared with conventional TCCS, the differentiation between artifact and real changes of the vessel anatomy is much easier. Furthermore, 3D-TCCS enables the investigator to reconstruct virtually any arbitrary view angle. Unfavorably located vessel segments, such as the carotid siphon, can be insonated in transversal planes and may be assessed after 3D reconstruction. The possibility of repeated postprocessing and analysis of a 3D-TCCS data set by different investigators improves reliability and objectivity of TCCS.

TCCS and 3D-TCCS are not suitable as screening methods because of their moderate sensitivity to detect small aneurysms, and aneurysms in certain locations. However, routine TCCS allows the incidental detection of asymptomatic intracranial aneurysms and raise the possibility of treating these before rupture. Further clinical applications of TCCS and 3D-TCCS are in monitoring progressive intra-aneurysmal thrombosis following coil embolization and follow-up of untreatable fusiform aneurysms. Embolization material, consisting of platinum coils, and the adjacent thrombotic material appear homogeneously highly echogenic, but without echo-shadowing. Turner et al. [12] and Schuknecht et al. [8] were able do detect residual intra-aneurysmal flow after coil embolization with a sensitivity of 100% and a specificity of 97%. Thus, TCCS is a reliable and noninvasive follow-up tool for the investigation of cerebral aneurysms.

Cerebral Arteriovenous Malformations

Using TCCS, large (>4 cm) cerebral arteriovenous malformations (AVMs) can be depicted by B-mode imaging as echodense areas interspersed with zones of lower echo intensity (table 1). The color-coded illustration of intravascular flow phenomena allows the distinct identification of the major feeding vessels, venous drainage, and vascular convolution of the AVM (fig. 4). Information on hemodynamics, such as the blood supply of the angioma, may be obtained by analysis of the Doppler spectrum, in addition to color-coded identification of flow direction [13–17].

Dramatic changes of cerebral hemodynamics occur during transcatheter treatment of cerebral AVMs. In AVMs with more than one feeding artery, for example, embolization of one of the feeders may cause recruitment of blood flow from another, yet untreated, feeding artery. In addition to increased perfusion of untreated feeders and steal effects, intracerebral hemorrhage or perifocal edema may develop as a result of an imbalance of arterial inflow and venous drainage. During treatment, feeders and draining veins change their

Table 1. Main and additional diagnostic criteria for the depiction of cerebral aneurysms, arteriovenous malformations, and dural arteriovenous fistulae

	Main diagnostic criterion	Additional diagnostic criteria
Cerebral aneurysm	A color-coded appendix connected with a vessel in transcranial color-coded duplex sonography (TCCS)	(1) A red *and* a blue zone within the lumen of the suspected lesion (in larger lesions with slim neck) (2) A circular echogenic structure in B-mode imaging (3) Aneurysms with thrombosed components: echogenic shell which surrounds the less echogenic thrombosed portions
Arteriovenous malformation	Echo-dense areas interspersed with zones of lower echo intensity in B-mode and color-coded nidus (serpiginous vascular structure) in TCCS	Identification of (1) Feeding vessels (increased blood flow velocity, reduced pulsatility) (2) Draining vessels (increased blood flow velocity) (3) Collaterals
Dural arteriovenous fistula	Extracranial depiction of increased blood flow velocity and reduced pulsatility in a neck artery (commonly in external carotid artery, less common in vertebral artery or internal carotid artery) *and* detection of increased venous blood flow velocity in TCCS	Detection of (1) Reverse venous flow (2) Veins or sinuses, which commonly are not depictable by TCCS

flow characteristics, making a repeated identification of these vessels by means of TCD, both difficult and unreliable. However, a noninvasive monitoring system for follow-up examinations during stepwise treatment of AVMs is undoubtedly useful.

Klötzsch et al. [14] studied the ability of TCCS to detect AVMs with different size and location in 41 patients, and furthermore, investigated the capability of this method to estimate hemodynamic changes during stepwise embolization. In this study, the AVM and the main feeding arteries were demonstrable in 29 of 41 consecutive patients (71%). Anatomic limitations of the temporal bone window with restricted insonation angles constrain sufficient

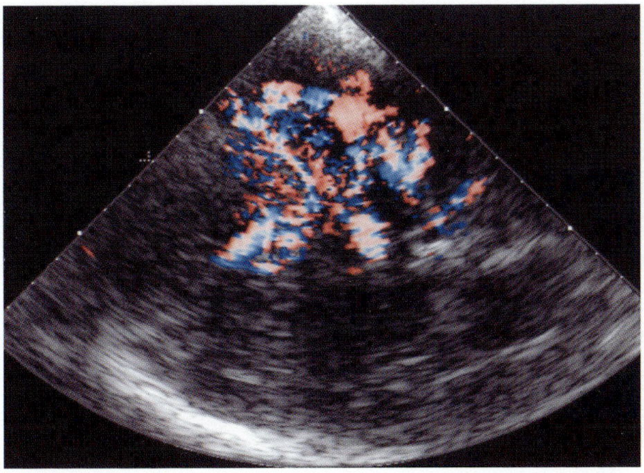

Fig. 4. Arteriovenous malformation, transverse. Transversal insonation through the temporal bone reveals a large arteriovenous malformation with convolutes of arterial and venous vessels in the temporal lobe and the basal ganglia. Aliasing phenomena reflect increased flow velocities in all vessels. The echo-intense (bright) signal at the bottom of the figure is caused by the contralateral temporal bone.

visualization of malformations with parieto-occipital or superficial localization. Moreover, in AVMs located in the posterior fossa, differentiation of feeding arteries is unreliable because of the close proximity of the vessels. Additional meningeal or choroidal feeders cannot be visualized as a consequence of their small diameter and/or close location to the skull. The spectral analysis of small micro-fistulous AVMs is impaired by the low shunt volume and slightly elevated peak flow velocities in the feeding arteries. As a noninvasive bedside test, TCCS is suitable as a quickly applicable screening method for AVMs in patients with cryptogenic intracranial hemorrhage; however, a negative TCCS examination certainly does not exclude an AVM.

In case all feeding vessels of an AVM can be identified sonographically, TCCS offers the unique possibility to quantitatively evaluate the hemodynamic changes occurring after transcatheter treatment of cerebral supratentorial AVMs [14]. The untreated feeders show an increase in peak flow velocities as a result of increased collateral flow. In contrast to TCD, TCCS allows repeated insonation of a vessel under visual control at the same depth and with the same insonation angle. TCCS also enables detecting an increase in flow velocity in untreated feeders or newly recruited feeders. This information may well be instrumental in the decision of which feeder should be treated next.

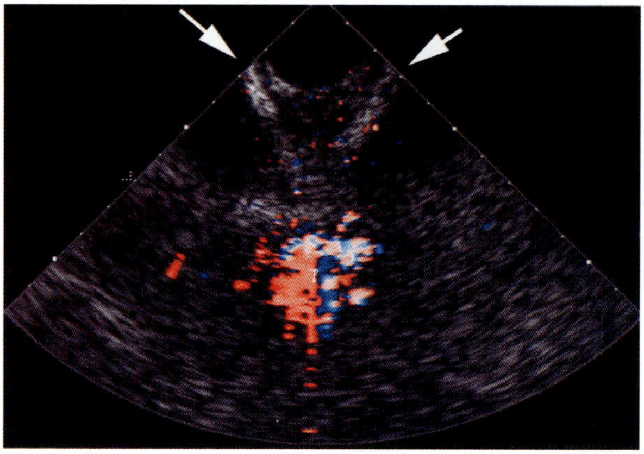

Fig. 5. Carotid-cavernous fistula, transorbital. Transorbital insonation of a direct (type A) carotid cavernous fistula caused by the rupture of a cavernous aneurysm: the fistula exhibits a mosaic color-coded pattern, which results from aliasing phenomena.

Dural Arteriovenous Fistulae

Extracranial Doppler or color-coded duplex sonography has long been applied for arterial investigation of dural arteriovenous fistulae (DAVF) [18]. Decrease of the resistance index of the external carotid artery is the most important Doppler sonographic parameter for the indirect identification of intracranial dural AVFs.

A number of studies have described imaging of pathologically increased arterial and venous flow velocities of carotid-cavernous fistulae (CCF) [19–22]. Direct visualization of the CCF using transorbital color-coded sonography can be achieved in patients with direct CCF depicting heterogeneous mosaic flashes, which result from high flow velocities and turbulences (fig. 5). Abnormal flow patterns reflecting venous drainage can be detected in both, direct CCF and indirect (dural) CCF. The transorbital and -foraminal windows demonstrate arterialized blood flow directed towards the probe in the dilated retrograde superior ophthalmic vein. In the nidus, pulse-wave Doppler shows bidirectional blood flow spectra along with high-frequency signals, the so-called musical murmur or seagull's cry. The combination of carotid color-coded duplex sonography and transcranial (transorbital) color-coded sonography provides a noninvasive method for accurate hemodynamic studies and direct imaging of CCF. Occipital DAVF are commonly located in the posterior cranial fossa, and some of them may have developed after sinus thrombosis.

Venous drainage usually comprises of the transverse and sigmoid sinus, occasionally involving contralateral sinuses. Drainage into cortical veins carries a high risk of intracranial hemorrhage, nonhemorrhagic neurological deficit, and death.

For the detection of a DAVF, a TCCS set-up with a high sensitivity for low venous blood flow needs to be applied; therefore, the pulse repetition frequency should be reduced, a low wall filter should be selected, and the color gain needs to be increased taking interindividual differences, such as quality of the temporal bone window and contrast effect, into account. Transtemporally, the deep middle cerebral vein, the basal vein of Rosenthal, the straight sinus, the posterior part of the superior sagittal sinus, and the contralateral transverse sinus can commonly be assessed in up to 90% of cases [24].

TCCS-based diagnosis of a DAVF [23] is established when at least one of the following criteria is present: detection of increased venous blood flow velocity according to the criteria published by Baumgartner et al. [24], the detection of reverse venous flow, or the detection of sinuses, which commonly are not depictable by TCCS (sigmoid sinus, superior/inferior petrosal sinus, inferior sagittal sinus). Insonation of these is attempted in each case via the contralateral temporal bone window using the transverse sinus and the petrous bone as anatomical lead for the sigmoid sinus, and again the petrous bone as leading structure for the superior/inferior petrosal sinus, with stronger downward tilt for depiction of the inferior petrosal sinus.

Harrer et al. [23] included 24 patients to determine the value of contrast-enhanced frequency-based TCCS for the direct investigation of hemodynamic changes in DAVF before and after transcatheter embolization. By means of TCCS, twenty-five of twenty-seven draining veins/sinuses (93%) could be detected. The superior sagittal sinus, sigmoid sinus, and superior petrosal sinus could only be depicted in patients who exhibited fistula drainage into these particular sinuses. Abnormally increased blood flow velocities compared with normal values were found in all patients in at least one cerebral vein or sinus. Analysis of flow velocities of draining veins as well as veins not contributing to the drainage of the DAVF showed an increase of flow velocities from cranial to caudal veins/sinuses. Flow velocities in draining veins decreased significantly after embolization when compared with pretreatment values. According to this study, any venous peak systolic flow velocity exceeding 50 cm/s should be regarded as pathological and lead to further neuroradiological investigations.

A certain drawback of TCCS for this application is the failure to depict additional cortical venous drainage, especially because drainage into cortical veins implies a significantly increased risk of cerebral hemorrhage due to venous hypertension. However, experienced investigators will detect typical ultrasonographic features in cases where a DAVF is present in a regular TCCS investigation of the intracranial arteries. Because application of a routine set-up for investigation of the arterial system will not allow demonstration of normal cerebral veins and sinuses, depiction of these would require spectral analysis to clarify whether increased venous blood flow is present in the respective vessels. This is also true for the depiction of reverse flow in cerebral veins and sinuses, indicating venous collateral flow.

References

1 Becker G, Greiner K, Kaune B, Winkler J, Brawanski A, Warmuth-Metz M, Bogdahn U: Diagnosis and monitoring of subarachnoidal hemorrhage by transcranial colour-coded real-time sonography. Neurosurgery 1991;28:814–820.

2 Baumgartner RW, Mattle HP, Kothbauer K, Schroth G: Transcranial colour-coded Duplex sonography in cerebral aneurysms. Stroke 1994;25:2429–2434.

3 Wardlaw JM, Cannon JC: Colour transcranial power Doppler ultrasound of intracranial aneurysms. J Neurosurg 1996;84:459–461.

4 Klötzsch C, Nahser HC, Fischer B, Henkes H, Kühne D, Berlit P: Visualization of intracranial aneurysms by transcranial duplex sonography. Neuroradiology 1996;38:555–559.

5 Lindner A, Shambal S, Georgiadis D, Becker G: Transcranial color-coded duplex ultrasound in interventional therapy of cerebral aneurysms. Ultraschall Med 1997;18:148–152.

6 Griewing B, Motsch L, Piek J, Schminke U, Brassel F, Kessler C: Transcranial power mode Doppler duplex sonography of intracranial aneurysms. J Neuroimaging 1998;8:155–158.

7 Fischer B, Klötzsch C, Nahser HC, Henkes H, Kühne D, Berlit P: Klinische Anwendung der TCCS zum Nachweis intrakranieller Aneurysmen. Nervenarzt 1998;69:671–677.

8 Schuknecht B, Chen JJ, Valavanis A: Transcranial color-coded Doppler sonography of intracranial aneurysms before and after endovascular occlusion with Guglielmi detachable coils. AJNR Am J Neuroradiol 1998;19:1659–1667.

9 Percival J, Wardlaw JM, Cannon J: Observer variability in the measurement of the size of intracranial aneurysms using power TCD. J Neuroimaging 1998;8:75–77.

10 Klötzsch C, Bozzato A, Lammers G, Mull M, Lennartz B, Noth J: Three-dimensional transcranial color-coded sonography of cerebral aneurysms. Stroke 1999;30:2285–2290.

11 White PM, Wardlaw JM, Teasdale E, Sloss S, Cannon J, Easton V: Power transcranial Doppler ultrasound in the detection of intracranial aneurysms. Stroke 2001;32:1291–1297.

12 Turner CL, Higgins JN, Kirkpatrick PJ: Assessment of transcranial color-coded duplex sonography for the surveillance of intracranial aneurysms treated with Guglielmi detachable coils. Neurosurgery 2003;53:866–872.

13 Martin PJ, Gaunt ME, Naylor AR, Hope DT, Orpe V, Evans DH: Intracranial aneurysms and arteriovenous malformations: Transcranial colour-coded sonography as a diagnostic aid. Ultrasound Med Biol 1994;20:689–698.

14 Klötzsch C, Henkes H, Nahser HC, Kühne D, Berlit P: Transcranial color-coded duplex sonography in cerebral arteriovenous malformations. Stroke 1995;26:2298–2301.

15 Baumgartner RW, Mattle HP, Schroth G: Transcranial colour-coded duplex sonography of cerebral arteriovenous malformations. Neuroradiology 1996;38:734–737.

16 el-Saden SM, Grant EG, Sayre J, Vinuela F, Duckwiler G: Transcranial color Doppler imaging of brain arteriovenous malformations in adults. J Ultrasound Med 1997;16:327–334.

17 Kaspera W, Majchrzak H: Evaluation of blood supply dynamics and possibilities of cerebral arteriovenous malformations (AVM) imaging by means of transcranial color-coded duplex sonography (TCCS). Neurol Neurochir Pol 2002;36:735–748.

18 Tsai LK, Jeng JS, Wang HJ, Yip PK, Liu HM: Diagnosis of intracranial dural arteriovenous fistulas by carotid duplex sonography. J Ultrasound Med 2004;23:785–791.

19 Chen YW, Jeng JS, Liu HM, Yip PK, Hwang BS, Lin WH, Chang YC, Tu YK: Diagnosis and follow-up of carotid-cavernous fistulas by carotid duplex sonography and transcranial color Doppler imaging. Ultrasound Med Biol 1996;22:1155–1162.
20 Chen YW, Jeng JS, Liu HM, Hwang BS, Lin WH, Yip PK: Carotid and transcranial color-coded duplex sonography in different types of carotid cavernous fistula. Stroke 2000;31:701–706.
21 Kawaguchi S, Sakaki T, Morimoto T, Uranishi R: Colour Doppler flow imaging of the superior ophthalmic vein in dural arteriovenous fistulas before and after surgery. J Clin Neurosci 2000;7: 42–46.
22 Kawaguchi S, Sakaki T, Uranishi R: Color Doppler flow imaging of the superior ophthalmic vein in dural arteriovenous fistulas. Stroke 2002;33:2009–2013.
23 Harrer JU, Popescu O, Henkes HH, Klötzsch C: Assessment of dural arteriovenous fistulae by transcranial color-coded duplex sonography. Stroke 2005;36:976–979.
24 Baumgartner RW, Gönner F, Arnold M, Müri RM: Transtemporal power- and frequency-based color-coded duplex sonography of cerebral veins and sinuses. AJNR Am J Neuroradiol 1997; 18:1771–1781.

Prof. Dr. Christof Klötzsch
Akutneurologie der Kliniken Schmieder, Allensbach,
und Neurologische Abteilung des Hegau-Klinikums Singen
Zum Tafelholz 8
DE–78476 Allensbach (Germany)
Tel. +49 7533 808 1332, Fax +49 7533 808 1376
E-Mail c.kloetzsch@kliniken-schmieder.de

Baumgartner RW (ed): Handbook on Neurovascular Ultrasound.
Front Neurol Neurosci. Basel, Karger, 2006, vol 21, pp 182–193

Cerebral Veins and Sinuses

Erwin Stolz

Department of Neurology, Justus-Liebig-University, Giessen, Germany

Abstract

Transcranial ultrasonography is an established and reliable method for the evaluation of the arteries of the circle of Willis, even at the patient's bedside. Examination of cerebral veins and sinuses is a new application, which has been developed during the recent years. The ultrasound anatomy, examination technique, findings in cerebral venous thrombosis, and the application of transcranial ultrasonography in nonvenous cerebrovascular diseases is reviewed. While transcranial ultrasonography is an established and reliable method for the diagnostic evaluation of disturbed arterial blood flow, the venous side of circulation has long been neglected. Reasons for this late interest may be the relatively lower incidence of primary intracranial venous disease and the low spatial resolution and limited low flow capability of early transcranial ultrasound systems. It was not until the mid-1990s that venous transcranial ultrasound in adults was systematically developed. In the following the examination technique and clinical applications of this technique are summarized.

Ultrasound Anatomy

A distinct characteristic of the intracranial venous system is the lack of valves. This implies that the flow direction in cerebral veins and dural sinuses is governed solely by the current pressure gradient. Further, in the deep white matter a venous watershed exists, which separates a centrifugal drainage directed towards the dural sinuses and a centripetal drainage towards the Galenic system.

The superficial cerebral veins cannot be imaged with ultrasound methods. However, usually, three of the surface veins of the brain appear dominant and may serve as important collaterals. Their recruitment can be assumed by indirect ultrasound findings. The superficial middle cerebral vein connects to the sphenoparietal (SPaS) or cavernous sinus (60%), or to the pterygoid plexus (14%) [1, 2]. The superior anastomotic (Trolard's) vein drains towards the superior sagittal sinus (SSS) and the inferior anastomotic (Labbé's) vein joins the transverse sinus (TS).

The SSS is a fairly constant vascular structure and receives blood predominantly from ascending veins, including the superior anastomotic vein. Variants include hypoplasia of the anterior third and a doubling of the posterior third of the vessel [3, 4]. The SSS ends in the confluens sinuum, which splits into the paired TS, serving as the major outflow channel towards the internal jugular vein via the sigmoid sinus. In more than 50% of the cases right-sided caliber dominance is present [5, 6]. Aplasia is found in about 4%.

The cavernous sinus is a paired structure connected by the intercavernous sinuses [7]. It comprises an important alternative runoff via the ophthalmic veins and the basilar plexus. Only its major tributaries, the SPaS and the superior petrosal sinus (SPS), can be depicted by ultrasound. The SPaS usually originates in a frontal lacuna of the SSS, forms an extension of the middle meningeal vein over the convexity, follows the lesser wing of the sphenoid bone and empties into the anterior angle of the cavernous sinus [8]. The SPS runs in a groove on the posterosuperior margin of the pyramid of the sphenoid bone. It connects the cavernous sinus with the sigmoid sinus. A further collateral connection is provided by the inferior petrosal sinus (IPS), which occupies the petrooccipital suture and expands from the cavernous sinus to the internal jugular vein. At the origin it runs in close neighborhood of the basilar artery.

The deep middle cerebral vein (dMCV) is formed by insular veins, follows a medial course in close proximity to the middle cerebral artery (MCA) within the lateral sulcus, and empties into the basal vein (BV) (of Rosenthal). It is present in more than 80% of cases [9]. The BV has a slightly ascending course around the mesencephalon and is divided into a striatal, a peduncular, and postpeduncular segment [10]. Whereas the postpeduncular segment is a constant anatomical structure in a slightly cranial and lateral position of the P2-segment of the posterior cerebral artery (PCA), the remaining segments are subject to variation in the embryological formation and course. Together with the internal cerebral veins (ICV) the BV usually joins the great cerebral vein (GCV) (vein of Galen). The GCV originates above the pineal gland, describes a convex arch around the splenium of the corpus callosum, and joins the straight sinus (SRS). The SRS runs in the apex of the cerebellar tentorium to end in the confluens sinuum. The venous anatomy relevant to transcranial ultrasonography is summarized in figures 1a and 2.

Examination Technique

Transcranial Doppler Sonography

For transtemporal transcranial Doppler sonography (TCD) examination of the venous system, the main segments of the circle of Willis are important landmarks. The dMCV is insonated in close proximity to the MCA mainstem, the BV is found slightly superior of the P2-segment of the PCA [11]. The leading structure towards the SPaS and SPS is the carotid siphon [12]. However, a clear distinction between both sinuses is not possible by TCD alone. The aforementioned venous vessels show a flow directed away from the transducer. In a depth of 9–10 cm the basilar artery serves as the leading structure to the IPS, which is found lateral to the artery, with a flow towards the probe when the transforaminal approach is used [13]. The ophthalmic window can be used to examine the superior ophthalmic vein and the parasellar region [12], whereas the occipital bone window provides access to the SRS [14]. The relationship of these venous structures to the arteries is illustrated in figure 2a, b. Due to the low venous flow velocities (vFVs), the pulse repetition frequency needs to be reduced and a small sample volume has to be used to prevent masking of the venous signal by the arterial Doppler spectrum. Sometimes it may be necessary to ascertain the venous origin of a Doppler signal by the prompt reactivity to a brief Valsalva maneuver.

Transcranial Color-Coded Duplex Sonography

In principal transcranial color-coded duplex sonography (TCCS) used the same acoustic bone windows as TCD. However, the clear advantage of TCCS over TCD is that it represents a true imaging method with depiction of parenchymal structures simultaneous with the blood flow information. In order to examine intracranial veins and sinuses a low-flow sensitive color program with a low wall filter setting has to be used and the pulse repetition frequency needs to be reduced. The color gain is increased to the artifact threshold. As shown in figure 1b, venous TCCS examination starts in the mesencephalic examination plane. The dMCV is found adjacent to the MCA and is best insonated in the transition of the M1- to the M2-segments. Flow is directed away from the probe. In excellent insonation conditions the peduncular segment

Fig. 1. ***a–f*** Venous ultrasound anatomy and examination technique with transcranial color-coded duplex sonography (TCCS). ***a*** Ultrasound anatomy, ***b–f*** examination technique, and typical TCCS appearance and characteristic venous Doppler spectrum (for details, see text). The blue plane represents the examination plane, light blue the examination plane of previous step. The red arrows indicate the movement of the transducer and the resultant change of the insonation plane. The vessels marked in red are the ones that can be examined in the given examination plane. dMCV = Deep middle cerebral vein; ICV = internal cerebral vein; SSS = superior sagittal sinus; GCV = great cerebral vein (of Galen); SRS = straight sinus; SPS = superior petrosal sinus; BV = basal vein (of Rosenthal); SPaS = sphenoparietal sinus; MCA = middle cerebral artery; ACA = anterior cerebral artery; TS = transverse sinus; ipsil. = ipsilateral; contral. = contralateral.

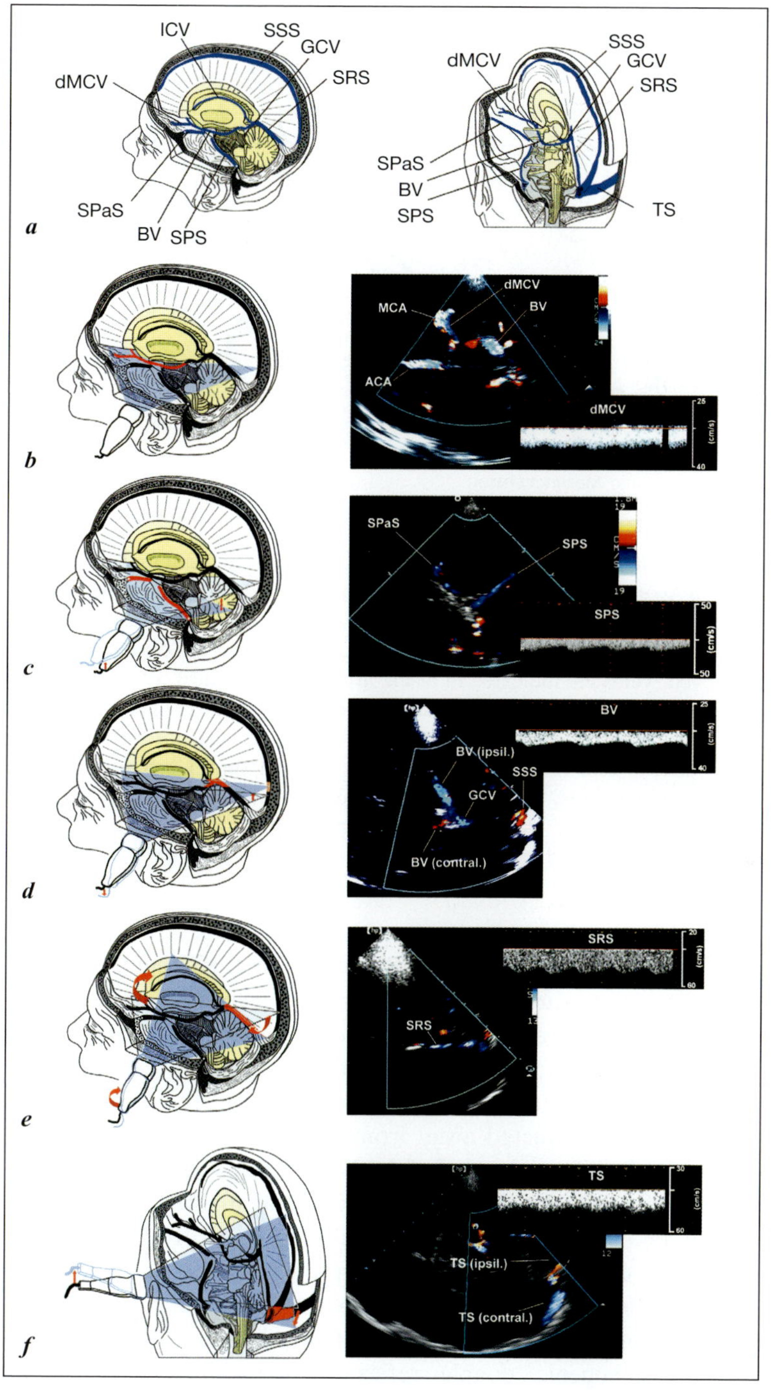
ICV
SSS
GCV
dMCV
SRS
SPaS
BV
SPS
TS
a
b
c
d
e
f
MCA
ACA
dMCV
BV
SPaS
SPS
BV (ipsil.)
SSS
GCV
BV (contral.)
SRS
TS
TS (ipsil.)
TS (contral.)
(cm/s)

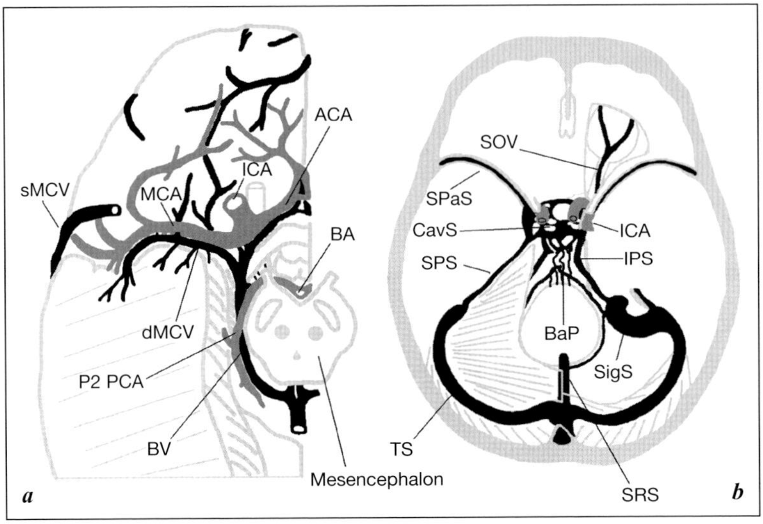

Fig. 2. ***a, b*** Topographic anatomy of cerebral arteries and veins relevant for transcranial Doppler sonography. ***a*** Anatomy of the deep cerebral veins. In the schematic drawing, part of the temporal lobe has been removed. ***b*** Anatomy of the cavernous sinus inflow region. In the drawing on the right side, part of the bony structures of the cranial base and cerebellar tentorium have been removed. Veins are indicated in black, arteries in gray. dMCV = Deep middle cerebral vein; BV = basal vein; MCA = middle cerebral artery; ICA = internal cerebral artery; ACA = anterior cerebral artery; P2 PCA = P2-segment of the posterior cerebral artery; BA = basilar artery; sMCV = superficial middle cerebral vein; CavS = cavernous sinus; SPaS = sphenoparietal sinus; SPS = superior petrosal sinus; IPS = inferior petrosal sinus; SOV = superior ophthalmic vein; BaP = basilar plexus; TS = transverse sinus; SigS = sigmoid sinus; SRS = straight sinus.

of the BV can be visible in close proximity to the proximal P2-segment of the PCA with a flow directed towards the transducer. The cavernous sinus inflow region is imaged by a downward tilt of the transducer to the cranial base. Landmark structure for insonation of the SPaS is the echogenic lesser wing and for the SPS the echogenic pyramid of the sphenoid bone (fig. 1c). Normal flow direction of both sinuses is directed away from the probe. Using the mesencephalon as reference plane for depiction of the BV, the transducer is angulated upwards towards the diencephalic plane. The BV is found slightly cranial to the P2-segment of the PCA, which both display a flow away from the probe (fig. 1d). The vein can easily be identified by its low pulsatile Doppler spectrum. Then the B-mode depth is increased, so that the contralateral skull becomes visible. Prominent midline structures of the diencephalic insonation plane comprise the echogenic double reflex of the third ventricle and echogenic pineal gland. The GCV is found immediately behind the pineal gland, with a flow away from the transducer. In this examination plane the rostral part of the SSS may be visible (fig. 1d). In order to examine the SRS the anterior tip of the transducer needs to be rotated upwards to align the insonation plane with the plane of the apex of the cerebellar tentorium (fig. 1e), which possesses an increased echogenicity. The course of the SRS is directed away from the transducer towards the confluens sinuum. Proceeding from this transducer position the probe is angulated downwards again to depict the contralateral TS (fig. 1f). For examination of the IPS the same approach is used as for TCD. They can be used to examine the midline venous vessels (ICV, GCV, SRS).

Normal Values

Normal values and detection rates based on cohorts of presumably healthy adults of more than 40 subjects are summarized in table 1. Venous Doppler signals display a low pulsatility with a constant outwards flow, unlike peripheral veins. vFVs are higher in women than in men and decrease with advancing age [11, 15–17]. Detection rates decrease with age and are comparable with those of the circle of Willis for the deep cerebral veins. For sinuses, detection rates are lower and vary among different research groups. This is most likely due to differences in the low flow detection sensitivity of the ultrasound systems used. Reproducibility of vFV measurements is high and comparable to measurements in the arterial system [18].

Cerebral Venous Thrombosis

Based on the current literature the following ultrasound criteria support the diagnosis of cerebral venous thrombosis (CVT):

- Visibility of numerous prominent veins due to high vFV in collaterals when an arterial presetting of the ultrasound system is used.
- Pathological vFVs as a result of a collateral venous outflow defined as greater than mean plus two standard deviations [15, 19–21]. The extent of the increase of vFVs ascertained by ultrasonography depends on the anatomical location, the ability of venous wall distension, the original caliber of the collateral, and the volume flow in relation to the total collateral volume flow. False-positive results may arise when vFVs in SPaS and SPS are measured in proximity to the cavernous sinus, because of the gradual tapering of the diameter, so that measurements should be performed more distally from the cavernous entrance [22].

Table 1. Flow velocities and detection rates in presumably healthy adults

Reference		[15]	[17]	[16]	[39]	[11]	[13]	[12]
		TCCS				TCD		
		TBW	TBW	OBW	FBW	TBW	TFBW	TBW
N		120	130	120	75	60	80	43
ø Age		60 ± 18	46 ± 17	50 ± 17	45 ± 17	42 ± 15	38 ± 15	32 ± 10
Vessel								
dMCV	FV	10 (4–15)/ 7 (3–11)	8.7 ± 2.9/ 5.8 ± 1.9	–	–	11 ± 3	–	–
	DR	53–93%	55–95%	–	–	22%	–	–
BV	FV	13 (7–19)/ 9 (5–14)	12.2 ± 3.8/ 8.7 ± 2.8	–	–	10 ± 2	–	–
	DR	86–100%	85–96%	–	–	97%	–	–
GCV	FV	–	11.9 ± 3.6/ 7.7 ± 2.8	23 (12–34)/ 16 (7–26)	–	–	–	–
	DR	–	84–94%	20–34%	–	–	–	–
SRS	FV	26 (12–39)/ 17 (7–27)	12.1 ± 4.7/ 8.6 ± 3.7	35 (7–64)/ 23 (2–43)	–	–	–	–
	DR	23–73%	57–82%	50–81%	–	–	–	–
TS	FV	32 (9–56)/ 21 (5–38)	14.0 ± 5.9/ 9.7 ± 4.8	–	–	–	–	–
	DR	20–54%	46–84%	–	–	–	–	–

SSS	FV	–	9.8 ± 3.6/ 6.1 ± 2.5	–	–	–	–	–
	DR	–	38–67%	–	–	–	–	–
IPS	FV	–	–	–	–	–	20 ± 9	–
	DR	–	–	–	–	–	78%	–
ICV	FV	–	7.2 ± 1.7/ 4.9 ± 1.1	14 (10–18)/ 10 (5–15)	13.6 ± 4.1/ 9.9 ± 2.9	–	–	–
	DR	–	23%	13–34%	30–60%	–	–	–
SPaS + SPS	FV	–	–	–	–	–	–	27 ± 17
	DR	–	–	–	–	–	–	84%

The table summarizes studies of cohorts of more than 40 subjects. TCCS = Transcranial color-coded duplex sonography; TCD = transcranial Doppler sonography; TBW = temporal bone window; OBW = occipital bone window; FBW = frontal bone window; TFBW = transforaminal bone window; N = cohort size; ø Age = average age in years; dMCV = deep middle cerebral vein; BV = basal vein (of Rosenthal); GCV = great cerebral vein (of Galen); SRS = straight sinus; TS = transverse sinus; SSS = superior sagittal sinus; IPS = inferior petrosal sinus; ICV = internal cerebral vein; SPaS = sphenoparietal sinus; SPS = superior petrosal sinus; FV = flow velocity in cm/s; DR = detection rate in percentage. Flow velocities are given as peak systolic/end-diastolic velocities, otherwise as mean velocities. Data in brackets indicate the range, values given as plus/minus show the standard deviation. When a range is given for detection rates, this indicates the variation in different age groups.

- Pathological flow direction in the BVs is typically found in SRS occlusion [15, 20, 23]. In the proximal part of the TS flow reversal can be observed when the sinus is distally occluded. The SPS may show a reversed flow when the pressure gradient is directed towards the TS [23].
- Significant side differences (>50%) for the dMCV and BV were not observed in normal subjects [17]. Due to the considerable rate of hypoplasias or caliber differences, side differences of vFV in paired sinuses have only a diagnostic relevance when vFVs are pathologically increased.
- Direct criteria comprise the lack of color signal within a dural sinus after application of echo contrast agents [19, 24, 25]. However, thrombotic occlusion or partial thrombosis cannot be differentiated from aplasia or hypoplasia by ultrasound alone.

Reported rates of pathological ultrasound findings in acute CVT, where the examiners were not blinded to the diagnosis, range from 50 to 100% [19–21]. In two studies limited to the examination of the TS after application of an echo contrast agent a sensitivity of 73–100% and a specificity of 65–80% are reported [24, 25]. In both studies patients thought to have CVT based on clinical symptoms were examined using magnetic resonance imaging and angiography as reference. Based on this data and due to the fact that large parts of the SSS nor cortical veins can be examined, venous transcranial ultrasound examination is not capable of excluding CVT. On the other hand, transcranial ultrasound provides information on venous hemodynamics, which is not offered by computed tomography angiography and conventional time-of-flight magnetic resonance angiography, and is therefore complementary to these methods.

Venous TCD and duplex sonography are particularly suitable for follow-up examinations. In our own prospective study of 26 patients with acute CVT, an initially normal venous ultrasound examination or normalization within 90 days were significantly associated with an excellent outcome (modified Rankin scale score 0 or 1) [23]. In contrast, in 37 prospectively studied patients with CVT, recanalization of occluded dural sinuses was frequently observed as early as 22 days after diagnosis using magnetic resonance imaging; however, even early recanalization was not associated with the outcome [26]. This highlights the importance of hemodynamic factors for the long-term outcome of CVT, which cannot be assessed by current routine computed tomography and magnetic resonance angiography.

Other Applications of Transcranial Venous Ultrasound

Because of the tight relationship between intracranial pressure (ICP) and cerebral venous pressure, changes in vFVs can be expected in any disorders with disturbed ICP. About 70 to 80% of the intracranial blood volume is located in the venous system, so that it represents an important reserve space in brain volume shifts [27].

Although a close correlation of vFVs and the ICP has been described by Schoser et al. [28], so far these results have not been confirmed [29–31].

In patients with head trauma or subarachnoid hemorrhage, vFVs correlated better with the clinical outcome than arterial blood flow velocities (FVs) [29–31]. This has been attributed to a tighter correlation of vFVs with the cerebral blood flow as compared with arterial FVs, which was found in 14 patients with subarachnoid hemorrhage using the Kety-Schmidt method [30]. However, before venous transcranial ultrasound monitoring in head trauma or subarachnoid hemorrhage can be recommended as a prognostic tool, further studies are necessary.

In a group of 21 patients with ischemic stroke and developing space-occupying brain edema, vFVs were monitored prospectively [32]. FVs in the BV ipsilateral to the lesion were significantly lower in those patients with a fatal course on days 1–5. Presumably as an effect of brain tissue dislocation, a significant increase of FV in the GCV and SRS was observed exclusively in patients who died of brain stem herniation. While arterial FVs did not show a specific pattern discriminating patients who survive or are of danger to die of herniation, monitoring of vFVs might have a prognostic implication.

The selective examination of arteries and cerebral veins supplying the brain enables the analysis of temporal aspects of brain circulation by measurement of the arterio-venous transit time (a-vTT). The principle of a-vTT measurements is based on the time latency of the intensity increase in artery and vein after intravenous application of an echo-contrast-enhancing agent [33–35]. Suitable pairs of artery and vein are the internal carotid artery and internal jugular vein or the P2-segment of the PCA and GCV. Significantly shortened a-vTTs were observed in arteriovenous malformations, however, without correlation to their size [35]. In patients with ischemic stroke compared to matched controls significantly increased a-vTTs were found [36]. No correlation with the functional outcome was found after one year. The most promising application for measurement of a-vTTs currently seems to be the work-up of demented patients. A-vTTs were significantly increased in patients with CADASIL and vascular dementia, whereas patients with Alzheimer's type of dementia did not differ from matched controls [34, 37, 38].

References

1 Rhoton AL: The cerebral veins. Neurosurgery 2002;51(suppl 1):159–205.

2 Lang J, Jensen HP, Schröder F: Venen und Sinus durales; in Lang J, Wachsmuth W (eds): Praktische Anatomie. Ein Lehr- und Hilfsbuch der anatomischen Grundlagen ärztlichen Handelns.

Kopf. Teil 1A. Übergeordnete Systeme. Begründet von T. von Lanz und W. Wachsmuth, fortgeführt und herausgegeben von J. Lang und W. Wachsmuth. Unveränderter Nachdruck der ersten Auflage 1985. Berlin/Heidelberg/New York/Tokio, Springer, 2004, pp 578–633.

3 Kaplan HA, Bowder A, Bowder EJ: Nasal venous drainage and the foramen caecum. Laryngoscope 1974;83:327–329.

4 Huang YP, Okudera T, Ohta T, Robbins A: Anatomic variations of the dural venous sinuses; in Kapp JP, Schmidek HH (eds): The Cerebral Venous System and Its Disorders. London, Orlando, Grune and Stratton, 1984, pp 109–167.

5 Bono F, Lupo MR, Lavano A, Mangono L, Fera F, Pardatscher K, Quattrone A: Cerebral MR venography of transverse sinuses in subjects with normal CSF pressure. Neurology 2003;61: 1267–1270.

6 Durgun B, Ilgit ET, Cizmeli MO, Atasever A: Evaluation by angiography of the lateral dominance of the drainage of the dural venous sinuses. Surg Radiol Anat 1993;15:125–130.

7 Zenker W: Die Blutgefässe des Zentralnervensystems; in Zenker W (ed) unter Mitarbeit von Akert K, Firbas W, Fritsch O, Gruber H, Mayr R, Neuhuber W, Petsche H, Rager G: Benninghoff. Markroskopische und mikroskopische Anatomie des Menschen. 3. Band. Nervensystem, Haut und Sinnesorgane. 13./14. völlig neubearbeitete Auflage. München/Wien/Baltimore, Urban und Schwarzenberg, 1985, pp 181–202.

8 Oka K, Rhoton AL, Barry M, Rodruigez R: Microsurgical anatomy of the superficial veins of the cerebrum. Neurosurgery 1985;17:711–748.

9 Ono M, Rhoton AL, Peace D, Rodriguez RJ: Microsurgical anatomy of the deep venous system of the brain. Neurosurgery 1984;15:621–657.

10 Salamon G, Huang YP: Radiologic Anatomy of the Brain. Berlin/Heidelberg/New York, Spinger, 1976.

11 Valdueza JM, Schmierer K, Mehraein S, Einhäupl KM: Assessment of normal flow velocity in basal cerebral veins: A transcranial Doppler ultrasound study. Stroke 1996;27:1221–1225.

12 Valdueza JM, Hoffmann O, Doepp F, Lehmann R, Einhäupl KM: Venous Doppler ultrasound assessment of parasellar region. Cerebrovasc Dis 1998;8:113–117.

13 Doepp F, Hoffmann O, Lehmann R, Einhäupl KM, Valdueza JM: The inferior petrosal sinus: Assessment by transcranial Doppler ultrasound using the suboccipital approach. J Neuroimaging 1999;9:193–197.

14 Aaslid R, Lindegaard KF, Sorteberg W, Nornes H: Cerebral autoregulation dynamics in humans. Stroke 1989;20:45–52.

15 Baumgartner RW, Gönner F, Arnold M, Müri RM: Transtemporal power- and frequency-based color-coded duplex sonography of cerebral veins and sinuses. AJNR Am J Neuroradiol 1997;18:1771–1781.

16 Baumgartner RW, Nirkko AC, Müri RM, Gönner F: Transoccipital power-based color-coded duplex sonography of cerebral sinuses and veins. Stroke 1997;28:1319–1323.

17 Stolz E, Kaps M, Dorndorf W: Transcranial color-coded duplex sonography of intracranial veins and sinuses in adults. Reference data from 130 volunteers. Stroke 1999;30:1070–1075.

18 Stolz E, Babacan SS, Bödeker RH, Gerriets T, Kaps M: Interobserver and intraobserver reliability of venous transcranial color-coded flow velocity measurements. J Neuroimaging 2001;11: 385–392.

19 Stolz E, Kaps M, Dorndorf W: Assessment of intracranial venous hemodynamics in normals and patients with cerebral venous thrombosis. Stroke 1999;30:70–75.

20 Valdueza JM, Hoffmann O, Weih M, Mehraein S, Einhäupl KM: Monitoring of venous hemodynamics in patients with cerebral venous thrombosis by transcranial Doppler ultrasound. Arch Neurol 1999;56:229–234.

21 Canhão P, Batista P, Ferro JM: Venous transcranial Doppler in acute dural sinus thrombosis. J Neurol 1998;245:276–279.

22 Schreiber SJ, Stolz E, Valdueza JM: Transcranial ultrasonography of cerebral veins and sinuses. Eur J Ultrasound 2002;16:59–72.

23 Stolz E, Gerriets T, Bödeker RH, Hügens-Penzel M, Kaps M: Intracranial venous hemodynamics is a factor related to a favorable outcome in cerebral venous thrombosis. Stroke 2002;33: 1645–1620.

24 Delcker A, Häussermann P, Weimar C: Effect of echo contrast media on the visualization of transverse sinus thrombosis with transcranial 3-D duplex sonography. Ultrasound Med Biol 1999;25: 1063–1068.

25 Ries S, Steinke W, Neff KW, Hennerici M: Echocontrast-enhanced transcranial color-coded sonography for the diagnosis of transverse sinus thrombosis. Stroke 1997;28:696–700.

26 Stolz E, Trittmacher S, Rahimi A, Gerriets T, Röttger C, Siekmann R, Kaps M: Influence of recanalization on outcome in dural sinus thrombosis: A prospective study. Stroke 2004;35: 544–547.

27 Schmidek HH, Auer L, Kapp JP: The cerebral venous system. Neurosurgery 1985;17:663–678.

28 Schoser BG, Riemenschneider N, Hansen HC: The impact of raised intracranial pressure on cerebral venous hemodynamics: A prospective venous transcranial Doppler ultrasonography study. J Neurosurg 1999;91:744–749.

29 Mursch K, Müller CA, Buhre W, Lang JK, Vatter H, Behnke-Mursch J: Blood flow velocities in the basal cerebral vein after head trauma: A prospective study in 82 patients. J Neuroimaging 2002;12:325–329.

30 Mursch K, Wachter A, Radke K, Buhre W, Al-Sufi S, Behnke-Mursch J, Kolenda H: Blood flow velocities in the basal vein after subarachnoid haemorrhage. A prospective study using transcranial duplex sonography. Acta Neurochir (Wien) 2001;143:793–800.

31 Niesen WD, Rosenkranz M, Schummer W, Weiller C, Sliwka U: Cerebral venous flow velocity predicts poor outcome in subarachnoid hemorrhage. Stroke 2004;35:1873–1878.

32 Stolz E, Gerriets T, Babacan SS, Jauss M, Kraus J, Kaps M: Intracranial venous hemodynamics in patients with midline dislocation due to postischemic brain edema. Stroke 2002;33:479–485.

33 Hoffmann O, Weih M, Schreiber S, Einhäupl KM, Valdueza JM: Measurement of cerebral circulation time by contrast-enhanced Doppler sonography. Cerebrovasc Dis 2000;10:142–146.

34 Puls I, Hauck K, Demuth K, Horowski A, Schliesser M, Dörfler P, Scheel P, Toyka KV, Reiners K, Schöning M, Becker G: Diagnostic impact of cerebral transit time in the identification of microangiopathy in dementia: A transcranial ultrasound study. Stroke 1999;30:2291–2295.

35 Schreiber SJ, Kauert A, Doepp F, Valdueza JM: Measurement of global cerebral circulation time using power duplex echo-contrast bolus tracking. Cerebrovasc Dis 2003;15:129–132.

36 Ruprecht-Dörfler P, Brechtelsbauer D, Schliesser M, Puls I, Becker G: Prognostic and diagnostic value of global cerebral blood flow volume and cerebral transit time in acute stroke. Ultrasound Med Biol 2002;28:1405–1411.

37 Puls I, Becker G, Maurer M, Müllges W: Cerebral arteriovenous transit time (CTT): A sonographic assessment of cerebral microcirculation using ultrasound contrast agents. Ultrasound Med Biol 1999;25:503–507.

38 Liebetrau M, Herzog J, Kloss CU, Hamann GF, Dichgans M: Prolonged cerebral transit time in CADASIL: A transcranial ultrasound study. Stroke 2002;33:509–512.

39 Stolz E, Kaps M, Dorndorf W: Frontal bone windows for transcranial color-coded duplex sonography. Stroke 1999;30:814–820.

Erwin Stolz, MD
Department of Neurology, Justus-Liebig-University
Am Steg 14
DE–35385 Giessen (Germany)
Tel. +49 641 99 45310, Fax +49 641 99 45309
E-Mail Erwin.Stolz@neuro.med.uni-giessen.de

Baumgartner RW (ed): Handbook on Neurovascular Ultrasound.
Front Neurol Neurosci. Basel, Karger, 2006, vol 21, pp 194–205

Detection of Microembolic Signals with Transcranial Doppler Ultrasound

Dimitrios Georgiadis[a], *Mario Siebler*[b]

[a]Department of Neurology, University of Zürich, Zürich, Switzerland; [b]Department of Neurology, University of Düsseldorf, Düsseldorf, Germany

Abstract

Detection of microembolic signals (MES) with transcranial Doppler was introduced in the late 1980s; several animal and in vitro models reported a high sensitivity and specificity with this technique. Monitoring for MES in various patient groups has provided valuable insights on stroke pathophysiology, although its clinical value remains a matter of debate. Diagnosis of imminent occlusion of the internal carotid artery following carotid endarterectomy, selection of high-risk patients with asymptomatic carotid disease, and evaluation of drug efficacy constitute potential applications of this technique.

High-intensity signals were initially observed during intraoperative transcranial Doppler monitoring in patients undergoing carotid endarterectomy. Several experimental models have since demonstrated that these are caused by (micro)embolic material [1, 2], so that the term microembolic signals (MES) was adapted. MES detection was also shown to be a highly sensitive technique, able to detect formed or gaseous embolic material with a minimal diameter of 40 or 10 μm, respectively [3]. Results of clinical studies on MES detection and potential applications of this technique will be discussed in this chapter.

Methodological Aspects

MES detection is commonly performed by continuous transtemporal insonation of the middle cerebral artery (MCA). Recommended monitoring duration varies between 30–60 min, with the transducer fixed to the skull with dedicated devices to minimize movement artifacts.

Identification of MES and rejection of artifact signals, caused by tiny probe movements, patient coughing, speaking, or chewing etc, remains a methodological challenge. Following criteria were established during the 9th International Conference on Cerebral Hemodynamics [4]:

(1) Short duration (usually <300 ms).
(2) Amplitude usually at least 3 dB higher than that of the background blood flow signal, depending on the characteristics of the individual MES.
(3) Unidirectional signal within the Doppler velocity spectrum, provided that the signal intensity is within the appropriate dynamic range of bidirectional Doppler equipment.
(4) Characteristic acoustic qualities, usually 'snap', 'chirp', or 'moan', depending on the equipment used and the velocity of the underlying embolus.

These criteria, though, are subjective; furthermore, the fact that a human observer is still considered the golden standard in MES detection significantly increases the temporary requirements and costs of this method. Therefore, various approaches for automated MES detection were introduced. Siebler et al. [5] proposed the use of a neuronal network. First results were encouraging, but a study comparing the neuronal network with human observes merely rendered a sensitivity of 67% [6]. The 'bigate' approach, initially proposed by R. Aaslid, is based on simultaneous insonation of two segments of the same vessel; embolic material should ideally be detected in the different sample volumes with a temporary delay depending on blood flow velocity; artifact signals on the other hand should be detected simultaneously in both sample volumes (fig. 1). This method produced promising results when evaluated off-line [7, 8], but unfortunately not when used as 'stand alone' system [9, 10]. Further approaches (reference-gate method [10], 'narrow band' method [11], automated detection using 'frequency filtering' [12]) also failed to reach the sensitivity and specificity levels required for a routine use. The human observer, therefore, remains the golden standard for MES detection.

Differentiation between gaseous and formed underlying embolic material constitutes a further methodological issue in MES detection. Existing methods (analysis of Doppler spectrum [13], 'time domain analysis' [14], insonation with two separate frequencies [15], 'matching pursuit' method [16], analysis of frequency variations of MES [17]) were either unable to produce reproducible results, or have not been sufficiently validated.

MES-Monitoring during Cardiac Surgery

MES incidence during cardiac surgery is quite high (80–100%), whereby only a small portion of the generated embolic material (3.9–18.1%)

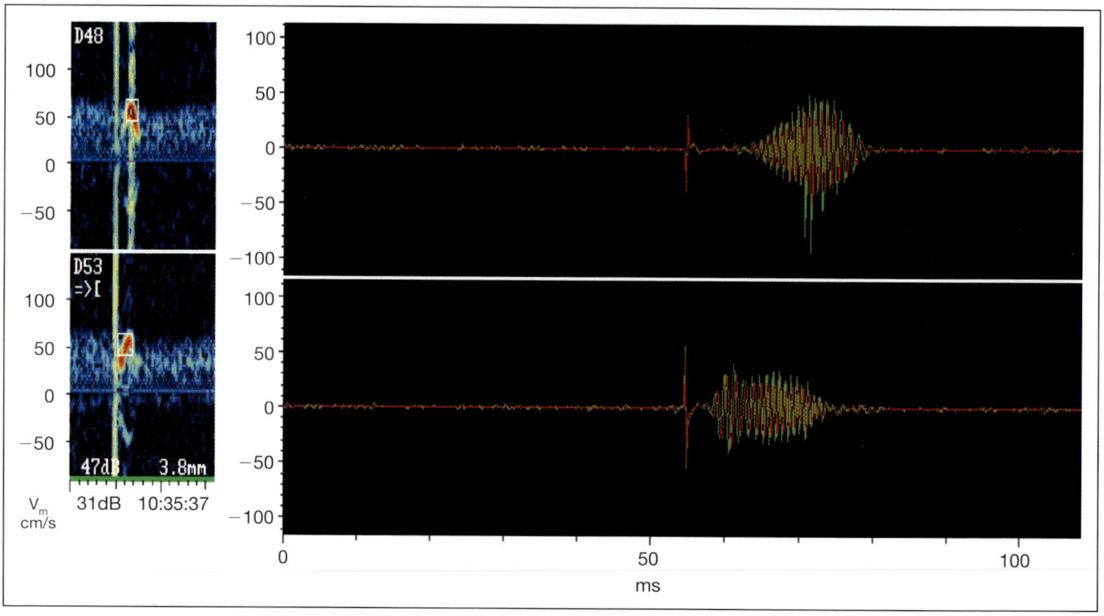

Fig. 1. MES detection with the bigate method. Marked temporary delay in the appearance of the embolic signal between the distal (upper; depth of 48 mm) and the proximal (lower; depth of 53 mm) sample volume. The artifact signal preceding the MES appears simultaneously in both sample volumes.

reaches the cerebral circulation [18]. MES counts strongly depend on the operation stage, with most MES detected during aortic clamping and its release [19].

Several studies described a relation between MES counts and postoperative neuropsychological deficit [20–22]. Barbut et al. [23] described significantly higher MES counts in patients with postoperative ischemic stroke, but this observation was based on merely 4 symptomatic patients, and was not confirmed by a later study [20].

Serial pre- and postoperative magnetic resonance imaging examinations in 41 patients demonstrated that patients with new ischemic lesions on magnetic resonance imaging had significantly higher MES counts during the preincision phase as compared to remaining patients. The incidence of postoperative neuropsychological deficit though, was related to the total count of intraoperatively detected MES [21]. This study suggests that the mechanism of MES generation (and probably their underlying material) significantly influences their impact. Jacobs et al. [24] examined the cerebral glucose metabolism in 19 patients undergoing elective cardiac surgery using both, pre- and postoperative PET scanning, and found no correlation between global or regional changes in glucose metabolism and MES counts. On the other hand, a significant correlation between (1) the total count of intraoperatively detected MES and length of postoperative hospital stay [23] and (2) MES count during aortic cannulation and serum levels of S-100β [25] were demonstrated. It thus appears probable that MES count constitutes a marker for adverse outcome following cardiac surgery, although it does not provide prognostic information for individual patients. Evaluation of the count of MES generated during various operative approaches, therefore, appears justified. Up to date, studies have shown that (1) cannulation of the distal instead of the ascending portion of the aorta [26], (2) coronary bypass operations without use of extracorporeal circulation [27], and (3) anterograde instead of retrograde cerebral perfusion [28], but not smaller diameters of the aortic cannula [29], are associated with significantly lower MES counts.

Monitoring during Carotid Surgery and Angioplasty

Detection of MES during carotid endarterectomy was initially described by Padayachee et al. [30] in 1986 and their clinical relevance confirmed through several studies [31–34]. Three studies examined the influence of intraoperatively detected MES on new postoperative hyperintense lesions in T2- or diffusion-weighted magnetic resonance imaging: two demonstrated a clear-cut relationship [33, 34], while the third was negative, whereby this could be due to the fact that it only included 2 patients with new diffusion-weighted imaging lesions [35].

MES detected during the first postoperative hours following carotid endarterectomy possess a high predictive value for perioperative stroke [36] or imminent thrombotic occlusion on the carotid endarterectomy site; their counts can be significantly reduced with dextran infusions [37]. Postoperative monitoring for MES was shown to reduce the incidence of postoperative complications due to internal carotid artery (ICA) thrombosis from 2.7 to 0% [38].

MES counts during carotid angioplasty are significantly higher, as compared to those detected during carotid endarterectomy [39], although the incidence of neuropsychological deficits after both interventions is similar [40]. The low number of patients monitored during carotid angioplasty in the currently available studies allows no definitive statements concerning the clinical relevance of MES in this setting.

Monitoring during Invasive Cardiological or Angiological Procedures

Detection of clinically silent MES was described during cardiac catheterization [41], carotid angiography [42], cardiac ablation [43], and transmyocardial revascularization [44]. Their relevance remains unclear, mainly due to the small number of patients monitored.

Patients with Prosthetic Heart Valves

Detection of MES in patients with prosthetic heart valves was initially described by Berger et al. [45] in 1990. The causative role of the valve implant has been equivocally proven by serial pre- and postoperative monitoring [46]. Type of prosthetic valve, but no further clinical or hematological parameters (including INR) significantly influences MES counts [47–49]. Influence of MES counts on the prevalence of ischemic stroke was reported in two initial studies, based on a total of 21 symptomatic patients [48, 50], but not confirmed by subsequent reports [47, 49]. Influence of MES counts on neuropsychological deficit was only examined in two studies, which did not have the size necessary for definitive conclusions on this issue [51, 52].

Observations from various studies (and particularly the significant reduction of MES counts under inhalation of 100% oxygen [53] and their significant increase under hyperbaric oxygenation [54]) point at nitrogen bubbles as most probable underlying embolic material. Formation of cavitation bubbles is a common feature of prosthetic heart valves in in vitro models [55].

In summary, detection of MES in patients with prosthetic heart valves is not associated with any clinical consequences and should be limited to clinical studies.

Patients with Potential Cardioembolic Source

Two studies examining a total of 311 patients with potential cardioembolic source described an MES prevalence of 15–43%, but no relationship between MES counts and prevalence of ischemic stroke or patients' medication [56, 57]. Similar results were reported by Cullinane et al. [58], who examined 111 patients with nonrheumatic atrial fibrillation. Nadareishvilli et al. [59] examined 100 patients with acute (within 72 h of symptom onset) myocardial infarction and demonstrated a relation between MES prevalence and (1) left ventricular ejection fraction and (2) presence of akinetic segments in the left ventricle or intraventricular thrombi. Prevalence of ischemic stroke was higher in MES-positive patients, though this result was based on merely 3 symptomatic cases. Nabavi et al. [60] and Moazami et al. [61] examined 6 and 14 patients with 'left ventricular assist devices', respectively, and described an MES prevalence of 84% (143/170 monitoring sessions) and 26% (9/35 monitoring sessions), respectively. Nabavi et al. [60] also observed significantly higher MES counts in days, during which the patients experienced symptoms of cerebral ischemia, as compared to remaining days.

In summary, detection of MES in patients with potential cardioembolic source has no clinical relevance. Further studies are probably warranted in patients with left ventricular assist devices, but these patients are relatively rare, and the performance of a large-scale study is thus rather difficult.

Patients with Patent Foramen Ovale

Transcranial Doppler monitoring for MES possesses a high sensitivity and specificity for identification of patients with patent foramen ovale, as compared to transesophageal echocardiography [62, 63]. A recently published paper provided guidelines for the performance of this examination and the quantification of the shunt, based on the counts of detected MES [64]. This simple bedside method is not associated with any complications and should be routinely established in acute stroke units.

Patients with Stenotic Lesions in Brain Supplying Arteries

Detection of MES in patients with carotid disease was first described by Spencer et al. [65] and Siebler et al. [66] in 1990 and 1992, respectively. Up to date, studies have demonstrated that (1) MES prevalence and counts in patients with symptomatic carotid disease are significantly higher when compared to those with asymptomatic carotid disease [67], (2) MES counts decline with increasing temporary distance from the acute cerebral ischemic event [67], (3) MES counts are significantly reduced or abolished after carotid endarterectomy [68, 69], and (4) MES counts in patients with symptomatic carotid disease depend on the morphology of plaques [70].

Prognostic value of MES in patients with asymptomatic carotid disease was evaluated in three studies: the first examined 42 patients, who were subsequently followed-up for 258 ± 247 days; prevalence of MES in the MCA ipsilateral to the stenosed ICA was 29%. During follow-up, one patient suffered an ischemic stroke and one a transient ischemic attack. A significant association between presence of MES and subsequent ischemic event was noted [71]. The second study examined 64 patients; mean follow-up time was 72 weeks. A microembolic rate of ≥2 per hour was associated with a substantially increased risk of developing ischemia of the corresponding carotid territory [72]. A recently published study failed to reproduce these results: 202 patients were monitored for MES; follow-up time was 5 years. MES were not found to be significant predictors of ischemic events in the territory supplied by the stenosed ICA [73]. This issue is currently being examined in a prospective multicenter study (ACES, principal investigator HR Markus).

Two studies examined the MES prevalence in patients with MCA stenosis (total of 72 patients, 92 stenosed MCAs). MES was detected in only 2 patients, with acute ischemic symptoms in the territory of the affected vessel [74, 75]. The hypothesis that MES can be used to evaluate the embolic activity of an MCA stenosis remains to be evaluated.

Srinivasan et al. [76] described a 59% MES prevalence in 17 patients with traumatic or spontaneous carotid dissection, a significantly higher incidence of ischemic stroke in MES-positive patients and a gradual decline of MES counts after initiation of antiplatelet treatment or oral anticoagulation.

Summing up, MES detection provides interesting pathophysiological insights into patients with symptomatic ICA stenosis, but possesses no clinical relevance. Their clinical relevance in patients with asymptomatic ICA stenosis or MCA stenosis remains unclear.

Acute Stroke Patients

Studies in patients with acute ischemic stroke have demonstrated that MES prevalence and counts depend on the etiology of stroke [77] and progressively decline in the days poststroke [78]. Two studies including a large patient population were unable to provide any evidence for a clinical significance of the detected signals [78, 79]. Therefore, MES detection in this patient group does not appear justified.

Patients with Autoimmune Diseases

Up to date, MES were detected in patients with Sneddon's syndrome [80], systemic lupus erythematosus [81], and Behcet's disease [82]. Initial results suggest that MES could provide information on the activity of these autoimmune diseases and, in particular, on the affection of the central nervous system.

Evaluation of Treatment Efficacy

Siebler et al. [83] and Georgiadis et al. [84] reported results of serial transcranial Doppler monitoring for MES in a patient with acutely symptomatic MCA and ICA stenosis, respectively. MES counts appeared to be influenced by intravenous heparin administration in the first, but not in the second study. Goertler et al. [85, 86] examined 82 patients with acute ischemic stroke and described an influence of aspirin on MES counts; unfortunately, the methodology applied for MES detection was not compatible with current guidelines. Markus and colleagues [87] observed significant differences in MES counts in 42 patients monitored after carotid endarterectomy, depending on postoperative treatment (i.v. *L*-arginine, *S*-nitrosoglutathinone, or placebo). Finally, Junghans and Siebler [88] reported a reversible elimination of MES in patients with symptomatic ICA stenosis following infusion of GPIIb/IIIa inhibitors (tirofiban). These studies suggest that MES detection can play an important role in evaluating the efficacy of various antithrombotic agents.

References

1 Moehring MA, Klepper JR: Pulse Doppler ultrasound detection, characterisation and size estimation of emboli in flowing blood. IEEE Trans Biomed Eng 1994;41:35–44.

2 Russell D, Madden KP, Clark WM, Sandset PM, Zivin JA: Detection of arterial emboli using Doppler ultrasound in rabbits. Stroke 1991;22:253–258.

3 Russell D, Brucher R: The size of cerebral microemboli in prosthetic heart valve patients (abstract). Stroke 1995;26:733.

4 Consensus Committee of the Ninth International Cerebral Hemodynamics Symposium: Basic identification criteria of Doppler microembolic signals. Stroke 1995;26:1123–1124.

5 Siebler M, Rose G, Sitzer M, Bender A, Steinmetz H: Real-time identification of cerebral microemboli with US feature detection by a neural network. Radiology 1994;192:739–742.

6 van Zuilen EV, Mess WH, Jansen C, Van der Tweel I, Van Gijn J, Ackerstaff GA: Automatic embolus detection compared with human experts. A Doppler ultrasound study. Stroke 1996;27: 1840–1843.

7 Georgiadis D, Goeke J, Hill M, Konig M, Nabavi DG, Stogbauer F, Zunker P, Ringelstein EB: A novel technique for identification of doppler microembolic signals based on the coincidence method: In vitro and in vivo evaluation. Stroke 1996;27:683–686.

8 Smith JL, Evans DH, Fan L, Bell PR, Naylor AR: Differentiation between emboli and artefacts using dual-gated transcranial Doppler ultrasound. Ultrasound Med Biol 1996;22: 1031–1036.

9 Georgiadis D, Wenzel A, Zerkowski HR, Zierz S, Lindner A: Automated intraoperative detection of Doppler microembolic signals using the bigate approach. Stroke 1998;29:137–139.

10 Georgiadis D, Uhlmann F, Astler M, Cencetti S, Zierz S: Automated identification of Doppler microembolic signals: Comparison of two techniques. Neurol Res 2000;22:738–740.

11 Roy E, Abraham P, Montresor S, Baudry M, Saumet JL: The narrow band hypothesis: An interesting approach for high-intensity transient signals (HITS) detection. Ultrasound Med Biol 1998;24:375–382.

12 Markus H, Cullinane M, Reid G: Improved automated detection of embolic signals using a novel frequency filtering approach. Stroke 1999;30:1610–1615.

13 Georgiadis D, Mackay TG, Kelman AW, Grosset DG, Wheatley DJ, Lees KR: Differentiation between gaseous and formed embolic materials in vivo. Application in prosthetic heart valve patients. Stroke 1994;25:1559–1563.

14 Smith JL, Evans DH, Bell PR, Naylor AR: Time domain analysis of embolic signals can be used in place of high-resolution Wigner analysis when classifying gaseous and particulate emboli. Ultrasound Med Biol 1998;24:989–993.

15 Russell D, Brucher R: Multifrequency Doppler discriminates between gaseous and solid microemboli (abstract). Cerebrovasc Dis 1999;9(suppl 1):81.

16 Devuyst G, Vesin JM, Despland PA, Bogousslavsky J: The matching pursuit: A new method of characterizing microembolic signals? Ultrasound Med Biol 2000;26:1051–1056.

17 Smith JL, Evans DH, Naylor AR: Analysis of the frequency modulation present in Doppler ultrasound signals may allow differentiation between particulate and gaseous cerebral emboli. Ultrasound Med Biol 1997;23:727–734.

18 Barbut D, Lo YW, Gold JP, Trifiletti RR, Yao FS, Hager DN, Hinton RB, Isom OW: Impact of embolization during coronary artery bypass grafting on outcome and length of stay. Ann Thorac Surg 1997;63:998–1002.

19 Barbut D, Hinton RB, Szatrowski TP, Hartman GS, Bruefach M, Williams-Russo P, Charlson ME, Gold JP: Cerebral emboli detected during bypass surgery are associated with clamp removal. Stroke 1994;25:2398–2402.

20 Clark RE, Brillman J, Davis DA, Lovell MR, Price TR, Magovern GJ: Microemboli during coronary artery bypass grafting. Genesis and effect on outcome. J Thorac Cardiovasc Surg 1995;109: 249–257.

21 Sylivris S, Levi C, Matalanis G, Rosalion A, Buxton BF, Mitchell A, Fitt G, Harberts DB, Saling MM, Tonkin AM: Pattern and significance of cerebral microemboli during coronary artery bypass grafting. Ann Thorac Surg 1998;66:1674–1678.

22 Harrison MJG, Pugsley W, Newman S, Paschalis C, Klinger L, Treasure T, Aspey B: Detection of middle cerebral emboli during coronary artery bypass surgery using transcranial Doppler sonography (letter). Stroke 1990;21:1512.

23 Barbut D, Yao FS, Lo YW, Silverman R, Hager DN, Trifiletti RR, Gold JP: Determination of size of aortic emboli and embolic load during coronary artery bypass grafting. Ann Thorac Surg 1997;63:1262–1267.

24 Jacobs A, Neveling M, Horst M, Ghaemi M, Kessler J, Eichstaedt H, Rudolf J, Model P, Bonner H, de Vivie ER, Heiss WD: Alterations of neuropsychological function and cerebral glucose metabolism after cardiac surgery are not related only to intraoperative microembolic events. Stroke 1998;29:660–667.

25 Grocott HP, Croughwell ND, Amory DW, White WD, Kirchner JL, Newman MF: Cerebral emboli and serum S100beta during cardiac operations. Ann Thorac Surg 1998;65:1645–1649.

26 Borger MA, Taylor RL, Weisel RD, Kulkarni G, Benaroia M, Rao V, Cohen G, Fedorko L, Feindel CM: Decreased cerebral emboli during distal aortic arch cannulation: A randomized clinical trial. J Thorac Cardiovasc Surg 1999;118:740–745.

27 Watters MP, Cohen AM, Monk CR, Angelini GD, Ryder IG: Reduced cerebral embolic signals in beating heart coronary surgery detected by transcranial Doppler ultrasound. Br J Anaesth 2000;84: 629–631.

28 Baker AJ, Naser B, Benaroia M, Mazer CD: Cerebral microemboli during coronary artery bypass using different cardioplegia techniques. Ann Thorac Surg 1995;59:1187–1191.

29 Benaroia M, Baker AJ, Mazer CD, Errett L: Effect of aortic cannula characteristics and blood velocity on transcranial doppler-detected microemboli during cardiopulmonary bypass. J Cardiothorac Vasc Anesth 1998;12:266–269.

30 Padayachee TS, Gosling RG, Bishop CC, Burnard KG, Browse NL: Monitoring middle cerebral artery blood flow velocity during carotid endarterectomy. Br J Surg 1986;73:98–100.

31 Ackerstaff RG, Moons KG, van de Vlasakker CJ, Moll FL, Vermeulen FE, Algra A, Spencer MP: Association of intraoperative transcranial Doppler monitoring variables with stroke from carotid endarterectomy. Stroke 2000;31:1817–1823.

32 Gaunt ME, Martin PJ, Smith JL, Rimmer T, Cherryman G, Ratliff DA, Bell PR, Naylor AR: Clinical relevance of intraoperative embolization detected by transcranial Doppler ultrasonography during carotid endarterectomy: A prospective study of 100 patients. Br J Surg 1994;81:1435–1439.

33 Ackerstaff RG, Jansen C, Moll FL, Vermeulen FE, Hamerlijnck RP, Mauser HW: The significance of microemboli detection by means of transcranial Doppler ultrasonography monitoring in carotid endarterectomy. J Vasc Surg 1995;21:963–969.

34 Muller M, Reiche W, Langenscheidt P, Hassfeld J, Hagen T: Ischemia after carotid endarterectomy: Comparison between transcranial Doppler sonography and diffusion-weighted MR imaging. AJNR Am J Neuroradiol 2000;21:47–54.

35 Barth A, Remonda L, Lovblad KO, Schroth G, Seiler RW: Silent cerebral ischemia detected by diffusion-weighted MRI after carotid endarterectomy. Stroke 2000;31:1824–1828.

36 Levi CR, O'Malley HM, Fell G, Roberts AK, Hoare MC, Royle JP, Chan A, Beiles BC, Chambers BR, Bladin CF, Donnan GA: Transcranial Doppler detected cerebral microembolism following carotid endarterectomy. High microembolic signal loads predict postoperative cerebral ischaemia. Brain 1997;120:621–629.

37 Lennard N, Smith J, Dumville J, Abbott R, Evans DH, London NJ, Bell PR, Naylor AR: Prevention of postoperative thrombotic stroke after carotid endarterectomy: The role of transcranial Doppler ultrasound. J Vasc Surg 1997;26:579–584.

38 Hayes PD, Lloyd AJ, Lennard N, Wolstenholme JL, London NJ, Bell PR, Naylor AR: Transcranial Doppler-directed Dextran-40 therapy is a cost-effective method of preventing carotid thrombosis after carotid endarterectomy. Eur J Vasc Endovasc Surg 2000;19:56–61.

39 Jordan WD Jr, Voellinger DC, Doblar DD, Plyushcheva NP, Fisher WS, McDowell HA: Microemboli detected by transcranial Doppler monitoring in patients during carotid angioplasty versus carotid endarterectomy. Cardiovasc Surg 1999;7:33–38.

40 Crawley F, Stygall J, Lunn S, Harrison M, Brown MM, Newman S: Comparison of microembolism detected by transcranial Doppler and neuropsychological sequelae of carotid surgery and percutaneous transluminal angioplasty. Stroke 2000;31:1329–1334.

41 Bladin CF, Bingham L, Grigg L, Yapanis AG, Gerraty R, Davis SM: Transcranial Doppler detection of microemboli during percutaneous transluminal coronary angioplasty. Stroke 1998;29: 2367–2370.

42 Gerraty RP, Bowser DN, Infeld B, Mitchell PJ, Davis SM: Microemboli during carotid angiography: Association with stroke risk factors or subsequent magnetic resonance imaging changes? Stroke 1996;27:1543–1547.

43 Georgiadis D, Hill M, Kottkamp H, Breithard G, Borggrefe M: Intracranial microembolic signals during radiofrequency ablation of accessory pathways. Am J Cardiol 1997;80:805–807.

44 von Knobelsdorff G, Brauer P, Tonner PH, Hanle F, Naegele H, Stube HM, Esch JS: Transmyocardial laser revascularisation induces cerebral microembolisation. Anesthesiology 1997;87:58–62.

45 Berger M, Davis D, Lolley D, Rams J, Spencer MP: Detection of subclinical microemboli in patients with prosthetic heart valves (abstract). J Cardiovasc Tech 1990;9:282–283.

46 Grosset DG, Georgiadis D, Stirling S, Coburn P, Faichney A, Lees KR: Subclinical embolism in patients undergoing cardiac valve implantation and coronary artery bypass surgery. Eur J Cardiothorac Surg 1994;8:63–66.

47 Georgiadis D, Grosset DG, Kellman AW, Faichney A, Lees KR: Prevalence and characteristics of intracranial microemboli signals in patients with different types of prosthetic cardiac valves. Stroke 1994;25:587–592.

48 Sliwka U, Diehl RR, Meyer B, Schönhube F, Noth J: Transcranial Doppler 'high-intensity transient signals' in the acute phase and long-term follow-up of mechanical heart valve implantation. J Stroke Cerebrovasc Dis 1995;5:139–146.

49 Sliwka U, Georgiadis D: Clinical correlations of Doppler microemboli signals in patients with prosthetic heart valves. Analysis of 580 cases. Stroke 1998;29:140–143.

50 Braekken KS, Russell D, Brucher R, Svennevig J: Incidence and frequency of cerebral embolic signals in patients with a similar bileaflet mechanical heart valve. Stroke 1995;26: 1225–1230.

51 Deklunder G, Roussel M, Lecroart JL, Prat A, Gautier C: Microemboli in cerebral circulation and alteration of cognitive abilities in patients with mechanical prosthetic heart valves. Stroke 1998;29:1821–1826.

52 Deklunder G, Prat A, Lecroart JL, Roussel M, Dauzat M: Can cerebrovascular microemboli induce cognitive impairment in patients with prosthetic heart valves? Eur J Ultrasound 1998;7: 47–51.
53 Georgiadis D, Wenzel A, Lehmann D, Lindner A, Zierz S, Spencer MP: Influence of oxygen ventilation on Doppler microemboli signals in patients with artificial heart valves. Stroke 1997;28:2189–2194.
54 Baumgartner RW, Frick A, Hermann M, Ochslin P, Russi E, Turina J, Georgiadis D: Microembolic signals in patients with artificial heart valves during hyperbaric exposure. J Thorac Cardiovasc Surg 2001;122:1142–1146.
55 Graf T, Fischer H, Reul H, Rau G: Cavitation potential of mechanical heart valve prostheses. Int J Artif Organs 1991;14:169–174.
56 Sliwka U, Job FP, Wissuwa D, Diehl RR, Flachskampf FA, Hanrath P, Noth J: Occurrence of transcranial Doppler high-intensity transient signals in patients with potential cardiac sources of embolism. A prospective study. Stroke 1995;26:2067–2070.
57 Georgiadis D, Lindner A, Manz M, Sonntag M, Zunker P, Zerkowski HR, Borggrefe M: Intracranial microembolic signals in 500 patients with potential cardiac or carotid embolic source and in normal controls. Stroke 1997;28:1203–1207.
58 Cullinane M, Wainwright R, Brown A, Monaghan M, Markus HS: Asymptomatic embolization in subjects with atrial fibrillation not taking anticoagulants. A prospective study. Stroke 1998;29:1810–1815.
59 Nadareishvili ZG, Choudary Z, Joyner C, Brodie D, Norris JW: Cerebral microembolism in acute myocardial infarction. Stroke 1999;30:2679–2682.
60 Nabavi DG, Georgiadis D, Mumme T, Schmid C, Mackay TG, Scheld HH, Ringelstein EB: Clinical relevance of intracranial microembolic signals in patients with left ventricular assist devices. A prospective study. Stroke 1996;27:891–896.
61 Moazami N, Roberts K, Argenziano M, Catanese K, Mohr JP, Rose EA, Oz MC: Asymptomatic microembolism in patients with long-term ventricular assist support. ASAIO J 1997;43:177–180.
62 Jauss M, Kaps M, Keberle M, Haberbosch W, Dorndorf W: A comparison of transesophageal echocardiography and transcranial Doppler sonography with contrast medium for detection of patent foramen ovale. Stroke 1994;25:1265–1267.
63 Klotzsch C, Janssen G, Berlit P: Transesophageal echocardiography and contrast-TCD in the detection of a patent foramen ovale: Experiences with 111 patients. Neurology 1994;44:1603–1606.
64 Jauss M, Zanette E: Detection of right-to-left shunt with ultrasound contrast agent and transcranial Doppler sonography. Cerebrovasc Dis 2000;10:490–496.
65 Spencer MP, Thomas GI, Nicholls SC, Sauvage LR: Detection of middle cerebral artery emboli during carotid endarterectomy using transcranial Doppler ultrasonography. Stroke 1990;21:415–423.
66 Siebler M, Sitzer M, Steinmetz H: Detection of intracranial emboli in patients with symptomatic extracranial carotid artery disease. Stroke 1992;23:1652–1654.
67 Forteza AM, Babikian VL, Hyde C, Winter M, Pochay V: Effect of time and cerebrovascular symptoms of the prevalence of microembolic signals in patients with cervical carotid stenosis. Stroke 1996;27:687–690.
68 Siebler M, Sitzer M, Rose G, Bendfeldt D, Steinmetz H: Silent cerebral embolism caused by neurologically symptomatic high-grade carotid stenosis. Event rates before and after carotid endarterectomy. Brain 1994;116:1005–1015.
69 van Zuilen EV, Moll FL, Vermeulen FE, Mauser HW, Van Gijn J, Ackerstaff RG: Detection of cerebral microemboli by means of transcranial Doppler monitoring before and after carotid endarterectomy. Stroke 1995;26:210–213.
70 Valton L, Larrue V, Arrue P, Geraud G, Bes A: Asymptomatic cerebral embolic signals in patients with carotid stenosis. Correlation with appearance of plaque ulceration on angiography. Stroke 1995;26:813–815.
71 Molloy J, Markus HS: Asymptomatic embolization predicts stroke and TIA risk in patients with carotid artery stenosis. Stroke 1999;30:1440–1443.
72 Siebler M, Nachtmann A, Sitzer M, Rose G, Kleinschmidt A, Rademacher J, Steinmetz H: Cerebral microembolism and the risk of ischemia in asymptomatic high-grade internal carotid artery stenosis. Stroke 1995;26:2184–2186.

73 Abbott AL, Chambers BR, Stork JL, Levi CR, Bladin CF, Donnan GA: Embolic signals and prediction of ipsilateral stroke or transient ischemic attack in asymptomatic carotid stenosis: A multicenter prospective cohort study. Stroke 2005;36:1128–1133.
74 Nabavi DG, Georgiadis D, Mumme T, Zunker P, Ringelstein EB: Detection of microembolic signals in patients with middle cerebral artery stenosis by means of a bigate probe. A pilot study. Stroke 1996;27:1347–1349.
75 Sliwka U, Klotzsch C, Popescu O, Brandt K, Schmidt P, Berlit P, Noth J: Do chronic middle cerebral artery stenoses represent an embolic focus? A multirange transcranial Doppler study. Stroke 1997;28:1324–1327.
76 Srinivasan J, Newell DW, Sturzenegger M, Mayberg MR, Winn HR: Transcranial Doppler in the evaluation of internal carotid artery dissection. Stroke 1996;27:1226–1230.
77 Grosset DG, Georgiadis D, Abdulah I, Bone I, Lees KR: Doppler emboli signals vary according to stroke subtype. Stroke 1994;25:382–384.
78 Delcker A, Schnell A, Wilhelm H: Microembolic signals and clinical outcome in patients with acute stroke – A prospective study. Eur Arch Psychiatry Clin Neurosci 2000;250:1–5.
79 Lund C, Rygh J, Stensrod B, Sandset PM, Brucher R, Russell D: Cerebral microembolus detection in an unselected acute ischemic stroke population. Cerebrovasc Dis 2000;10:403–408.
80 Sitzer M, Sohngen D, Siebler M, Specker C, Rademacher J, Janda I, Aulich A, Steinmetz H: Cerebral microembolism in patients with Sneddon's syndrome. Arch Neurol 1995;52:271–275.
81 Specker C, Rademacher J, Sohngen D, Sitzer M, Janda I, Siebler M, Steinmetz H, Schneider M: Cerebral microemboli in patients with antiphospholipid syndrome. Lupus 1997;6:638–644.
82 Kumral E, Evyapan D, Oksel F, Keser G, Bereketoglu MA, Balkir K: Transcranial Doppler detection of microembolic signals in patients with Behcet's disease. J Neurol 1999;246:592–595.
83 Siebler M, Nachtmann A, Sitzer M, Steinmetz H: Anticoagulation monitoring and cerebral microemboli detection (letter). Lancet 1994;344:555.
84 Georgiadis D, Hill M, Zunker P, Stogbauer F, Ringelstein EB: Anticoagulation monitoring with transcranial Doppler (letter). Lancet 1994;344:1373–1374.
85 Goertler M, Baeumer M, Kross R, Blaser T, Lutze G, Jost S, Wallesch CW: Rapid decline of cerebral microemboli of arterial origin after intravenous acetylsalicylic acid. Stroke 1999;30:66–69.
86 Goertler M, Blaser T, Krueger S, Lutze G, Wallesch CW: Acetylsalicylic acid and microembolic events detected by transcranial doppler in symptomatic arterial stenoses. Cerebrovasc Dis 2001;11:324–329.
87 Kaposzta Z, Baskerville PA, Madge D, Fraser S, Martin JF, Markus HS: *L*-arginine and *S*-nitrosoglutathione reduce embolization in humans. Circulation 2001;103:2371–2375.
88 Junghans U, Sieber M: Cerebral microembolism is blocked by tirofiban, a selective nonpeptide platelet glycoprotein IIb/IIIa receptor antagonist. Circulation 2003;107:2717–2721.

Dr. Dimitrios Georgiadis
Department of Neurology, University Hospital
Frauenklinikstrasse 26
CH–8091 Zürich (Switzerland)
Tel. +41 1 255 55 65, Fax +41 1 255 88 64, E-Mail dimitrios.georgiadis@usz.ch

Baumgartner RW (ed): Handbook on Neurovascular Ultrasound.
Front Neurol Neurosci. Basel, Karger, 2006, vol 21, pp 206–215

Contrast-Enhanced Transcranial Doppler Ultrasound for Diagnosis of Patent Foramen Ovale

Krassen Nedeltchev[a], *Heinrich P. Mattle*[b]

[a]Institute of Diagnostic and Interventional Neuroradiology, and [b]Department of Neurology, University of Bern, Bern, Switzerland

Abstract

The suspected cause of clinical manifestations of patent foramen ovale (PFO) is a transient or a permanent right-to-left shunt (RLS). Contrast-enhanced transcranial Doppler ultrasound (c-TCD) is a reliable alternative to transesophageal echocardiography (TEE) for diagnosis of PFO, and enables also the detection of extracardiac RLS. The air-containing echo contrast agents are injected intravenously and do not pass the pulmonary circulation. In the presence of RLS, the contrast agents bypass the pulmonary circulation and cause microembolic signals (MES) in the basal cerebral arteries, which are detected by TCD. The two main echo contrast agents in use are agitated saline and *D*-galactose microparticle solutions. At least one middle cerebral artery (MCA) is insonated, and the ultrasound probe is fixed with a headframe. The monitored Doppler spectra are stored for offline analysis (e.g., videotape) of the time of occurrence and number of MES, which are used to assess the size and functional relevance of the RLS. The examination is more sensitive, if both MCAs are investigated. In the case of negative testing, the examination is repeated using the Valsalva maneuver. Compared to TEE, c-TCD is more comfortable for the patient, enables an easier assessment of the size and functional relevance of the RLS, and allows also the detection of extracardiac RLS. However, c-TCD cannot localize the site of the RLS. Therefore, TEE and TCD are complementary methods and should be applied jointly in order to increase the diagnostic accuracy for detecting PFO and other types of RLS.

In 1877, Cohnheim [1] described paradoxical embolism in association with patent foramen ovale (PFO). Since then, the clinical relevance of this cardiac anomaly has remained a matter of debate. Several case-control studies demonstrated a higher prevalence of PFO in patients with cryptogenic stroke than healthy subjects [2]. In addition, refractory hypoxemia following right-sided myocardial infarction or severe lung disease, the rare platypnea-orthodeoxia syndrome, and the neurological decompression illness in divers have also been attributed to patency of the foramen ovale [3–5]. Moreover, an association between migraine with aura and PFO has been reported [6].

A transient or a permanent right-to-left shunt (RLS) appears to be the common pathway of the manifold clinical manifestations of the PFO. The RLS permits thrombotic material originating from the deep leg or pelvic veins to bypass the pulmonary and reach the systemic circulation. Several cardiac (atrial and ventricular septum defects) and extracardiac (pulmonary arteriovenous malformations) conditions and abnormalities can also be associated with an RLS. Given its prevalence of at least 20% in the general population, the PFO is the most common type of RLS.

A PFO cannot be diagnosed on the basis of a clinical examination. Transesophageal echocardiography (TEE) enhanced by echo contrast agents is considered the 'gold standard' for the detection of cardiac RLS [7–11]. Cardiac RLS can also be identified by the use of contrast-enhanced transcranial Doppler ultrasound (c-TCD) [12–18]. Furthermore, c-TCD has proved its value for the diagnosis of an extracardiac RLS [12, 14, 19], and thus may be used to complement TEE.

Cardiac RLS have their origins in the embryonic development of the human heart. Therefore, basic anatomical and pathophysiological knowledge is a prerequisite to understand the examination technique using c-TCD.

Anatomical Basis

The development of the human heart begins in the third gestational week. In the fifth week, a functional cardiovascular system already exists. As a consequence of several external and internal transformations during the fifth and sixth week, the primary heart tube forms different cavities. Atrial septation starts with the development of a thin membrane, the septum primum, which grows from the posterosuperior wall towards the atrioventricular canal (fig. 1). Two orifices, the ostium primum and, after its obliteration, the ostium secundum, maintain a communication between the two atria. A second membrane, the septum secundum, then emerges on the right side of the septum primum. The septum secundum will cover the septum primum completely, except at the area close to the inferior vena cava (foramen ovale). Both the foramen ovale and the ostium secundum continue to allow blood passage from the right into the left atrium, since the two membranes do not fuse.

After birth, the left atrial blood pressure increases and pushes the thin left-sided septum primum against the thicker right-sided septum secundum.

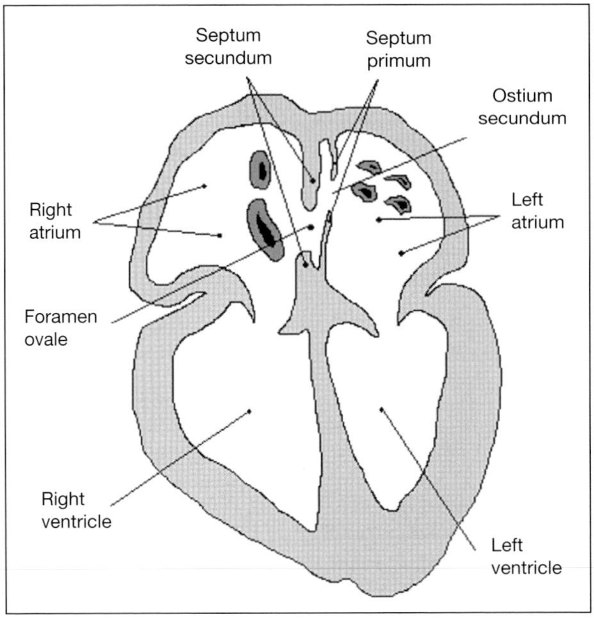

Fig. 1. The adult heart with a patent foramen ovale in cross-sectional plane. The structures involved in the right-to-left shunt are shown: septum primum and septum secundum, foramen ovale, and ostium secundum.

Thereby, the foramen ovale is functionally closed. Morphological closure follows later in infancy in the majority of people.

Pathophysiology

Elevation of the right atrial pressure in the abatement phase of a Valsalva maneuver (VM; i.e., coughing, defecation) can cause a transient RLS in patients with PFO. With severe lung disease or after a right ventricular infarction permanent right-to-left pressure gradients can occur. In such a situation there is hypoxemia that does not respond to oxygen therapy. With normal intracardiac pressure, the valve-like nature of the PFO permits short-lasting RLS during a single heart cycle, even without any provocation [20].

Local gas nucleation predominantly in adipose tissues and arterial gas embolism are considered to cause decompression illness and cerebral ischemic lesions in scuba divers. It is likely that paradoxical embolism of venous gas bubbles occurs in divers with PFO and increases the risk of decompression illness.

Paradoxical embolism and altered oxygen saturation might be the pathomechanisms in migraine attacks preceded by an aura [6, 21]. The exact pathogenic role of the RLS in the platypnea-orthodeoxia syndrome is not yet completely understood.

Examination Technique

The diagnosis of RLS using c-TCD is established using intravenously injected, air-containing echo contrast agents. Normally, the aforementioned contrast agents are unable to pass the pulmonary capillary bed. In the presence of an RLS, the contrast agent enters the systemic arterial circulation and produces microembolic signals (MES), which are detected by c-TCD.

An international Consensus Meeting established the performance criteria of c-TCD for the diagnosis of RLS [16]. The patients must be in supine position with the arm horizontal. An intravenous Daflon catheter (#18) is inserted into the antecubital vein and is connected to a 250-ml bottle with physiological solution by means of a flexible tube to maintain venous access. Insonation of at least one middle cerebral artery (MCA) using TCD is performed. The examination is more sensitive if bilateral TCD recording is used. The contrast agent is rapidly injected as a bolus with the patient at rest.

In the event of little or no detection of MES in the insonated MCA, the examination is repeated using the VM. The contrast agent is injected 5 s prior to the start of the VM; the overall duration of the VM is 10 s. The patients should start the VM on examiner's command. The strength of the VM can be controlled by peak velocity of the Doppler curve. The time when the first MES appears within the MCA will be noted. The relevance of cardiac RLS is related to size and functional factors that require quantification of RLS during the examination [22–25].

At present, there are two main contrast agents in use: agitated saline containing air bubbles and a *D*-galactose microparticle agent (Echovist®, Schering AG, Berlin, Germany) that, on dissolution and agitation in sterile water, generates air-filled microbubbles (MBs). The MBs are filtered in the pulmonary capillary circulation [26]. Both saline/air mixture and Echovist® are reliable with respect to sensitivity and specificity when used with VM (table 1). Sensitivity and specificity reached 100% by using both Echovist® and saline/air mixture. Direct comparisons between both contrast agents revealed no significant differences concerning sensitivity [17, 27]. However, both studies detected more MBs using Echovist® even when applied in a smaller dose (5 ml) than saline (10 ml). Echovist® contains more MB than saline/air mixture, a fact that should be taken into consideration when quantifying an RLS.

Table 1. Sensitivity and specificity of contrast-enhanced transcranial Doppler ultrasound for detection of a patent foramen ovale using different echo contrast agents and dosages using transesophageal echocardiography as standard of reference

Source	Dosage per injection	Echovist®		Saline/air mixture	
		Sensitivity %	Specificity %	Sensitivity %	Specificity %
Chimowitz et al. [43]				100	100
Nemec et al. [44]	6 ml saline, 0.2 ml air			100	
Di Tullio et al. [40]	10 ml saline, 0.5 ml air			68	100
Anzola et al. [30]	20 ml saline agitated			90	100
Zanette et al. [13][1]	10 ml saline/air			79	
Devyust et al. [14]	9 ml saline, 0.2 ml air			100	100
Jauss et al. [33]	5 ml Echovist®	93	100		
Klötzsch et al. [12]	5 ml Echovist®	91	94		
Schminke et al. [45]	5 ml Echovist®	91	81		
Horner et al. [34]	10 ml Echovist®	97	70		
Hamann et al. [38]	2.5 ml Echovist®	75	100		
Schwarze et al. [36]	5–10 ml Echovist®	100	97		
Droste et al. [27, 46]	10 ml Echovist®	up to 100	up to 85		
Blersch et al. [47]	10 ml Echovist	91	88		
Droste et al. [17]	5 ml Echovist®/ 9 ml saline, 1 ml air	95	75	95	75

[1]Injection of contrast agent before Valsalva maneuver was considered.

Extensive safety testing of Echovist® revealed no safety concerns at the recommended dose [28]. There are no reports on adverse effects after saline/air mixture administration. The Consensus Meeting recommend to use the saline/air mixture, since it is not subject to local approval rules and it has proved as effective in numerous studies [16].

The amount of saline/air mixture should be 10 ml (1 ml air and 9 ml saline) [16]. To minimize bacterial contamination, a bacterial filter should be used for air aspiration. A three-way stopcock will be connected to a 10-ml syringe I (containing 9 ml of 0.9% saline), a 10-ml syringe II (containing 1 ml air aspired through a bacterial filter), and the antecubital vein of the patient (using a short flexible tube of <10 cm length to minimize discomfort during the manipulation). An 18-gauge intravenous catheter should be preferred over a 20-gauge catheter to increase the sensitivity [29]. One milliliter of air (syringe I) and 9 ml of saline (syringe II) should be rapidly exchanged between the syringes at least ten times. Afterwards, the air/saline mixture should be injected into the patient as a bolus.

Time windows proposed between the intravenous injection of the contrast agent and its appearance in the insonated MCA are 6 heart beats [12], 10 [30], 15 [31], 20 [32], 22 [13], and 25 s [17, 33]. The time needed for the contrast agent to pass from the antecubital vein to the MCA is about 11 s for a passage through an intracardial shunt and about 14 s for a passage through a pulmonary shunt [34]. An overlap interval for cardiac and pulmonary shunts seems to exist and makes the distinction between the two conditions unreliable [35]. The strength and duration of the VM introduce additional variance into the passage times. Droste et al. [27] compared different cut-off limits with respect to concordant and discordant TEE findings and demonstrated that a rigid diagnostic time window does not exist. It is, therefore, of no value to consider any cut-off limit in the assessment of the MB test results. Instead, a quantitative assessment of the RLS size seems to be of clinical relevance [16].

Assessment of the RLS size can be achieved using c-TCD in a semi-quantitative manner by counting the number of MES in the MCA after injection of the contrast agent. A four-level categorization is accepted according to the number of MES in the TCD spectrum using uni- or bilateral (values in parentheses) MCA monitoring: (1) no occurrence of MES, (2) 1–10 (1–20) MES, (3) >10 (>20) MES, but no curtain, and (4) curtain, where a single MES cannot be discriminated within the TCD spectra [16]. In order to obtain comparable results, a strict standardization of the examination technique is required. The dosage of the contrast agent and the position of the patient can affect the number of MES [36, 37]. The MES count must be documented and evaluated separately for the baseline conditions and the VM. The Doppler spectra must be stored for offline analysis.

There is a general agreement that VM is necessary to increase the sensitivity of the detection of RLS using c-TCD [16]. The time of injection of the contrast agent in relation to the VM varies in the different studies. Injection before the VM [31, 33, 38], during the VM [34, 39, 40], or in the abatement phase of the VM [30] has been applied. Zanette et al. [13] compared the efficacy of the different procedures, and found that the highest number of patients with RLS, confirmed by TEE, was detected when the saline/air mixture was injected before the VM. Studies using Echovist® reported comparable results [18, 37]. It has been recommended to start the VM 5 s after the injection of the contrast agent and to maintain it for at least 5 s [16].

The strength of the VM is also a factor that should be controlled for. The use of a sphygmomanometer has the advantage of a quantitative assessment of the VM strength and allows a visible feedback for the patient [23]. Unfortunately, the sphygmomanometer cannot distinguish between intrathoracic pressure and a high pressure due to palatal closure and may erroneously indicate a sufficient VM. The

Table 2. Sensitivity and specificity of contrast-enhanced transcranial Doppler ultrasound using different Valsalva maneuvers (VMs) for detection of a patent foramen ovale using transesophageal echocardiography (TEE) as standard of reference

Source	Mode of injection	Sensitivity, %		Specificity, %	
		VM	No VM	VM	No VM
Teague and Sharma [39][1]	during VM	100	100	76	79
Jauss et al. [33]	before VM	93	47	100	100
Zanette et al. [13][2]	before, during, and after VM	79	53		
Hamann et al. [38][3]	before VM	75	40	100	100
Droste et al. [27][4]	before VM	90	55	85	88
Uzuner et al. [48][5]	during VM	100	58		

[1]Gold standard was transthoracic echocardiography instead of TEE.
[2]Only patients with positive TEE were included in the study.
[3]Injection of contrast agent at the antecubital site was considered.
[4]Using 22 s as a time window.
[5]Injection of galactose-based contrast agent was considered.

decrease of the envelope curve of the TCD spectrum reflects the hemodynamic effects of the VM [12]. The combination of pressure measurements using a sphygmomanometer and monitoring the TCD envelope allows an optimal control of the VM. The VM should be trained with the patient before the examination.

Numerous studies emphasized the role of the VM to increase the sensitivity of c-TCD for the detection of RLS (table 2). The VM should not be performed, if the test has revealed a 'curtain pattern' at basal conditions. Otherwise, the possibility of air embolism during VM exists in principle.

To improve the sensitivity of the c-TCD, it is recommended to change the position of the patient in the case of a first negative test. Telman et al. [15] used c-TCD to examine 34 patients with TEE-proved PFO. Examinations were done in both the sitting and supine positions in random order. Patients' positions and the sequence of testing did not affect the number of MES detected. However, for each individual, one of the two positions was more sensitive.

Recent studies revealed a significant association between the distribution of MES during c-TCD testing and the clinical cerebrovascular syndromes in stroke patients with PFO [41, 42]. The authors suggest that the distribution of MES is similar to the clinical situation when real emboli reach the cerebral vasculature, and has a possible predictive value for future strokes. On the other hand, c-TCD recordings from the territory of the cerebrovascular symptoms in symptomatic patients may increase the sensitivity of the examination.

Bilateral recordings of the MCA or repetition of the TCD examination also increase the sensitivity compared with unilateral recordings or single examinations [13, 17, 34].

There is evidence suggesting an increased sensitivity to detect a PFO, if the contrast agent is injected into the femoral vein [38]. The difference between femoral and antecubital injections may be caused by different inflow patterns to the right atrium: inferior vena cava flow is directed to the right atrial septum, whereas superior vena cava flow is directed to the tricuspid valve.

References

1 Cohnheim J: Thrombose und Embolie; in Cohnheim J. (ed.): Vorlesung über Allgemeine Pathologie. Berlin, Hirschwald, 1877, pp 134.

2 Overell JR, Bone I, Lees KR: Interatrial septal abnormalities and stroke: A meta-analysis of case-control studies. Neurology 2000;55:1172–1179.

3 Wilmshurst PT, Byrne JC, Webb-Peploe MM: Relation between interatrial shunts and decompression sickness in divers. Lancet 1989;2:1302–1306.

4 Seward JB, Hayes DL, Smith HC, Williams DE, Rosenow EC, Reeder GS, Piehler JM, Tajik AJ: Platypnea-orthodeoxia: Clinical profile, diagnostic workup, management, and report of seven cases. Mayo Clin Proc 1984;59:221–231.

5 Silver MT, Lieberman EH, Thibault GE: Refractory hypoxemia in inferior myocardial infarction from right-to-left shunting through a patent foramen ovale: A case report and review of the literature. Clin Cardiol 1994;17:627–630.

6 Del Sette M, Angeli S, Leandri M, Ferriero G, Bruzzone GL, Finocchi C, Gandolfo C: Migraine with aura and right-to-left shunt on transcranial Doppler: A case-control study. Cerebrovasc Dis 1998;8:327–330.

7 Belkin RN, Pollack BD, Ruggiero ML, Alas LL, Tatini U: Comparison of transesophageal and transthoracic echocardiography with contrast and color flow Doppler in the detection of patent foramen ovale. Am Heart J 1994;128:520–525.

8 Chen WJ, Kuan P, Lien WP, Lin FY: Detection of patent foramen ovale by contrast transesophageal echocardiography. Chest 1992;101:1515–1520.

9 Pearson AC, Labovitz AJ, Tatineni S, Gomez CR: Superiority of transesophageal echocardiography in detecting cardiac source of embolism in patients with cerebral ischemia of uncertain etiology. J Am Coll Cardiol 1991;17:66–72.

10 Hausmann D, Mugge A, Becht I, Daniel WG: Diagnosis of patent foramen ovale by transesophageal echocardiography and association with cerebral and peripheral embolic events. Am J Cardiol 1992;70:668–672.

11 Sun JP, Stewart WJ, Hanna J, Thomas JD: Diagnosis of patent foramen ovale by contrast versus color Doppler by transesophageal echocardiography: Relation to atrial size. Am Heart J 1996;131: 239–244.

12 Klotzsch C, Janssen G, Berlit P: Transesophageal echocardiography and contrast-TCD in the detection of a patent foramen ovale: Experience with 111 patients. Neurology 1994;44: 1603–1606.

13 Zanette EM, Mancini G, De Castro S, Solaro M, Cartoni D, Chiarotti F: Patent foramen ovale and transcranial Doppler. Comparison of different procedures. Stroke 1996;27:2251–2255.

14 Devuyst G, Despland PA, Bogousslavsky J, Jeanrenaud X: Complementarity of contrast transcranial Doppler and contrast transesophageal echocardiography for the detection of patent foramen ovale in stroke patients. Eur Neurol 1997;38:21–25.

15 Telman G, Kouperberg E, Sprecher E, Yarnitsky D: The positions of the patients in the diagnosis of patent foramen ovale by transcranial Doppler. J Neuroimaging 2003;13:356–358.
16 Jauss M, Zanette EM: Detection of right-to-left shunt with ultrasound contrast agent and transcranial Doppler sonography. Cerebrovasc Dis 2000;10:490–496.
17 Droste DW, Reisener M, Kemeny V, Dittrich R, Schulte-Altedorneburg G, Stypmann J, Wichter T, Ringelstein EB: Contrast transcranial Doppler ultrasound in the detection of right-to-left shunts: Reproducibility, comparison of 2 agents, and distribution of microemboli. Stroke 1999;30: 1014–1018.
18 Droste DW, Lakemeier S, Wichter T, Stypmann J, Dittrich R, Ritter M, Moeller M, Freund M, Ringelstein EB: Optimizing the technique of contrast transcranial Doppler ultrasound in the detection of right-to-left shunts. Stroke 2002;33:2211–2216.
19 Heckmann JG, Niedermeier W, Brandt-Pohlmann M, Hilz MJ, Hecht M, Neundorfer B: Detection of patent foramen ovale. Transesophageal echocardiography and transcranial Doppler sonography with ultrasound contrast media are 'supplementary, not competing, diagnostic methods'. Med Klin (Munich) 1999;94:367–370.
20 Strunk BL, Cheitlin MD, Stulbarg MS, Schiller NB: Right-to-left interatrial shunting through a patent foramen ovale despite normal intracardiac pressures. Am J Cardiol 1987;60:413–415.
21 Anzola GP, Magoni M, Guindani M, Rozzini L, Dalla Volta G: Potential source of cerebral embolism in migraine with aura: A transcranial Doppler study. Neurology 1999;52:1622–1625.
22 Steiner MM, Di Tullio MR, Rundek T, Gan R, Chen X, Liguori C, Brainin M, Homma S, Sacco RL. Patent foramen ovale size and embolic brain imaging findings among patients with ischemic stroke. Stroke 1998;29:944–948.
23 Serena J, Segura T, Perez-Ayuso MJ, Bassaganyas J, Molins A, Davalos A: The need to quantify right-to-left shunt in acute ischemic stroke: A case-control study. Stroke 1998;29:1322–1328.
24 Schuchlenz HW, Weihs W, Horner S, Quehenberger F: The association between the diameter of a patent foramen ovale and the risk of embolic cerebrovascular events. Am J Med 2000;109:456–462.
25 De Castro S, Cartoni D, Fiorelli M, Rasura M, Anzini A, Zanette EM, Beccia M, Colonnese C, Fedele F, Fieschi C, Pandian NG: Morphological and functional characteristics of patent foramen ovale and their embolic implications. Stroke 2000;31:2407–2413.
26 Butler BD, Hills BA: The lung as a filter for microbubbles. J Appl Physiol 1979;47:537–543.
27 Droste DW, Kriete JU, Stypmann J, Castrucci M, Wichter T, Tietje R, Weltermann B, Young P, Ringelstein EB: Contrast transcranial Doppler ultrasound in the detection of right-to-left shunts: Comparison of different procedures and different contrast agents. Stroke 1999;30:1827–1832.
28 Schlief R, Schurman R, Niendorf HP: Basic properties and results of clinical trials of ultrasound contrast agents based on galactose. Ann Acad Med Singapore 1993;22:762–767.
29 Khan KA, Yeung M, Shuaib A: Comparative study of 18 gauge and 20 gauge intravenous catheters during transcranial Doppler ultrasonography with saline solution contrast. J Ultrasound Med 1997;16:341–344.
30 Anzola GP, Renaldini E, Magoni M, Costa A, Cobelli M, Guindani M: Validation of transcranial Doppler sonography in the assessment of patent foramen ovale. Cerebrovasc Dis 1995;5: 194–198.
31 Job FP, Ringelstein EB, Grafen Y, Flachskampf FA, Doherty C, Stockmanns A, Hanrath P: Comparison of transcranial contrast Doppler sonography and transesophageal contrast echocardiography for the detection of patent foramen ovale in young stroke patients. Am J Cardiol 1994;74:381–384.
32 Yeung M, Khan KA, Shuaib A: Transcranial Doppler ultrasonography in the detection of venous to arterial shunting in acute stroke and transient ischaemic attacks. J Neurol Neurosurg Psychiatry 1996;61:445–449.
33 Jauss M, Kaps M, Keberle M, Haberbosch W, Dorndorf W: A comparison of transesophageal echocardiography and transcranial Doppler sonography with contrast medium for detection of patent foramen ovale. Stroke 1994;25:1265–1267.
34 Horner S, Ni XS, Weihs W, Harb S, Augustin M, Duft M, Niederkorn K: Simultaneous bilateral contrast transcranial Doppler monitoring in patients with intracardiac and intrapulmonary shunts. J Neurol Sci 1997;150:49–57.

35 Horner S, Schuchlenz S, Harb S, Weihs W, Ni XS, Fazekas F, Duft M, Kleinert G, Niederkorn K: Contrast transcranial Doppler monitoring in stroke patients with pulmonary right-to-left shunts (abstract). Cerebrovasc Dis 1998;8(suppl 3):7.
36 Schwarze JJ, Sander D, Kukla C, Wittich I, Babikian VL, Klingelhofer J: Methodological parameters influence the detection of right-to-left shunts by contrast transcranial Doppler ultrasonography. Stroke 1999;30:1234–1239.
37 Schwarze JJ, Klingelhofer J, Sander D, Kukla C, Wittich I: Factors influencing the sensitivity of contrast-TCD method in the detection of right-to-left shunts; in Klingelhofer J, Bartels E, Ringelstein EB (eds): New Trends in Cerebral Hemodynamics and Neurosonology. Amsterdam, Elsevier, 1997, pp 475–482.
38 Hamann GF, Schatzer-Klotz D, Frohlig G, Strittmatter M, Jost V, Berg G, Stopp M, Schimrigk K, Schieffer H: Femoral injection of echo contrast medium may increase the sensitivity of testing for a patent foramen ovale. Neurology 1998;50:1423–1428.
39 Teague SM, Sharma MK: Detection of paradoxical cerebral echo contrast embolization by transcranial Doppler ultrasound. Stroke 1991;22:740–745.
40 Di Tullio M, Sacco RL, Venketasubramanian N, Sherman D, Mohr JP, Homma S: Comparison of diagnostic techniques for the detection of a patent foramen ovale in stroke patients. Stroke 1993;24:1020–1024.
41 Klingelhofer J, Schwarze JJ, Sander D, Kukla C, Wittich I: Distribution of ultrasonic medium predicts the territory of cerebral infarction; in Klingelhöfer J, Bartels E, Ringelstein EB (eds): New Trends in Cerebral Hemodynamics and Neurosonology. Amsterdam, Elsevier 1997, pp 494–499.
42 Telman G, Kouperberg E, Sprecher E, Goldsher D, Yarnitsky D: Distribution of artificial cerebral microemboli in stroke patients with patent foramen ovale. Neurol Res 2005;27:109–111.
43 Chimowitz MI, Nemec JJ, Marwick TH, Lorig RJ, Furlan AJ, Salcedo EE: Transcranial Doppler ultrasound identifies patients with right-to-left cardiac or pulmonary shunts. Neurology 1991;41:1902–1904.
44 Nemec JJ, Marwick TH, Lorig RJ, Davison MB, Chimowitz MI, Litowitz H, Salcedo EE: Comparison of transcranial Doppler ultrasound and transesophageal contrast echocardiography in the detection of interatrial right-to-left shunts. Am J Cardiol 1991;68:1498–1502.
45 Schminke U, Ries S, Daffertshofer M, Staedt U, Hennerici M: Patent foramen ovale: A potential source of cerebral embolism. Cerebrovasc Dis 1995;5:133–138.
46 Droste DW, Silling K, Stypmann J, Grude M, Kemeny V, Wichter T, Kuhne K, Ringelstein EB: Contrast transcranial Doppler ultrasound in the detection of right-to-left shunts: Time window and threshold in microbubble numbers. Stroke 2000;31:1640–1645.
47 Blersch WK, Draganski BM, Holmer SR, Koch HJ, Schlachetzki F, Bogdahn U, Holscher T: Transcranial duplex sonography in the detection of patent foramen ovale. Radiology 2002;225: 693–699.
48 Uzuner N, Horner S, Pichler G, Svetina D, Niederkorn K: Right-to-left shunt assessed by contrast transcranial Doppler sonography: New insights. J Ultrasound Med 2004;23:1475–1482.

Dr. Krassen Nedeltchev
Inselspital
Freiburgstrasse 4
CH–3010 Bern (Switzerland)
Tel. +41 31 63 29522, Fax +41 31 63 24872, E-Mail krassen.nedeltchev@insel.ch

Baumgartner RW (ed): Handbook on Neurovascular Ultrasound.
Front Neurol Neurosci. Basel, Karger, 2006, vol 21, pp 216–228

Cerebral Autoregulation and Vasomotor Reactivity

Rune Aaslid

Hemodynamics AG, Bern, Switzerland

Abstract

Various aspects of the cerebral blood-flow regulation can be assessed by transcranial Doppler (TCD). This chapter describes and discusses the approaches that have been reported in the literature. The steady-state characteristics of the cerebral autoregulation can be determined by changing the blood pressure level, and calculating the response of the vasomotors. Moreover, the lower limit of the autoregulatory 'plateau' can be investigated after lowering the blood pressure by pharmacological means. The excellent time-resolution of the TCD technique also facilitates the determination of the quasi-stationary and dynamic aspects of the autoregulatory response. The leg-cuff method shows that regulatory action is very fast, compensating for a sharp drop in blood pressure within seconds. Less intrusively, the autoregulatory characteristics can be assessed from recordings of spontaneous variations in blood pressure. Transfer function methods describe the faster aspects of the mechanism, while correlation techniques reveal the quasi-stationary characteristics. However, the repeatability and accuracy of methods based on spontaneous fluctuations are probably less than those of stimulus–response tests. In this chapter, the various CO_2 and acetazolamide approaches that determine vasomotor reactivity are described and discussed.

Cerebral Blood-Flow Control

The cerebral circulation delivers oxygen and nutrients to the brain tissue for its metabolic activity. The blood-flow transport system also removes the waste products – the most important being carbon dioxide. The cerebral blood-flow (CBF) is regulated by a complex system influenced by multiple factors, such as cerebral perfusion pressure (CPP), brain metabolic activity, autonomic innervation, vasodilators (CO_2, nitric oxide), and drugs (acetazolamide, papaverine). The classic concept [1] of what is called 'cerebral autoregulation' is graphically illustrated in figure 1. The CBF is kept relatively constant within

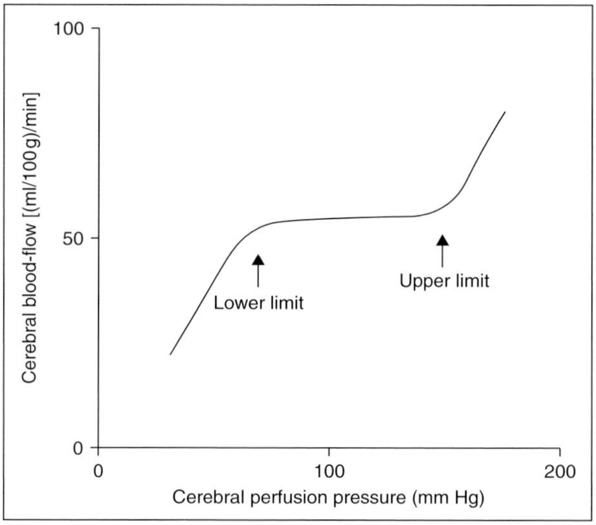

Fig. 1. The relationship between cerebral perfusion pressure (CPP) and cerebral blood flow (CBF) when regulated by an intact cerebral autoregulation mechanism.

a wide range of the CPP (the driving force). Above the upper and below the lower limits of autoregulation, the regulation mechanism is exhausted and hyper-respective hypoperfusion is possible.

Theoretically, considering the law of Poiseuille, regulatory action is most effective in the vessels with the smallest calibers – the precapillary sphincters and the smallest arterioles. The conductance arteries from the Circle of Willis to the larger arterioles play a minor role in CBF regulation. From a macro-perspective, the pressure–flow relationship is controlled by both the slope and the pressure axis intercept (critical closing pressure) [2].

Three different mechanisms can be hypothesized to contribute to cerebral autoregulation as illustrated in figure 2:

(1) *Metabolic regulation*. This hypothesis assumes that the balance between cerebral metabolism (demand) and oxygen delivery via the CBF (supply) is the input to a controlling mechanism that acts via a vasoactive substance. In principle, this is a negative feedback control system that seeks to balance CBF to demand.

(2) *Myogenic regulation*. The effect of transmural blood pressure changes are directly detected by the vascular smooth muscle (probably via a stress sensing mechanism) and the calibers are adjusted accordingly to keep blood-flow constant.

(3) *Neurogenic regulation*. The vascular smooth muscle actuators in the resistance vessels are controlled via sympathetic innervation, receiving the

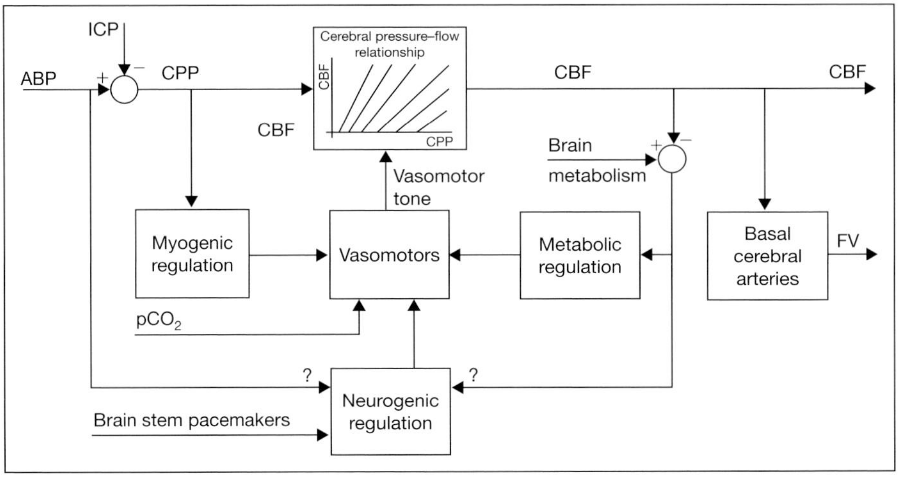

Fig. 2. Illustration of different hypothesis of cerebral autoregulation. ABP = Arterial blood pressure; CBF = cerebral blood flow; CPP = cerebral perfusion pressure; FV = flow velocity measured by TCD; ICP = intracranial pressure.

inputs from the appropriate brainstem autonomous control center. Nitric oxide (NO) released by parasympathetic fibers may also play a role.

The cerebral vasculature is profoundly affected by the partial pressure of CO_2 (pCO_2) in arterial blood. The precise definition of where the interaction between pCO_2 and vasodilation/constriction takes place in this physiological model is simplified in figure 2 as a direct effect on the vascular smooth muscle actuators. But, it is entirely possible that the vasoactive effect of CO_2 is mediated/augmented through NO or even other vasoactive substances.

Since more than 20 years, transcranial Doppler (TCD) has been used extensively to study CBF regulation [3–22] and vasomotor reactivity [23–27] in normal subjects as well as in patients with various forms of cerebrovascular disease. Since TCD measures flow velocity (FV) and not CBF per se, only assessment of changes in flow rather than absolute values can be made [3]. Since determinations of vasomotor reactivity or autoregulatory effectiveness are based on stimulus–response principles; absolute values are not as important as reliable and repeatable recordings with short (beat-to-beat) time resolution. For this purpose TCD is a well-suited technique both in the investigational and the clinical setting.

Steady-State (Static) Cerebral Autoregulation

The steady-state or static pressure-flow relationship of the cerebral vascular bed shown in figure 1 is quite remarkable. Indices of static autoregulation

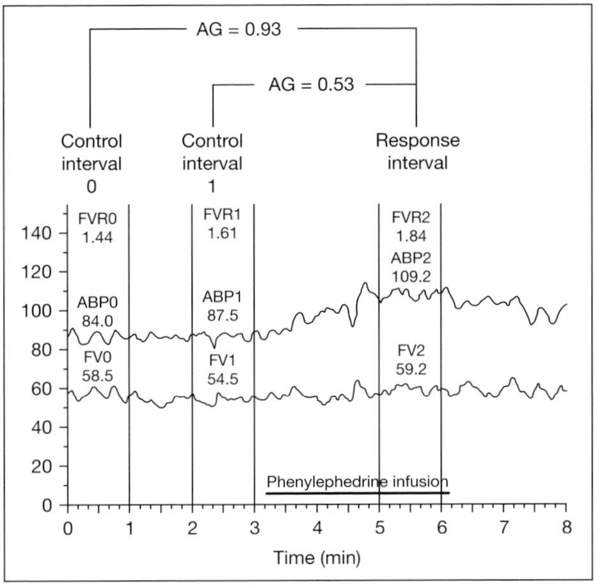

Fig. 3. Steady-state cerebral autoregulation test using infusion of phenylephedrine to raise blood pressure (ABP). Note the different autoregulatory gain (AG) results due to changes in flow velocity (FV) between the two control intervals. The flow velocity resistance (FVR) is calculated by FVR = ABP/FV.

are related to the 'flatness' of the plateau between the lower and upper limits [4–6].

The stimulus-response method consists of inducing a change in mean arterial blood pressure (ABP), typically by drug administration, and calculating the corresponding change in flow velocity resistance (FVR). The FVR (FVR = ABP/FV) is assumed to be proportional to volume flow resistance, the premise being that the changes in vessel lumen area are small [3]. This approach is illustrated in figure 3, where the patient's blood pressure was increased from its control value ABP1 to ABP2 after the infusion of phenylephedrine. A commonly used index is the autoregulatory gain (AG) (also called the static autoregulation index–sARI [4]), based on the normalized change in FVR divided by the normalized change in blood pressure:

$$AG = ((FVR2-FVR1)/FV1)/((ABP2-ABP1)/ABP1)$$

An AG of 0 means no autoregulation (flow and pressure are proportionally related, therefore FVR does not change). An AG of 1 means perfect autoregulation where FV remains constant and changes in FVR and ABP are equal.

A problem with this method is that some variations in blood-flow are not related to ABP. Significant changes in FV may also be related to variations in arterial pCO_2, brain metabolism, functional activation, and intrinsic pacemakers (B-waves). The possible influence of such uncontrolled factors on the accuracy of the AG determination is illustrated in figure 3. Using control interval 0 will result in a quite different value of AG than using control interval 1. In the ideal setting, this variability could be reduced by repeating the test many times and averaging the results. However, the clinical setting being limiting on such repetitive interventions, the results of a single steady-state autoregulation test must be interpreted with caution because of uncertainty of the influence of spontaneous non-ABP related variability.

It should also be mentioned that TCD is well suited to determine the lower limit of cerebral autoregulation [7].

Quasi-Steady-State Cerebral Autoregulation

The spontaneous fluctuations approach is based on calculating the Pearson correlation coefficient (Mx) between paired observations of mean ABP (or CPP if the intracranial pressure – ICP is recorded) and mean FV [8–10]. A sampling interval of 3 s is typically used to calculate the paired mean values. Clearly, for this approach to be valid, the ABP has to change spontaneously by some nontrivial amount during the observation period. If this is the case, a lower Mx is interpreted to signify better autoregulation. Higher values of Mx mean that changes in FV are correlated to changes in ABP and therefore indicate poor autoregulation. The correlation coefficient approach has also been applied to recordings of systolic (Sx) and diastolic (Dx) values but it is questionable if these add any value over the Mx.

The same caution with regard to the influence of blood-flow variability as discussed under the stimulus–response method also applies to the Mx method. The influence of such random noise might be even more pronounced because the ABP changes are typically less. However, this method has the advantage of being nonintrusive, and can be applied over long-time series. Therefore multiple readings can be averaged and some discarded if the ABP does not exhibit enough variability to obtain meaningful correlations.

The Mx method is essentially an intermediate approach between the steady-state stimulus–response evaluation and the true dynamic methods described in the next section. On one hand, it is related to the steady-state regulation, because it neglects frequency components higher than 0.1 Hz (due to sampling rate of 0.2 Hz), and because it does not take into account the phase relationship in the autoregulatory response. On the other hand, it does account for slow dynamic components of the cerebral autoregulation.

Dynamic Cerebral Autoregulation

Using TCD, with its excellent time resolution compared to techniques used to estimate CBF, the dynamic aspects of cerebral autoregulation can be explored; and such methods have been added to the clinical neurovascular armamentarium [9–21]. As with steady-state autoregulation, both stimulus–response and spontaneous fluctuations method have been reported.

The leg-cuff method was introduced in 1989 [11], with the purpose of producing a rapid step-like decrease in ABP to challenge the autoregulatory mechanism. This approach has been shown in numerous studies to give reproducible estimates of dynamic autoregulation in patients as well as in normal subjects [11–18]. It also correlates well with steady-state autoregulatory indices [4, 5].

A few simple precautions will optimize the application of this test in the clinical routine and the ICU: (1) The leg cuffs should be wider than the standard leg cuff used for BP measurements as shown in figure 4a. Cuffs as normally supplied for leg use are far too narrow and are indeed painful for the subject. Wider cuffs can be obtained from the suppliers of plethysmographic equipment, figure 4b and cause only mild pressure discomfort. (2) The cuff must be rapidly deflated (within a fraction of a second). Only leg cuffs with wide bore tubes can be deflated so as to give an adequate step-like stimulus in the ABP. A commercial cuff inflator/deflator (Model E20 with large leg cuff CC22 from Hokanson, Bellevue) is useful for this type of testing. (3) The leg cuff inflation period should be about 2 min to produce a step of sufficient duration and magnitude. (4) At least two tests should be made to avoid inaccuracies due to random fluctuations in FV.

An example of the dynamic autoregulation test is shown in figure 5.

The upper trace represents the ABP. At the vertical gray line there is a precipitous drop in ABP when the leg cuffs deflate (marked by the lower trace). This is followed by approximately 8 s of constant low ABP, and a slow recovery towards control over the next 15 s. The middle trace shows the FV. It recovers much faster. Clearly, dynamic autoregulation is present in this normal subject, and it is quite fast in its actions.

How can we quantify dynamic autoregulation? Early attempts used a rate of regulation (RoR) index [11]. It is also possible to use half-recovery times [12]. An even more promising approach is the use of mathematical models and parameter estimation [4, 5, 13–18]. This procedure may sound complicated, but the technique is in fact quite similar to statistical regression analysis, which also fits a model to the data. The difference is that differential equations are used in parameter estimation instead of the static equations of regression analysis. The principle of minimizing an error (least mean square) to fit the data is similar for

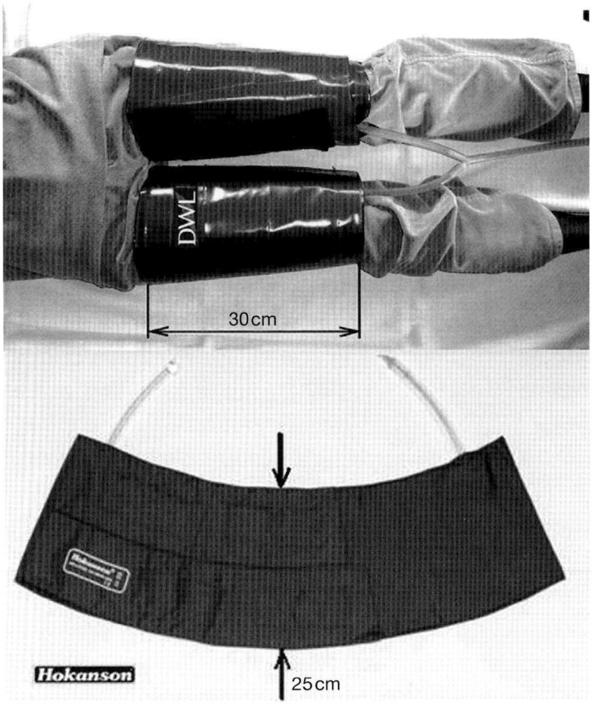

a

b

Fig. 4. Placement of leg cuffs for dynamic autoregulation test (***a***). Note large cuffs with generous tube caliber for fast deflation. Contoured leg cuffs suitable for use in the leg-cuff test (***b***).

the two. The second order differential equation system used in the autoregulation model is described in detail in [4].

Figure 5a shows an example of using the second order model to quantify the dynamic response. Both ABP and FV signals were low-pass filtered at 0.5 Hz to remove most of the pulsatility from the tracings. This process does not distort the phase or amplitude relationship between the measurements. The upper ABP tracing is used as an input to the differential equation model. The fit between the measured FV (solid line) and the velocity predicted by the model (shown as the dotted tracing) is good. The actual parameters of the model equations as determined by least mean square error parameter estimation are listed in figure 3. The autoregulation was intact with the gain better than 0.8 (gain of 1.0 is the perfect autoregulation) and a time constant of 3 s.

The leg-cuff technique causes a drop in ABP of about 20 mm Hg. However, since the hypotensive episode is of short lasting, ischemia is not a serious concern. The clear contraindication to this method is leg vascular disease or

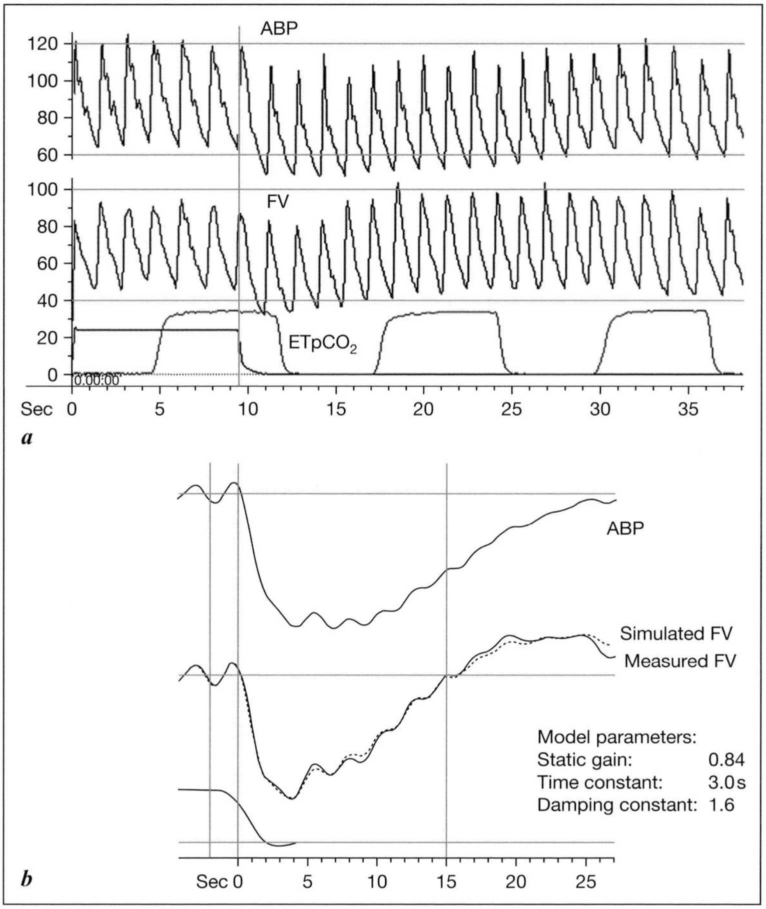

Fig. 5. Recordings of blood pressure (ABP) and flow velocity (FV) before and after release of leg-cuff pressure (***a***). Low-pass filtered tracings of ABP and FV with the simulated output of the second order differential equation model used for evaluating the autoregulatory dynamics superimposed (***b***).

fractures. Moreover, in patients with unstable ICP, the test should be avoided if there is a chance of triggering a plateau-waves (A-waves).

Other nonpharmacological stimuli such as common carotid compression have also been used to assess dynamic autoregulation [12]. Though easy and fast to perform, the procedure involves a certain risk of emboli generation. Moreover, the test is rather uncomfortable for the patient and this limits repeat measurements. Dynamic stimuli can also be generated using a tilt-table or the Valsalva maneuver. Unfortunately, these techniques are not so-well suited for routine clinical use, especially not in the ICU.

The transfer function method, like the Mx approach described above, is based on spontaneous fluctuations in the ABP [9, 10, 19–21]. But in contrast to the quasi-static Mx correlation coefficient, a dynamic transfer function is estimated over the frequency range from about 0 Hz to about 0.5 Hz. The transfer function of the cerebral pressure–flow relationship is usually expressed as two frequency-dependent characteristics:

(1) The phase relationship between ABP and FV is modified by the cerebral autoregulation. Typically, with an intact mechanism, the phase of the FV leads that of the ABP by between 20° and 60° below about 0.2 Hz. At high frequencies, the phase difference is reduced and it is unclear that if this higher range is useful for characterizing the response.

(2) The amplitude or gain relationship FV/ABP is also modified by intact autoregulation. One would expect the fluctuations in FV to be damped out, especially at low frequencies. However, as expected from control theory, the effects of autoregulation on amplitude are less pronounced than on phase. An attenuation of velocity fluctuations is only seen at very low frequencies (<0.07 Hz). At high frequencies the amplitude of the transfer function may even be greater than one, which means that the autoregulation actually augments fluctuations in FV. From a control systems viewpoint, this is expected, negative feedback systems often have such characteristics, as have the second order mathematical model used for the time-series analysis of the leg cuff data. This predicts a maximum in the gain at frequencies of 0.15–0.2 Hz.

Phase and amplitude relationships can also be assessed using stimulus such as forced rhythmic breathing [22]. This method limits the observation to a single line in the frequency spectrum; and furthermore, the technique may be difficult to implement in the low-frequency range where the autoregulatory response is most effective.

Choosing which dynamic autoregulation method is the best to use in a clinical setting or investigational study depends on what are all the aims of the test procedure.

The attractiveness of the transfer function approach is its potential of quantifying dynamic autoregulation without inducing artificial stimuli to change the blood pressure. However, this is also its disadvantage because the individual may not exhibit enough blood pressure variation input compared to noise and intrinsic variability in CBF and FV [21] to make accurate determinations of dynamic autoregulation in the individual case. Therefore, this method is probably best suited for investigational studies where general characteristics of groups or the influence of drugs are studied. Using statistical averaging methods, individual inaccuracies can be averaged and reduced in the group results because the standard error of the mean is lower: $SEM = SD/\sqrt{(n-1)}$ than the standard deviation. If an induced stimulus such as forced breathing [22] is used, the accuracy of the transfer function method can probably be improved so that meaningful determinations can be made in the individual case.

In spite of the disadvantage of adding leg cuffs to the setup and using a sharp ABP reduction as stimulus, the leg-cuff method should be considered preferable (to spontaneous fluctuation methods) in the clinical setting where the dynamic autoregulation response of an individual subject is assessed. The responses are highly reproducible, and the deviation of normal values in a population is small [13, 18] so that assessment of abnormal response can be made with acceptable certainty.

Vasomotor Reactivity (VMR) of the Cerebral Circulation

Carbon dioxide (CO_2) and acetazolamide are very potent vasodilators of the cerebral vasculature. Their effects are primarily confined to the arterioles and the precapillary sphincters. The basal cerebral arteries are only lightly affected, and therefore, velocity measured by TCD will be approximately proportional to CBF. TCD is therefore a convenient alternative to rCBF indicator techniques for determining the VMR of the cerebral circulation, and Doppler methods [23] were found to give similar results as described in previous reports using indicator techniques.

The VMR tests are applied to test the compensatory potential of the brain blood-flow regulating vessels, and are particularly useful for determining the hemodynamic severity of carotid artery disease [24]. The method has also been applied in the ICU to determine VMR in traumatic brain injury [14]. In such and other applications where the ICP is high or unstable, the test should not be carried out by increasing the pCO_2 or giving acetazolamide because of the danger of reducing the CPP. Therefore temporarily decreasing the pCO_2 is the only alternative to determine VMR in this setting.

VMR tests may be set up with varying degrees of complexity and accuracy. In addition to the TCD instrument, a device for sampling the expired air is typically used to measure the pCO_2. From this measurement (fig. 5a) the end-tidal partial pressure ($ETpCO_2$) is derived. It is assumed that this correspond to the alveolar CO_2 partial pressure, which in turn is close to the arterial pCO_2. The two most common approaches to VMR determination are illustrated in figure 6.

The VMR range (VMRr) approach was introduced by Ringelstein et al. [24] and involves subjecting the patient to various concentrations of mixtures of CO_2 in air (or sometimes in oxygen) up to 7%. Moreover, the subjects also hyperventilate, so that the entire physiological range of $ETpCO_2$ is covered. Paired measurements of $ETpCO_2$ and normalized FV are plotted as shown in figure 6a. (The FV is expressed as percentage of the FV at normal respiration.)

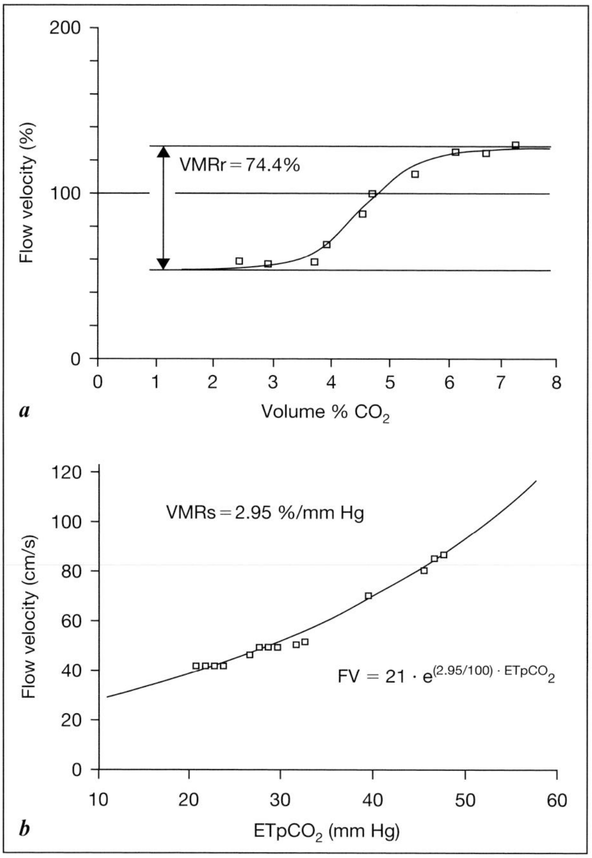

Fig. 6. Determination of the vasomotor reactivity range (VMRr) using a bi-asymptotic curve fit to the data (***a***). Redrawn from data in [24]. Determination of the vasomotor reactivity slope (VMRs) using exponential regression analysis (***b***). Redrawn from data in [23].

A bi-asymptotic curve (a tangent–hyperbolic function) is then fitted to the data. The distance between the upper and lower asymptotes is defined as cerebral vasomotor reactivity range (VMRr). In a simpler setting, this type of approach can also be used without monitoring the CO_2, then the VMRr is simply the difference between the highest and lowest normalized FV recorded when the patient is subjected to normo, hypo and hypercapnia.

The VMR slope (VMRs) method also exposes the patient to a wide range of $ETpCO_2$; and paired measurements are plotted as shown in figure 6b. The maximum concentration of CO_2 in air used in this test is typically 5% or less; higher concentrations may cause considerable discomfort. In this range, it was found that the relationship between $ETpCO_2$ and FV was best approximated with an exponential function [23]:

$$FV = FV_0 \cdot e^{(VMRs/100) \cdot ETpCO_2}$$

The parameters FV_0 and VMRs can be determined by nonlinear regression analysis of the data, and VMRs expresses the percentage change in FV per unit (mm Hg) change in $ETpCO_2$. A simplified version of this approach, often used in clinical routines, is to use only two (or three) points to determine VMRs. Since VMRr cannot be determined in head trauma patients, the VMRs is the only practical method to use, especially since most cases already are being monitored with regard to $ETpCO_2$. If the estimate of VMRs is based only on two paired determinations of FV and $ETpCO_2$, the same problems with intrinsic variability in FV as in the steady-state autoregulation test will surface. If accurate determination of VMR is required, multiple data points such as shown in figure 6b should be used along with exponential data fitting. Using this accurate approach, it could be shown that women have significantly higher VMR (3.7 ± 0.8) than men (3.0 ± 1.0) [25].

VMR determined from breath holding may be a useful screening test [26]. The patient is asked to hold the breath for at least 30 s. The rate of increase in mean FV during this period is calculated.

VMR based on acetazolamide injection is also a widely used method – presumable because its instrumentation setup is simpler than with a CO_2 test. However, the repeatability and accuracy of this approach is somewhat questionable because of the large standard deviation of the velocity response in normal subjects [27]. One reason for this could be that the drug may induce moderate hyperventilation in some individuals, which would counteract the vasodilatory effect of acetazolamide. Therefore, this approach should be considered inferior to a properly applied VMRs or VMRr test.

References

1 Lassen NA: Cerebral blood flow and oxygen consumption in man. Physiol Rev 1959;39:183–238.

2 Aaslid R, Lash SR, Bardy GH, Gild WH, Newell DW: Dynamic pressure–flow velocity relationships in the human cerebral circulation. Stroke 2003;34:1645–1649.

3 Newell DW, Aaslid R, Lam A, Mayberg TS, Winn HR: Comparison of flow and velocity during dynamic autoregulation testing in humans. Stroke 1994;25:793–797.

4 Tiecks FP, Lam AM, Aaslid R, Newell DW: Comparison of static and dynamic cerebral autoregulation measurements. Stroke 1995;26:1014–1019.

5 Strebel S, Lam AM, Matta B, Mayberg TS, Aaslid R, Newell DW: Dynamic and static cerebral autoregulation during isoflurane, desflurane, and propofol anesthesia. Anesthesiology 1995;83:66–76.

6 Jansen GF, Krins A, Basnyat B, Bosch A, Odoom JA: Cerebral autoregulation in subjects adapted and not adapted to high altitude. Stroke 2000;31:2314–2318.

7 Larsen FS, Olsen KS, Hansen BA, Paulson OB, Knudsen GM: Transcranial Doppler is valid for determination of the lower limit of cerebral blood flow autoregulation. Stroke 1994;25: 1985–1998.

8 Czosnyka M, Smielewski P, Kirkpatrick P, Menon DK, Pickard JD: Monitoring of cerebral autoregulation in head-injured patients. Stroke 1996;27:1829–1834.
9 Panerai RB, Kelsall AW, Rennie JM, Evans DH: Cerebral autoregulation dynamics in premature newborns. Stroke 1995;26:74–80.
10 Reinhard M, Roth M, Muller T, Czosnyka M, Timmer J, Hetzel A: Cerebral autoregulation in carotid artery occlusive disease assessed from spontaneous blood pressure fluctuations by the correlation coefficient index. Stroke 2003;34:2138–2144.
11 Aaslid R, Lindegaard K-F, Sorteberg W, Nornes H: Cerebral autoregulation dynamics in humans. Stroke 1989;20:45–52.
12 Aaslid R, Newell DW, Stooss R, Sorteberg W, Lindegaard K-F: Assessment of cerebral autoregulation dynamics from simultaneous arterial and venous transcranial Doppler recordings in humans. Stroke 1991;22:1148–1154.
13 Mahony P, Panerai R, Deverson S, Hayes P, Evans D: Assessment of the thigh cuff technique for measurement of dynamic cerebral autoregulation. Stroke 2000;31:476–480.
14 Newell DW, Aaslid R, Stooss R, Seiler RW, Reulen HJ: Evaluation of hemodynamic responses in head injury patients with transcranial Doppler monitoring. Acta Neurochir (Wien) 1997;139: 804–817.
15 Junger EC, Newell DW, Grant GA, Avellino AM, Ghatan S, Douville CM, Lam AM, Aaslid R, Winn HR: Cerebral autoregulation following minor head injury. J Neurosurg 1997;86:425–432.
16 Doering TJ, Aaslid R, Steuernagel B, Brix J, Niederstadt C, Breull A, Schneider B, Fischer GC: Cerebral autoregulation during whole-body hypothermia and hyperthermia stimulus. Am J Phys Med Rehabil 1999;78:33–38.
17 Vavilala MS, Newell DW, Junger E, Douville CM, Aaslid R, Rivara FP, Lam AM: Dynamic cerebral autoregulation in healthy adolescents. Acta Anaesthesiol Scand 2002;46:393–397.
18 Park CW, Sturzenegger M, Douville CM, Aaslid R, Newell DW: Autoregulatory response and CO_2 reactivity of the basilar artery. Stroke 2003;34:34–39.
19 Zhang R, Zuckerman JH, Giller CA, Levine BD: Transfer function analysis of dynamic cerebral autoregulation in humans. Am J Physiol 1998;274:H233–H241.
20 Zhang R, Zuckerman JH, Levine BD: Spontaneous fluctuations in cerebral blood flow: Insight from extended-duration recordings in humans. Am J Physiol 2000;278:H1848–H1855.
21 Giller CA, Mueller M: Linearity and non-linearity in cerebral hemodynamics. Med Eng Phys 2003;25:633–646.
22 Diehl RR, Linden D, Lucke D, Berlit P: Phase relationship between cerebral blood flow velocity and blood pressure: A clinical test of autoregulation. Stroke 1995;26:1801–1804.
23 Markwalder TM, Grolimund P, Seiler RW, Roth F, Aaslid R: Dependency of blood flow velocity in the middle cerebral artery on end-tidal carbon dioxide partial pressure – A transcranial ultrasound Doppler study. J Cereb Blood Flow Metab 1984;4:368–372.
24 Ringelstein EB, Sievers C, Ecker S, Schneider PA, Otis SM: Noninvasive assessment of CO_2-induced cerebral vasomotor response in normal individuals and patients with internal carotid artery occlusions. Stroke 1988;19:963–969.
25 Kastrup A, Thomas C, Hartmann C, Schabet M: Sex dependency of cerebrovascular CO_2 reactivity in normal subjects. Stroke 1997;28:2353–2356.
26 Markus HS, Harrison MJ: Estimation of cerebrovascular reactivity using transcranial Doppler, including the use of breath-holding as the vasodilatory stimulus. Stroke 1992;23:668–673.
27 Dahl A, Russell D, Rootwelt K, Nyberg-Hansen R, Kerty E: Cerebral vasoreactivity assessed with transcranial Doppler and regional cerebral blood flow measurements: Dose, serum concentration, and time course of the response to acetazolamide. Stroke 1995;26:2302–2306.

Dr. Rune Aaslid
Hemodynamics AG
Surbekstrasse 39, Postfach 668
CH–3000 Bern 31 (Switzerland)
Tel. +41 31 941 3830, Fax +41 31 941 3836, E-Mail rune@hemodynamic.com

Baumgartner RW (ed): Handbook on Neurovascular Ultrasound.
Front Neurol Neurosci. Basel, Karger, 2006, vol 21, pp 229–238

Cerebral Circulation Monitoring in Carotid Endarterectomy and Carotid Artery Stenting

Rob G. A. Ackerstaff

Department of Clinical Neurophysiology, St. Antonius Hospital, Nieuwegein (Utrecht), The Netherlands

Abstract

In the near future it is likely that surgeons, anesthesiologists, and interventional radiologists and cardiologists will care for increasing numbers of patients undergoing carotid endarterectomy (CEA) and carotid angioplasty and stenting (CAS). Perhaps the most important factor in assuring technically acceptable interventions is the availability of an experienced team with demonstrable low periprocedural morbidity and mortality and a proper understanding of both vascular principles and cerebral physiology. Although different monitoring techniques have proven successful during both surgical and endovascular carotid interventions, the advantages of periprocedural transcranial Doppler (TCD) monitoring, such as its sensitivity for recording blood flow velocities and microembolism in real-time, are convincing. Because of its high temporal resolution, it provides additional information about the cerebral circulation, especially during cross-clamping, clamp release, and balloon inflation and deflation, respectively. If made audible during the procedure, it also provides unique information concerning cerebral micro-embolization. In CEA, TCD monitoring gives a better understanding of the pathophysiology of complications and makes the operation safer. In CAS, it gives insight into the clinical relevance of cerebral embolism and the possible effects of protection devices.

Carotid endarterectomy (CEA) has been used to treat atherosclerotic carotid bifurcation disease for more than 50 years. Over this period of time, the surgical technique has undergone minor modifications and the indications for repair have been refined. This operation has held up to the scrutiny of several large multicenter randomized trials [1–4], and more CEAs are currently being performed than at any time in the history of this operation. However, during the past several years carotid angioplasty and stenting (CAS) is being assessed as an attractive alternative to CEA. Potential advantages of CAS over CEA include avoidance of general anesthesia, neck wound complications, nerve injuries, and an ability to dilate surgically inaccessible lesions such as high internal carotid artery stenoses. The main criticism of CAS is that atherosclerotic material dislodged during the procedure may embolize to the cerebral circulation and result in cerebral ischemia.

In the Antonius Hospital, Nieuwegein (Utrecht), The Netherlands, we analyzed clinical reports since 1990 whether cerebral embolism as detected by transcranial Doppler (TCD) during the different stages of CEA as well as CAS was associated with the occurrence of procedure-related adverse cerebral events. Additionally, we evaluated the association of TCD velocity variables during the procedures with cerebral outcome.

TCD Emboli and Velocity Variables in CEA and CAS

During CEA and CAS the same methods of TCD monitoring can be used [5–8]. Most of the newer TCD equipment provides fixed head probe systems so that the technician does not have to hold the probe in place during the procedure. Nevertheless, minor adjustments to the probe position may need to be made once the procedure has started. Particularly during CEA, however, one of the main problems has been the tendency for probe dislodgements, mostly because of the assistant's hand or elbow. This problem can be adequately prevented by using a semi-circular flat plate as a head guard [9]. This provides minimal inconvenience to the surgeon and the assistant now has a safe place to rest his or her elbow. Moreover, the anesthetist and vascular technologist can gain easy access to the endotracheal tube or TCD probe at any time of the operation. To optimize visualization of the intracranial vasculature during CAS, we developed a probe fixation system made of plastic.

During the last 15 years, the vascular community has become increasingly interested in the continuous online recording of middle cerebral artery (MCA) blood flow velocities during both CEA and CAS. The advantages of TCD monitoring during these vascular procedures include the ability to identify cerebral malperfusion, the need for shunting in CEA by measuring the decrease of MCA velocities during test clamping, the capacity to detect cerebral microemboli, and the ability to predict the possible occurrence of a postoperative hyperperfusion syndrome. Besides hemodynamic changes at cross-clamping and clamp release in CEA or during intraluminal manipulations and balloon inflation in CAS, special interest should be paid to the occurrence of embolic transients according to the criteria described by the consensus committees [10, 11].

Particularly in CAS, balloon deflation and stent deployment often result in showers of embolic signals that cannot be counted individually. In these occasions, the number of heartbeats with showers of microemboli are counted. In our studies, a macroembolus was defined as an embolus that partially or completely obstructs the MCA main stem for a period of several seconds to minutes [12]. Mostly, the Doppler spectra are observed in the operating theatre or the angiography suite by an experienced sonographer, and it is recommendable to make the audio Doppler signal audible throughout the entire procedure. For offline analysis, the Doppler signals should be recorded on digital audio tape or CD. With regard to the criteria for shunting or the prediction of a postoperative hyperperfusion syndrome in CEA, the following TCD velocity variables are clinically relevant: (1) decrease of peak systolic velocity (PSV) at cross-clamping, (2) increase of the PSV, and (3) increase of the Gosling pulsatility index (PI) of the Doppler signal at declamping at the end of the endarterectomy. These three velocity variables are computed from the envelope of the Doppler spectrum by the TCD equipment and calculated as the proportional change compared with the intraoperative preclamp values. Although most surgeons concentrate on prevention of hemodynamic failure during the clamp phase of CEA, the majority of operation-related strokes follow thromboembolism [13, 14]. In general, the most dangerous periods for intraoperative particulate embolization have been during dissection (skin preparation to carotid clamping) and during wound closure (termination of manipulation to the end of recording; ~30 min after final restoration of flow). Embolization during dissection warns the surgeon of a highly unstable plaque and a few discrete emboli without distortion of the Doppler waveform can be treated by adopting an even more gentle surgical technique with avoidance of dissection around the bifurcation. More frequent embolization warrants early cross-clamping of the internal carotid artery. Originally, it was shown that cerebral microemboli that occurred during the dissection stage of CEA were associated with minor cerebral deficits, for example, transient ischemic attacks and neuropsychological deterioration [15–17]. Moreover, Jansen et al. [18] demonstrated an association between multiple cerebral microemboli during dissection and new white matter lesions on magnetic resonance images of the brain made after surgery. However, in the majority of these patients the new magnetic resonance imaging lesions were clinically silent. These studies demonstrate that during CEA the incidence of TCD-detected microemboli far exceeds the morbidity and mortality rates for the operation. This, however, does not mean that TCD-detected microemboli are not clinically important. Cerebral complications that occur during the dissection stage of carotid surgery were reported before the introduction of TCD monitoring, but this was previously thought to be due to one large embolus. However, most research work on intraoperative emboli detection in carotid surgery using TCD ultrasonography suggests that multiple microembolization is the most likely mechanism. More recently, a pooled data analysis of individual patients of two major institutes in intraoperative TCD monitoring in CEA [19] revealed that microemboli that appeared during dissection and particularly during wound closure were statistically significantly associated with permanent cerebral deficits, i.e. intraoperative stroke and stroke-related death [odds ratio (OR): 2.3; 95% CI: 1.2–4.4, $p = 0.007$].

The Antonius Hospital in Nieuwegein is probably one of the few centers in the world that perform TCD monitoring during CAS on a structural basis. On the basis of our previous research on TCD monitoring during CAS [8], the following TCD emboli variables (isolated and showers) were thought to be associated with adverse cerebral outcome: (1) at predilation before stent placement, (2) at stent deployment, (3) at postdilation after stent placement, and (4) during introduction and removal of a filter protection device. Also evaluated for their impact on outcome were: (1) particulate macroembolism, (2) massive air embolism during balloon rupture, and (3) angioplasty-induced asystole of >15 s with significant hypotension (<80 mm Hg) in combination with a >70% reduction in MCA mean blood flow velocity. In a more recent study [21], we developed a multivariable prediction model based on some preoperative baseline clinical characteristics and various TCD velocity and emboli variables. We found that of all TCD microemboli variables quantified during the various stages of CAS, only the variable '>5 showers of microemboli at postdilation after stent deployment' was associated with transient and persistent retinal and cerebral deficits within 7 days (OR: 2.7; 95% CI: 1.4–5.0, $p = 0.003$). This association remained after taking into account three additional TCD emboli and velocity variables and various patient characteristics. The TCD emboli variables macroembolus and massive air embolism were associated with outcome independent of the TCD velocity variable (>70% reduction of MCA blood flow velocity during angioplasty-induced asystole with significant hypotension) and the patient characteristic preprocedural cerebral ischemia. This recently published study is an expansion of previous research from our group [8] by almost doubling the number of patients analyzed. In this perspective, it is important to underline that in the first study the variable 'multiple showers at postdilation after stent placement' only showed a statistically significant association with intraprocedural adverse cerebral outcome. Although in the enlarged study one third (21/63) of the cerebral events occurred with a symptom-free interval after the procedure, the variable '>5 showers of microemboli at postdilation after stent placement' now also showed a statistically significant association with adverse outcome within 7 days. Besides clear adverse events as macroembolism, and massive air embolism, microemboli that occur at postdilation after stent deployment are a major and independent risk factor for periprocedural cerebral deficit. Obviously, an uncovered stent squeezes plaque material from the vessel wall through the stent mesh that subsequently contributes to embolization in the cerebral circulation. To minimize the risk of these embolic events various protection strategies have been introduced, and in our institution in one third of the procedures (181/550), a filter wire protection device was used. However, former research from our group [20] on the impact of filtering protection devices on the cerebral embolic load showed that in all three stages of the stenting procedure (predilation, stent deployment, and postdilation) the number of TCD-detected microemboli was significantly higher in protected than in nonprotected procedures. As documented by others [22–24] we also found that transient, moderate hypotension occurs frequently during and after CAS and resolve spontaneously in the majority of patients. Although most of these events can be considered benign and self-limiting, hemodynamic instability due to asystole and severe hypotension may complicate CAS. In our institution, in 4% (22/550), asystole resulted in severe hypotension with a significant reduction of MCA blood flow velocities, and in 7 of these 22 patients this was related with adverse cerebral outcome. Most of these cases occurred during the first years of our study period. Undoubtedly, more aggressive use of vasopressor agents, adequate fluid balance, and advances in technique and equipment made the procedure safer in subsequent years.

Postoperative TCD Monitoring in CEA and CAS

Although Spencer et al. [5] was the first who observed that cerebral ischemia complicating CEA may be associated with the occurrence of frequent postoperative microemboli, most research on the clinical relevance of TCD monitoring for emboli detection during the first hours after CEA is performed in the United Kingdom (Leicester) and Australia (Melbourne) [25–32]. These studies showed that patients who developed signs and symptoms of cerebral ischemia in the recovery room after a symptom-free interval usually demonstrated either sustained TCD-detected microemboli from the endarterectomy zone or a postoperative thrombotic occlusion of the internal carotid artery [33]. Actually, patients do not develop a thrombotic stroke after CEA without first producing a significant number of microemboli. In general the vast majority of patients undergoing CEA have one or more TCD-detected microemboli within the first postoperative hours [34, 35]. However, only 5% of these patients will develop severe, sustained postoperative embolization. In most of these patients, the administration of a Dextran 40 or Rheomacrodex infusion was associated with a rapid decline in the rate of microemboli and did not progress onto a stroke due to carotid thrombosis. Several studies revealed a significantly higher number of postoperative microemboli in female patients [28, 36] or in patients who were preoperatively seropositive for *Chlamydia pneumoniae* [37]. On the contrary, traditional cardiovascular risk factors did not appear to influence embolization after CEA and only the presence of TCD-detected microemboli prior to the operation was significantly correlated with the occurrence of postoperative embolization [28]. The modern pathophysiological concept of sustained postoperative embolization in CEA assumes a more common pathway that underlies the tendency to form thrombus in both the pre- and postoperative periods. Probably, it is the patients inherent propensity to generate a thrombus in response to vascular injury.

So far, there is only one study [38] that investigated the rate of TCD-detected microemboli after CAS. In a very limited number of procedures (n = 10) late embolization after CAS occurred in 2 patients.

TCD and the Postoperative Hyperperfusion Syndrome

Fortunately, postoperative hyperperfusion with or without intracerebral bleeding after CEA is a relatively rare complication, although the outcome shows a high morbidity and mortality. The occurrence of the cascade of signs and symptoms of a postoperative hyperperfusion syndrome is unpredictable and often unexpected. Moreover, currently there are no therapeutic modalities that prevent further deterioration once clear clinical symptoms, such as confusion, seizures, and focal cerebral deficits, are recognized. It is, therefore, of utmost importance that all efforts should be directed towards identification of patients who are at risk of this devastating complication.

Performing CEA with intraoperative assessment of cerebral blood flow from clearance curves of intra-arterially injected xenon-133, a more than 200% increase of baseline blood flow in patients with a postoperative hyperperfusion syndrome was demonstrated [39]. An excessive increase of cerebral flow can also be evaluated by intraoperative TCD monitoring of ipsilateral MCA blood flow velocities [40]. These studies stimulated our group to retrospectively investigate in a cohort of 280 consecutive CEAs the occurrence of intracerebral hemorrhage [41]. In this study, intraoperative TCD monitoring was possible in 233 (83%) patients. We were especially interested in the changes in PSV and the Gosling PI of the MCA on the side of surgery. We measured PSV and PI one minute before test clamping and during a 3-min period after clamp release, on completion of the desobstruction. After an evaluation of different cut-off values for the PSV and the PI by a receiver operating characteristic analysis, the optimum threshold values for these two variables were calculated at 175 and 100%, respectively. For these thresholds, the positive predictive value, negative predictive value, sensitivity, and specificity of the test were 100, 99, 80, and 100%, respectively. Compared to the use of clinical variables as ipsilateral throbbing headache, hypertension, or both, the diagnostic gain increased from 22 to 98%. However, in one patient who developed an intracerebral hemorrhage after CEA, the intraoperative TCD monitoring did not accurately predict this complication. We, therefore, analyzed data of an additional 688 consecutive CEAs with adequate intraoperative TCD monitoring and re-evaluated the optimal threshold values of PSV and PI by receiver operating characteristic analysis [42]. In this second study we classified patients with a more than 100% increase of PSV, or more than 100% increase of PI, or both, as patients at risk for a postoperative hyperperfusion syndrome. Sixty-two patients (62/688 = 9%) fulfilled these TCD criteria. Patients identified as at risk for hyperperfusion were compared to a control group of 61 patients matched for age, sex, and date of operation. Patients at risk remained on the medium care unit for at least 24 h postoperatively and continuous invasive blood pressure monitoring was performed during this time. With strict control and treatment of hypertension in the selected group of patients, no intracerebral hemorrhage was identified postoperatively. Moreover, in the matched control group no patient exhibited clinical signs or symptoms of hyperperfusion. All patients clinically at risk were correctly identified. In the group of the 62 patients who fulfilled our TCD criteria and who were strictly monitored and treated after surgery, only 7 (11%) finally developed clinical signs and symptoms of a hyperperfusion syndrome. The low specificity of the test is a drawback: 8 out of 9 patients subjected to the more strict postoperative care showed no clinical features of hyperperfusion. We believe that the high morbidity and mortality of postoperative hyperperfusion after CEA outweighs the disadvantage of the low specificity. In conclusion, intraoperative TCD monitoring of ipsilateral MCA blood flow velocities is a simple, relatively cheap, and reliable test to identify patients who are at risk of postoperative hyperperfusion syndrome and intracerebral hemorrhage.

Cerebral hyperperfusion syndrome has been increasingly reported as a complication of CAS [43–46]. However, the incidence of cerebral hyperperfusion after endovascular revascularization procedures of the extracranial carotid artery has not been extensively studied, and therefore, remains unclear. Although CEA and CAS are technically different procedures, the resultant changes in vascular physiology are similar and the pathophysiological mechanisms of hyperperfusion between these two interventions probably are very equivalent. In addition to the well-known clinical and anatomical predictors, TCD probably also has the potential to predict which patients are at increased risk of hyperperfusion and intracerebral hemorrhage after CAS by measuring the proportional increase of ipsilateral MCA blood flow velocities. So far, however, no studies have been performed.

References

1 European Carotid Surgery Trialists' Collaborative Group: Randomised trial of endarterectomy for recently symptomatic carotid stenosis: Final results of the MRC European Carotid Surgery Trial (ECST). Lancet 1998;351:1379–1387.
2 Barnett HJ, Taylor DW, Eliasziw M, Fox AJ, Ferguson GG, Haynes RB, et al: Benefit of carotid endarterectomy in patients with symptomatic moderate or severe stenosis. N Engl J Med 1998;339:1415–1425.
3 Executive Committee for the Asymptomatic Carotid Atherosclerosis Study: Endarterectomy for asymptomatic carotid artery stenosis. JAMA 1995;273:1421–1428.
4 MRC Asymptomatic Carotid Surgery Trial (ACST) Collaborators: Prevention of disabling and fatal strokes by successful carotid endarterectomy in patients without recent neurological symptoms: Randomised controlled trial. Lancet 2004;363:1491–1502.
5 Spencer MP, Thomas GI, Nicholls SC, Sauvage LR: Detection of middle cerebral artery emboli during carotid endarterectomy using transcranial Doppler ultrasonography. Stroke 1990;21:415–423.
6 Jansen C, Moll FL, Vermeulen FE, Haelst JM, Ackerstaff RG: Continuous transcranial Doppler ultrasonography and electroencephalography during carotid endarterectomy: A multimodal monitoring system to detect intraoperative ischemia. Ann Vasc Surg 1993;7:95–101.
7 Ghali R, Palazzo EG, Rodriguez DI, Zammit M, Loudenback DL, DeMuth RP, et al: Transcranial Doppler intraoperative monitoring during carotid endarterectomy: Experience with regional or general anesthesia, with and without shunting. Ann Vasc Surg 1997;11:9–13.
8 Antonius Carotid Endarterectomy, Angioplasty, and Stenting Study Group: Transcranial Doppler monitoring in angioplasty and stenting of the carotid bifurcation. J Endovasc Ther 2003;10:702–710.
9 Naylor AR: Transcranial Doppler monitoring during carotid endarterectomy; in Hennerici M, Meairs SP eds: Cerebrovascular Ultrasound. Theory, Practice and Future Developments. Cambridge, Cambridge University Press, 2001, p 317–323.
10 Consensus Committee of the Ninth Cerebral Hemodynamic Symposium: Basic identification criteria of Doppler microembolic signals. Stroke 1995;26:1123.
11 Ringelstein EB, Droste DW, Babikian VL, Evans DH, Grosset DG, Kaps M, et al: Consensus on Microembolism Detection by TCD. International Consensus Group on Microembolus Detection. Stroke 1998;29:725–729.
12 Claus SP, Louwerse ES, Mauser HW, van der Mee M, Moll FL, Mess WH, et al: Temporary occlusion of middle cerebral artery by macroembolism in carotid surgery. Cerebrovasc Dis 1999;9:261–264.
13 Steed DL, Peitzman AB, Grundy BL, Webster MW: Causes of stroke in carotid endarterectomy. Surgery 1982;92:634–641.
14 Krul JMJ, van Gijn J, Ackerstaff RGA, Eikelboom BC, Theodorides T, Vermeulen FE: Site and pathogenesis of infarcts associated with carotid endarterectomy. Stroke 1989;20:324–328.
15 Jansen C: Static and dynamic risk factors in carotid endarterectomy. Results of logistic regression analysis in 301 patients: In Monitoring of Cerebral Function During Carotid Endarterectomy with Electroencephalography and Transcranial Doppler Ultrasonography. Utrecht, The Netherlands, 1994, p 77–92.
16 Ackerstaff RG, Jansen C, Moll FL, Vermeulen FE, Hamerlijnck RP, Mauser HW: The significance of microemboli detection by means of transcranial Doppler ultrasonography monitoring in carotid endarterectomy. J Vasc Surg 1995;21:963–969.
17 Gaunt ME, Martin PJ, Smith JL, Rimmer T, Cheerman G, Ratliff DA, et al: Clinical relevance of intraoperative embolization detected by transcranial Doppler ultrasonography during carotid endarterectomy: A prospective study of 100 patients. Br J Surg 1994;81:1435–1439.
18 Jansen C, Ramos LM, van Heesewijk JPM, Moll FL, van Gijn J, Ackerstaff RG: Impact of microembolism and hemodynamic changes in the brain during carotid endarterectomy. Stroke 1994;25:992–997.
19 Ackerstaff RG, Moons KG, van den Vlasakker CJW, Moll FL, Vermeulen FE, Algra A, et al: Association of intraoperative transcranial Doppler monitoring variables with stroke from carotid endarterectomy. Stroke 2000;31:1817–1823.

20 Vos JA, van den Berg JC, Ernst SM, Suttorp MJ, Overtoom TT, Mauser HW, et al: Carotid angioplasty and stenting in 509 cases: Comparison of transcranial Doppler data and clinical outcome with and without the use of filtering cerebral protection devices. Radiology 2005;234:493–499.
21 Ackerstaff RG, Suttorp MJ, van den Berg JC, Overtoom TT, Vos JA, Bal ET, et al: Prediction of early cerebral outcome by TCD monitoring in carotid bifurcation angioplasty and stenting. J Vasc Surg 2005;41:618–624.
22 Qureshi AI, Luft AR, Sharma M, Janardhan V, Lopes DK, Khan J, et al: Frequency and determinants of postprocedural hemodynamic instability after carotid angioplasty and stenting. Stroke 1999;30:2086–2093.
23 Mendelsohn FO, Weissman NJ, Lederman RJ, Crowley JJ, Gray JL, Phillips HR, et al: Acute hemodynamic changes during carotid artery stenting. Am J Cardiol 1998;82:1077–1081.
24 Howell M, Krajcer Z, Dougherty K, Strickman N, Skolkin M, Toombs B, et al: Correlation of periprocedural systolic blood pressure changes with neurological events in high-risk stent patients. J Endovasc Ther 2002;9:810–816.
25 Lennard N, Smith JL, Hayes P, Evans DH, Abbott RJ, London NJ, et al: Transcranial Doppler directed dextran therapy in the prevention of carotid thrombosis: Three hour monitoring is as effective as six hours. Eur J Vasc Endovasc Surg 1999;17:301–305.
26 Hayes PD, Lloyd AJ, Lennard N, Wolstenholme JL, London NJ, Bell PR, et al: Transcranial Doppler-directed Dextran-40 therapy is a cost-effective method of preventing carotid thrombosis after carotid endarterectomy. Eur J Vasc Endovasc Surg 2000;19:59–61.
27 Naylor AR: Regarding 'High embolic rate early after carotid endarterectomy is associated with early cerebrovascular complications, especially in women'. J Vasc Surg 2002;36:408–409.
28 Hayes PD, Payne DA, Evans NJ, Thompson MM, London NJ, Bell PR, et al: The excess of strokes in female patients after CEA is due to their increased thromboembolic potential – Analysis of 775 cases. Eur J Vasc Endovasc Surg 2003;26:665–669.
29 Levi CR, O'Malley HM, Fell G, Roberts AK, Hoare MC, Royle JP, et al: Transcranial Doppler detected cerebral microembolism following carotid endarterectomy. High microembolic signal loads predict postoperative cerebral ischaemia. Brain 1997;120:621–629.
30 Levi CR, Roberts AK, Fell G, Hoare MC, Royle JP, Chan A, et al: Transcranial Doppler microembolus detection in the identification of patients at high risk of perioperative stroke. Eur J Vasc Endovasc Surg 1997;14:170–176.
31 Levi CR, Bladin CF, Chambers BC, Donnan GA: Clinical role of transcranial Doppler embolus detection monitoring after carotid endarterectomy. Stroke 1997;28:1845.
32 Stork JL, Levi CR, Chambers BR, Abbott AL, Donnan GA: Possible determinants of early microembolism after carotid endarterectomy. Stroke 2002;33:2082–2085.
33 de Borst GJ, Moll FL, van de Pavoordt HD, Mauser HW, Kelder JC, Ackerstaff RG: Stroke from carotid endarterectomy: When and how to reduce perioperative stroke rate? Eur J Vasc Endovasc Surg 2001;21:484–489.
34 Lennard N, Smith J, Dumville J, Abbott R, Evans DH, London NJ, et al: Prevention of postoperative thrombotic stroke after carotid endarterectomy: The role of transcranial Doppler ultrasound. J Vasc Surg 1997;26:579–584.
35 van der Schaaf IC, Horn J, Moll FL, Ackerstaff RG: Transcranial Doppler monitoring after carotid endarterectomy. Ann Vasc Surg 2004;19:1–6.
36 Laman DM, Wieneke GH, van Duijn H, van Huffelen AC: High embolic rate early after carotid endarterectomy is associated with early cerebrovascular complications. J Vasc Surg 2002;36: 278–284.
37 Vainas T, Kurvers HA, Mess WH, Graaf R, Ezzahiri R, Tordoir JHM, et al: Chlamydia pneumoniae serology is associated with thrombosis-related but not with plaque-related microembolization during carotid endarterectomy. Stroke 2002;33:1249–1254.
38 Markus HS, Clifton A, Buckenham T, Brown MM: Carotid angioplasty: Detection of embolic signals during and after the procedure. Stroke 1994;25:2403–2406.
39 Sundt TM, Sharbrough FW, Piepgras DG, Kearns TP, Messick JM, O'Fallon WM: Correlation of cerebral blood flow and electroencephalographic changes during carotid endarterectomy with results of surgery and hemodynamics of cerebral ischemia. Mayo Clin Proc 1981;56:533–543.

40 Powers AD, Smith RR: Hyperperfusion syndrome after carotid endarterectomy: A transcranial Doppler evaluation. Neurosurgery 1990;26:56–60.
41 Jansen C, Sprengers AM, Moll FL, Vermeulen FE, Hamerlijnck RP, van Gijn J, et al: Prediction of intracerebral haemorrhage after carotid endarterectomy by clinical criteria and intraoperative transcranial Doppler monitoring: Results of 233 operations. Eur J Vasc Surg 1994;8:220–225.
42 Dalman JE, Beenakkers IC, Moll FL, Leusink JA, Ackerstaff RG: Transcranial Doppler monitoring during carotid endarterectomy helps to identify patients at risk of postoperative hyperperfusion. Eur J Vasc Endovasc Surg 1999;18:222–227.
43 Schoser BG, Heesen C, Eckert B, Thie A: Cerebral hyperperfusion injury after percutaneous transluminal angioplasty of extracranial arteries. J Neurol 1997;244:101–104.
44 Morrish W, Grahovac S, Douen A, Cheung G, Hu W, Farb R, et al: Intracranial hemorrhage after stenting and angioplasty of extracranial carotid stenosis. Am J Neuroradiol 2000;212:1911–1916.
45 Kaku Y, Yoshimura S, Kokuzawa J: Factors predictive of cerebral hyperperfusion after carotid angioplasty and stent placement. Am J Neuroradiol 2004;25:1403–1408.
46 Abou-Chebl A, Yadav JS, Reginelli JP, Bajzer CT, Bhatt D, Krieger DW: Intracranial hemorrhage and hyperperfusion syndrome following carotid artery stenting. Risk factors, prevention, and treatment. J Am Coll Cardiol 2004;43:1596–1601.

Rob G. A. Ackerstaff, MD, PhD
Department of Clinical Neurophysiology, St. Antonius Hospital
Koekoekslaan 1
NL–3435 CM Nieuwegein (Utrecht) (The Netherlands)
Tel. +31 30 609 2452, Fax +31 30 609 2327, E-Mail r.ackerstaff@antonius.net

Baumgartner RW (ed): Handbook on Neurovascular Ultrasound.
Front Neurol Neurosci. Basel, Karger, 2006, vol 21, pp 239–250

Syncope

Arto C. Nirkko[a], *Ralf W. Baumgartner*[b]

Department of Neurology, University Hospital, [a]Inselspital, Bern, [b]Zürich, Switzerland

Abstract

Syncope is defined as an acute, brief and transient loss of consciousness and postural tone with spontaneous and complete recovery. Neurovascular ultrasound has contributed to elucidate the underlying mechanism of different types of syncope. In routine diagnostic work-up of patients with syncope, however, neurovascular ultrasound is not among the first line tools. In particular, an ultrasound search for occlusive cerebro-vascular disease is of limited value because cerebral artery obstruction is a very rare and questionable cause of syncope. Transcranial Doppler sonography monitoring of the cerebral arteries is useful in the diagnostic work-up of patients with suspicion of postural related, cerebrovascular, cough and psychogenic syncope, and in some cases for differentiating focal epileptic seizures from transient ischemic attacks and migraine with aura.

A syncope is characterized by a sudden and short-lived loss of consciousness and postural tone with spontaneous, complete, and usually prompt recovery [1]. Most syncopes are caused by acute cardiovascular failure (e.g., postural related syncope), which lead to hypoperfusion of the ascending reticular activating system or the cerebral cortex, or both [2]. The other causes of syncope include neurological diseases, metabolic disorders, hyperventilation and intoxication, and psychiatric syncopes. In this chapter ultrasound findings associated with postural related, cerebrovascular, cough and psychogenic syncopes as well as epileptic seizures are discussed.

Cerebral Haemodynamics, Neurovascular Ultrasound, and Syncope

A sudden interruption of cerebral blood flow (CBF) for 6–8 s has been shown to be sufficient to cause a syncopal episode [3]. Tilt testing studies have found that a decrease in systolic blood pressure (BP) to 60 mm Hg reduces CBF to an extent that is associated with a loss of consciousness [4]. Furthermore, syncope may occur when regional cerebral tissue oxygen delivery is jeopardized [3]. Consequently, the integrity of several control mechanisms is crucial for maintaining adequate delivery of CBF, oxygen, and nutrients to the brain, including: (A) cerebrovascular autoregulation, which maintains CBF within certain limits of cerebral perfusion pressure (for details see the chapter by Aaslid, pp. 216–228) and which is mediated by (B) local metabolic and chemical control, enabling cerebral vasodilatation to counteract diminished BP, arterial pO_2 or elevated arterial pCO_2; (C) arterial baroreceptor-induced adjustments of heart rate, cardiac contractility, and systemic vascular resistance, which modify systemic circulatory dynamics to prevent CBF decrease; and (D) vascular volume regulation, in which renal and hormonal influences help to maintain central circulating volume. Transient failure of the aforementioned protective mechanisms, e.g., the reduction of systemic BP below the lower limit of cerebral autoregulation, may induce syncope. Furthermore, raised intracranial pressure (ICP) may cause a loss of consciousness, e.g., in cough syncope.

The relative change of Doppler flow velocity is proportional to the relative change of regional CBF in the area supplied by the insonated artery, as long as the diameter of the investigated vessel remains stable. Other factors such as hyperventilation, which may influence the results of transcranial Doppler sonography (TCD) monitoring, are discussed in the chapters by Aaslid, pp. 216–228, and Lohmann et al., pp. 251–260.

Postural Related Syncope

Postural related syncope can result from permanent autonomic failure (orthostatic hypotension) or from intermittent autonomic dysregulation (neurally mediated or vasovagal syncope). A rare variant induced by (mostly posturally elicited) irritation of baroreceptors is the carotid sinus syndrome, whereas a diminished baroreflex gain due to reduced baroreceptor sensitivity is more common.

A constant failure of the peripheral or central autonomic nervous system leads to orthostatic arterial hypotension and can thus result in syncope if the cerebrovascular autoregulation capacities are exceeded. To investigate the vasomotor response, we have developed a test using Doppler sonography of limb arteries. When an unspecific (electric, acoustic or breath hold) stimulus is applied as in sudomotor skin response (SSR) testing (which can be performed simultaneously using the same stimulus) diastolic flow in the radial or tibial arteries abruptly drops after a latency of 1–3 s (fig. 1). This test has proved to be more reliable than electrophysiological evaluation [5] and laser Doppler testing [6] in detecting peripheral autonomic dysfunction due to leprosy [7]. Because orthostatic syncope

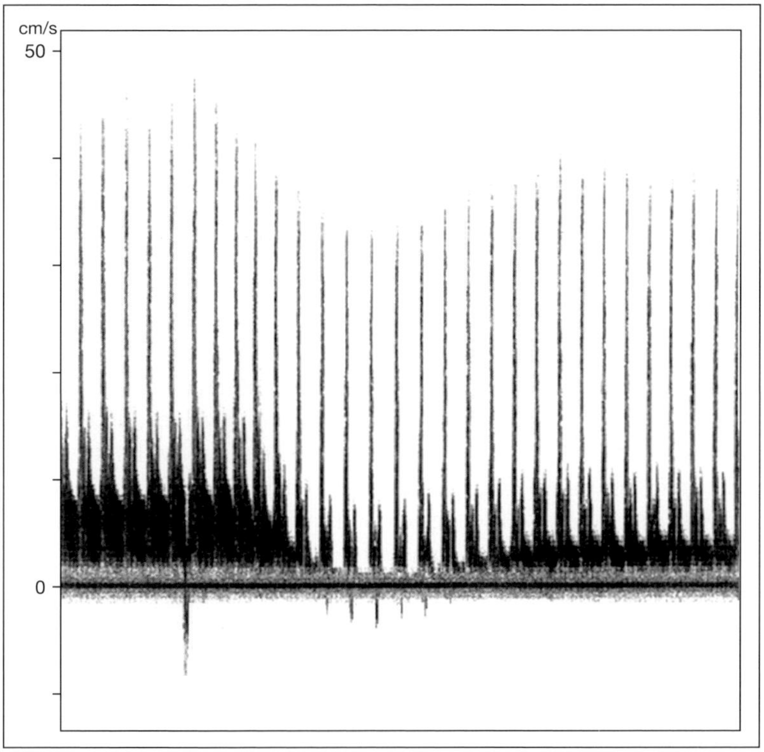

Fig. 1. Assessment of the vasomotor reflex response. Pulsed Doppler ultrasound recording of the radial artery at the wrist of a vasodilated warmed hand. The short backflow after the 6th systole is generated by the muscle twitch from the electrical median nerve stimulation and marks the stimulus time point. With a latency of 2–3 s, diastolic flow velocity is reduced due to stimulation-induced vasoconstriction.

is more related to vasomotor responses than to other autonomic features, Doppler ultrasound may be suitable for the assessment of early orthostatic failure, although no corresponding studies are yet available.

Neurally mediated (vasovagal) syncope is often elicited in susceptible, but otherwise healthy subjects by a combination of upright position, heat, and painful stimuli. Diagnostic testing relies on reproducing these conditions to elicit the breakdown of BP leading to the presyncopal or syncopal symptoms. Neurovascular ultrasound is not diagnostic, but helps to elucidate the temporal sequence and thresholds of symptom onset [8], and illuminates some pitfalls in interpretation. In neurally mediated syncope, a general pattern with an increase of the pulsatility index (with a decrease of diastolic, but unaltered systolic velocities) has been observed together with a decrease of mean flow velocity before the occurrence of hypotension or during presyncopal symptoms [9–12]. This has been interpreted as an increase of cerebrovascular resistance due to paradoxical cerebral vasoconstriction and has even led to the suggestion of a new type of 'cerebral syncope' [11]. However, detailed assessments have indicated that cerebrovascular autoregulation was preserved [13], whereas arterial pCO_2 was found to be decreased [14–16]. Simultaneous recording of breathing activity showed that this reflects subclinical hyperventilation during the episode [16]. Hyperventilation and resulting hypocapnia has long been known to produce these effects on flow velocities and cerebrovascular resistance [17]. Reduced flow velocities with increased pulsatility during hypocapnia thus merely confirm a preserved cerebrovascular autoregulation, but are not severe enough to explain syncope. Hyperventilation reduced antegrade flow velocity in the middle cerebral artery (MCA) to a third of baseline values, and a transient reverberating MCA flow was induced in some subjects without loss of consciousness or other neurologic symptoms (unpublished own data). Thus, the aforementioned modest decrease of velocities and increase of pulsatility before many types of syncope is probably due to an altered breathing pattern.

In carotid sinus syndrome, intermittent vasomotor dysregulation is induced by mechanical irritation of oversensitive baroreceptors in the carotid sinus, mainly during postural changes with compression by a neck collar or carotid massage. Mediated by the baroreflex, this results either in cardioinhibition and bradycardia or in direct vasodepression [18], both resulting in a drop of BP. As expected, TCD monitoring performed during carotid massage showed a 50% decrease of mean MCA flow velocity [18].

The opposite condition, a diminished baroreflex gain, is more frequent, especially among elderly people. It is one of the factors predisposing to orthostatic hypotension and syncope [19], by the mechanisms discussed in the previous section. Interestingly, baroreflex gain was independently related to elevated systolic BP in elderly subjects, and in the remaining subjects also to the mechanical stiffness of the carotid artery [19]. Another study assessed changes of BP and brachial blood flow velocity by Doppler ultrasonography during carotid baroreceptor loading/unloading by neck collar suction [20]. The authors found a latency of 14 s in early fainters and around 10 s in normal non-fainting patients and controls, suggesting that the delay of the baroreflex response might also play a pathogenic role [20].

Cardiac Syncope

The mechanism of cardiac syncope may be mechanical (e.g., aortic or mitral valve stenosis, atrial myxoma, hypertrophic subaortic stenosis) [21] and lead to exertion syncope, or arrhythmogenic (e.g., cardiac anomalies, coronary heart disease, cardiomyopathy) and manifest without warning [22]. Both mechanisms cause cerebral hypoperfusion with loss of consciousness. Ultrasound may elucidate the detailed mechanisms [15] and has been used to gain insights into the cerebral circulation during electrophysiological testing [10, 23], but plays no role in routine diagnosis of cardiac syncope.

Cerebrovascular Syncope

Neck hyperextension during stretching has been described as a cause of *adolescent stretch syncope* [24] or ischemic symptoms consistent with presyncope [25]. Head rotation and flexion did not elicit presyncope or syncope [24]. In a study [24], TCD monitoring of the posterior cerebral artery (PCA) revealed a rapid decrease of mean flow velocities to 28–41% of baseline values. Return to a neutral head position was associated with reactive hyperemia with flow velocity increases to 131–136% of baseline values [24]. The authors assumed that insufficient cross-flow through the posterior communicating artery due to bilateral hypoplasia in one patient and an accompanying stretching of the cervical internal carotid artery over the transverse process of the atlas in the other case were the additional prerequisites for syncope [24].

Unilateral mechanical compression of the vertebral artery during neck rotation (rotational vertebral artery occlusion), which was defined as zero diastolic flow velocity at duplex ultrasonography was observed in 5% of 1,108 patients [26]. None of these patients suffered a syncope during head rotation. The absence of syncope may be explained by the presence of a sufficient residual flow in the compressed vertebral artery, the development of collateral flow through the other vertebral artery, or the posterior communicating artery [27].

Loss of consciousness is very unusual during transient ischemic attacks [28] and it is thus unclear whether a syncope may be the only symptom of a transient ischemic attack. Yanagihara et al. [29] reported three patients with syncope and severe atherosclerotic stenosis or occlusion of both internal carotid arteries. Catheter angiography showed patent vertebrobasilar circulation and collaterals through both posterior communicating arteries to the carotid circulation. Clinical and extensive ancillary investigations showed no other possible etiology of the attacks of unconsciousness than occlusive cerebrovascular disease. Syncopes disappeared after carotid endarterectomy, and the authors assumed that bilateral hemispheric ischemia was the most likely cause.

Cough Syncope

In cough syncope, the underlying reduction of brain perfusion results from an acute increase of ICP, which is produced by congestion of venous backflow due to intrathoracic pressure increase in patients with obstruction of pulmonary airflow during coughing [30]. Most patients with cough syncope suffer also from chronic obstructive pulmonary disease, but also other causes like tracheomalacia may occur. An ultrasound study showed reduced flow velocities in the carotid arteries during cough syncope [31]. Another report described a patient with cough syncope and with critical carotid and vertebral artery occlusive disease, with resolution of syncopal attacks after vascular surgery [32]. In an own TCD study, we demonstrated cerebral circulatory arrest during cough syncope followed by reactive hyperemia (fig. 2) [30]. In our experience, healthy volunteers may produce reverberating flow in the MCA during maximally one heart cycle (fig. 3), but are not able to induce syncope.

Epileptic Seizures

In focal epileptic seizures, ictal hyperactivity causes a local increase of CBF and may thus be monitored by TCD. Systemic causes of CBF increase such as changes of BP, ICP, or arterial pCO_2, which can occur during altered breathing, have to be excluded. This is achieved by simultaneous TCD recording from another cerebral artery, which would also be influenced by systemic changes, but does not supply the brain region responsible for the focal symptoms. In a patient with recurring attacks of simple hallucinations of color patterns lasting around 20 s each, we used simultaneous recording with electroencephalography (EEG) and TCD of the PCA, which supplies the visual cortex. The MCA was monitored as reference artery (fig. 4) [33]. EEG showed desynchronization occurring simultaneously with the visual symptoms, but no epileptiform activity. Simultaneous TCD monitoring delineated an increase in PCA flow velocity at about 50%, whereas MCA flow velocity remained unchanged, excluding any contribution by systemic factors. This selective increase in PCA flow velocities and clinical presentation argued for an epileptic etiology of the symptoms and against ischemia or migraine. Other authors have subsequently used TCD monitoring for the localization of epileptic foci [34].

As mentioned above, parallel TCD recording of a cerebral artery not supplying the epileptic focus is used to exclude systemic influences in focal seizures [33]. This strategy, however, is not applicable in generalized seizures. Also, some types of generalized seizures might not necessarily be associated

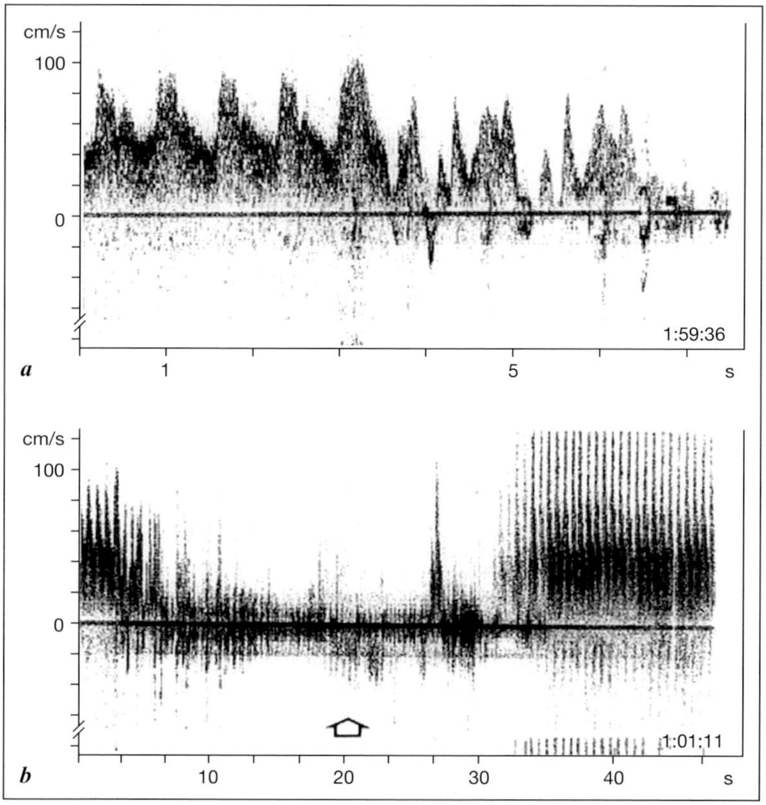

Fig. 2. Cerebral perfusion during cough syncope. Transcranial Doppler monitoring of the middle cerebral artery (MCA) in a patient with cough syncope. ***a*** Cerebral blood flow (CBF) velocity profile at the beginning of coughing. ***b*** CBF velocity profile before, during, and after the cough syncope. Fainting occurred 15–18 s after the onset of coughing (arrow). Reproduced from [30] with kind permission from Lippincott Williams & Wilkins.

with neuronal hyperactivity and consecutive hyperperfusion. While hyperperfusion was reproduced in partial motor [35] and generalized tonic and tonic–clonic seizures [36], early Doppler ultrasound studies of the carotid artery during absence seizures presented conflicting data [37]. Later TCD studies confirmed that blood flow velocities decreased during absence seizures [36, 38, 39]. To exclude all systemic influences remains difficult. In particular, autonomic dysfunction has also been shown to manifest in CBF velocity changes in epilepsy patients [40] as an initial increase was also found [41, 42], and because the subsequent CBF velocity decrease was shown to partially result

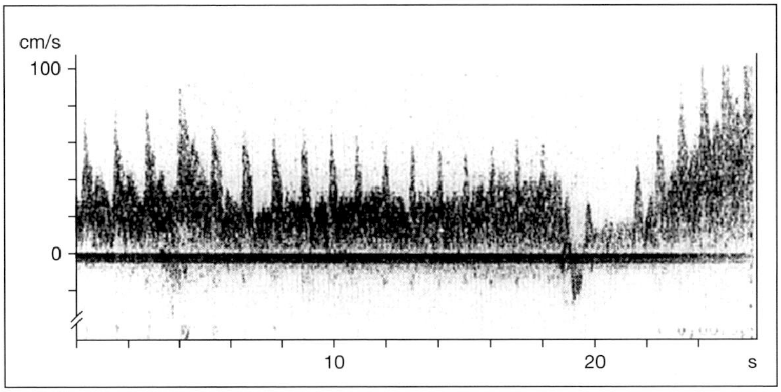

Fig. 3. Cerebral perfusion during an effort to reproduce cough syncope in a healthy volunteer. Transcranial Doppler monitoring of the MCA, while the volunteer performed a maximal expiratory Valsalva maneuver immediately followed by an 'inverse' Valsalva maneuver, keeping the glottis closed while changing to maximal inspiratory effort. This produced a reversal of flow over one cardiac cycle without fainting. Reproduced from [30], with kind permission from Lippincott Williams & Wilkins.

from hyperventilation-induced hypocapnia [42]. At least, with BP and pCO_2 monitoring, ictal BP dysregulation or premonitory hyperventilation could be excluded as the cause of the decrease of CBF velocity in absence epilepsy [39] so that a reduced metabolic demand seems the most likely explanation. The reason for the decrease of CBF velocities during primary absence seizures remains elusive, but one might speculate that it is due to an actual decrease of cortical neuronal activity during spike-wave activity mediated by inhibitory phenomena or withdrawal of activating inputs resulting from a non-cortical ('centrencephalic') origin of this type of primary generalized seizures, with the sum of their projections to the cortical surface resulting in electrical spike-wave activity and a net deactivation.

While the above findings are very informative about the underlying mechanism of epileptic seizures, TCD alone will rarely contribute in clinical routine for differentiating epilepsy from transient ischemic attack or migraine with aura.

Psychogenic Syncope

A study with head-upright tilt table testing found that BP, heart rate, TCD velocities, and EEG were normal during induced syncopes and seizures of psychogenic origin [43]. The authors stated 'patients who pass out or convulse during head-upright tilt without any change in physiologic parameters can be presumed psychogenic in origin and may be referred for psychiatric

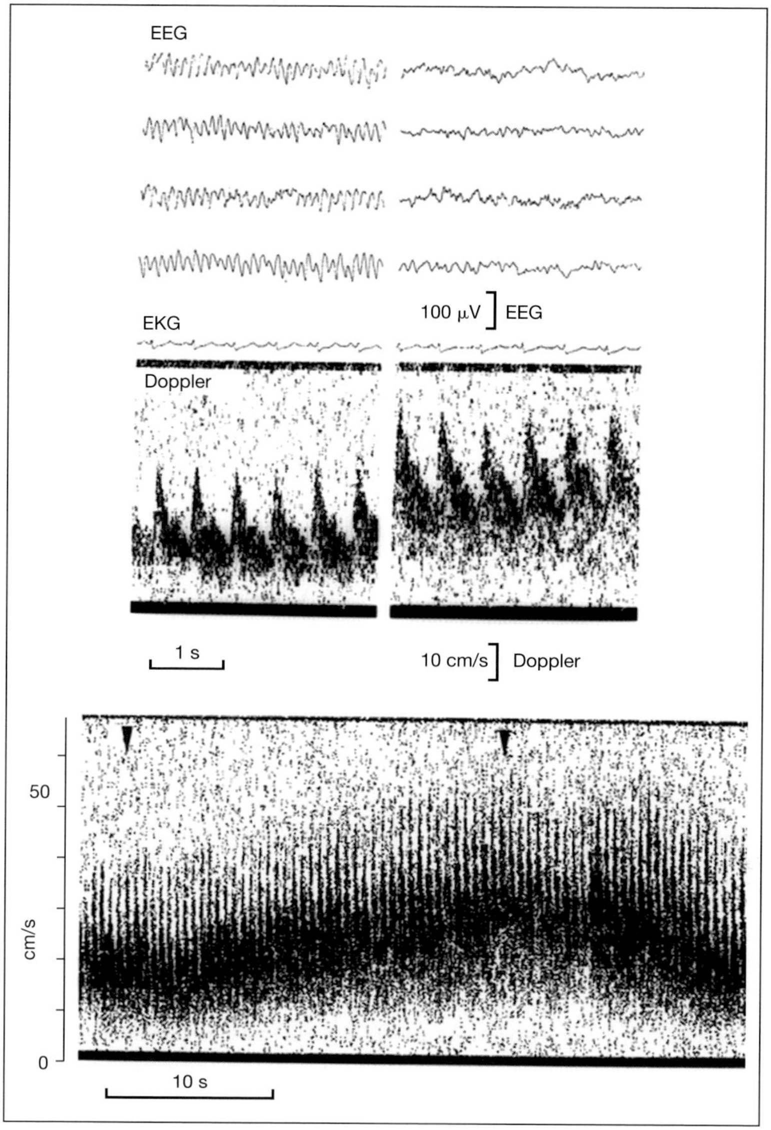

Fig. 4. Simultaneous electroencephalographic (EEG) and transcranial Doppler sonography (TCD) recordings during focal occipital epileptic seizures. Left upper panel: Baseline EEG and TCD of the posterior cerebral artery (PCA) in the symptom-free intervals between seizures. Right upper panel: EEG shows non-specific desynchronization during the visual symptoms, while TCD showed an increase of mean CBF velocity in the PCA by more than 50%. Lower panel: Time course of TCD in the PCA before, during, and after an occipital seizure. Arrows mark the beginning and end of visual symptoms. Note the hemodynamic delay of the cerebrovascular response. The MCA serving as the internal reference showed no changes (not shown). Reproduced from [33], with kind permission from Lippincott Williams & Wilkins.

evaluation'. A further report of a patient with recurrent syncope induced by head rotation [44] demonstrated the value of unaltered CBF velocities monitored by TCD during syncope, together with an unaltered EEG [44]. Besides monitoring of EEG and blood oxygenation during syncope, TCD is an important method since the absence of a change in CBF velocities excludes clinically relevant changes of many other parameters such BP, HR, venous backflow, and ICP.

References

1 European Society of Cardiology Task Force Report: Guidelines on management (diagnosis and treatment) of syncope. Eur Heart J 2001;22:1256–1306.

2 Kapoor WN: Syncope. N Engl J Med 2000;343:1098–1099.

3 Rossen R, Kabat H, Anderson JP: Acute arrest of cerebral circulation in man. Arch Neurol Psychiatr 1943;50:510–528.

4 Sheldon R, Killam S: Methodology of isoproterenol-tilt table testing in patients with syncope. J Am Coll Cardiol 1992;19:773–779.

5 Wilder-Smith AJ, Wilder-Smith EP: Electrophysiological evaluation of peripheral autonomic function in leprosy patients, leprosy contacts and controls. Int J Lepr Other Mycobact Dis 1996;64:433–440.

6 Wilder-Smith EP, Wilder-Smith AJ, Van Brakel WH, Egger M: Vasomotor reflex testing in leprosy patients, healthy contacts and controls: A cross-sectional study in western Nepal. Lepr Rev 1996;67:306–317.

7 Wilder-Smith EP, Wilder-Smith AJ, Nirkko AC: Skin and muscle vasomotor reflexes in detecting autonomic dysfunction in leprosy. Muscle Nerve 2000;23:1105–1112.

8 Njemanze PC: Critical limits of pressure-flow relation in the human brain. Stroke 1992;23: 1743–1747.

9 Grubb BP, Gerard G, Roush K, Temesy-Armos P, Montford P, Elliott L, Hahn H, Brewster P: Cerebral vasoconstriction during head-upright tilt-induced vasovagal syncope: A paradoxic and unexpected response. Circulation 1991;84:1157–1164.

10 Grubb ABP, Durzinsky D, Brewster P, Gbur C, Collins B: Sudden cerebral vasoconstriction during induced polymorphic ventricular tachycardia and fibrillation: Further observations of a paradoxic response. Pacing Clin Electrophysiol 1998;21:483–484.

11 Grubb ABP, Samoil D, Kosinski D, Wolfe D, Brewster P, Elliott L, Hahn H: Cerebral syncope: Loss of consciousness associated with cerebral vasoconstriction in the absence of systemic hypotension. Pacing Clin Electrophysiol 1998;21:652–658.

12 Krakow K, Ries S, Daffertshofer M, Hennerici M: Simultaneous assessment of brain tissue oxygenation and cerebral perfusion during orthostatic stress. Eur Neurol 2000;43:39–46.

13 Schondorf R, Stein R, Roberts R, Benoit J, Cupples W: Dynamic cerebral autoregulation is preserved in neurally mediated syncope. J Appl Physiol 2001;91:2493–2502.

14 Novak V, Spies JM, Novak P, McPhee BR, Rummans TA, Low PA: Hypocapnia and cerebral hypoperfusion in orthostatic intolerance. Stroke 1998;29:1876–1881.

15 Carey BJ, Eames PJ, Panerai RB, Potter JF: A case of arrhythmia-induced transient cerebral hyperemia. Cerebrovasc Dis 2000;10:330–333.

16 Lagi A, Cencetti S, Fattorini L, Georgiadis D, Bacalli S: Cerebral hemodynamics in vasovagal syncope induced by head-up tilt: A transcranial Doppler study. Circulation 2001;104:2694–2698.

17 Markwalder TM, Grolimund P, Seiler R, Roth F, Aaslid R: Dependency of blood flow velocity in the middle cerebral artery on end-tidal carbon dioxide partial pressure – A transcranial Doppler study. J Cereb Blood Flow Metab 1984;4:368–372.

18 Leftheriotis G, Rozak P, Dupuis JM, Victor J, Tadei A, Sumet JL: Cerebral hemodynamics during carotid massage in patients with carotid sinus syndrome. Pacing Clin Electrophysiol 1998;21: 1885–1892.
19 Mukai S, Gagnon M, Iloputaife I, Hamner JW, Lipsitz LA: Effect of systolic blood pressure and carotid stiffness on baroreflex gain in elderly subjects. J Gerontol A Biol Sci Med Sci 2003;58: 626–630.
20 Gulli G, Cooper VL, Claydon VE, Hainsworth R: Prolonged latency in the baroreflex mediated vascular resistance response in subjects with postural related syncope. Clin Auton Res 2005;15: 207–212.
21 Fiddler GI, Tajik AJ, Weidman W, McGoon DC, Ritter DG, Giuliani ER: Idiopathic hypertrophic subaortic stenosis in the young. Am J Cardiol 1978;42:793–799.
22 Dohrmann ML, Cheitlin MD: Cardiogenic syncope. Seizure versus syncope. Neurol Clin 1986;4:549–562.
23 Aaslid R, Lash SR, Bardy GH, Gild WH, Newell DW: Dynamic pressure – Flow velocity relationships in the human cerebral circulation. Stroke 2003;34:1645–1659.
24 Sturzenegger M, Newell DW, Douville CM, Byrd S, Schoonover KD, Nicholls SC: Transcranial Doppler and angiographic findings in adolescent stretch syncope. J Neurol Neurosurg Psychiatry 1995;58:367–370.
25 Fox MW, Piepgras DG, Bartleson JD: Anterolateral decompression of the atlantoaxial vertebral artery for symptomatic positional occlusion of the vertebral artery: Case report. J Neurosurg 1995;83:737–740.
26 Sakaguchi M, Kitagawa K, Hougaku H, Hashimoto H, Nagai Y, Yamagami H, Ohtsuki T, Oku N, Hashikawa K, Matsushita K, Matsumoto M, Hori M: Mechanical compression of the extracranial vertebral artery during neck rotation. Neurology 2003;61:845–847.
27 Frisoni GB, Anzola GP: Vertebrobasilar ischemia after neck motion. Stroke 1991;22:1452–1460.
28 Warlow CP, Dennis MS, van Gijn J, Hankey GJ, Sandercock PA, Bamford JM, Wardlaw JM: Is it a vascular event and where is the lesion? Identifying and interpreting the symptoms and signs of cerebrovascular disease; in Warlow CP, Dennis MS, van Gijn J, Hankey GJ, Sandercock PA, Bamford JM, Wardlaw JM (eds): Stroke: A Practical Guide to Management. Oxford, MA, USA, Blackwell Science, 2001, pp 28–105.
29 Yanagihara T, Klass DW, Piepgras DG, Houser OW: Brief loss of consciousness in bilateral carotid occlusive disease. Arch Neurol Psychiatr 1989;46:858–861.
30 Mattle HP, Nirkko AC, Baumgartner RW, Sturzenegger M: Transient cerebral circulatory arrest coincides with fainting in cough syncope. Neurology 1995;45:498–501.
31 Desser KB, Harris CL, Benchimol A: Carotid blood velocity during cough studies in man. Stroke 1976;7:416–418.
32 Linzer M, McFarland TA, Belkin M, Caplan L: Critical carotid and vertebral arterial occlusive disease and cough syncope. Stroke 1992;23:1017–1020.
33 Wilder-Smith EJ, Nirkko AC: Contribution of concurrent Doppler and EEG in differentiating occipital epileptic discharges from migraine. Neurology 1991;41:2005–2007.
34 Knake S, Haag A, Pilgramm G, Reis J, Klein KM, Hoeffken H, Bartenstein P, Oertel WH, Hamer HM, Rosenow F: Ictal functional TCD for the lateralization of the seizure onset zone – A report of two cases. Epilepsy Res 2004;62:89–93.
35 Niehaus L, Wiesmann UC, Meyer B: Changes in cerebral hemodynamics during simple partial motor seizures. Eur Neurol 2000;44:8–11.
36 Bode H: Intracranial blood flow velocities during seizures and generalized epileptic discharges. Eur J Pediatr 1992;151:706–709.
37 Shimizu H, Futagi Y, Mimaki T: Cerebral blood flow measured by Doppler flow meter during petit mal seizure. Brain Dev 1983;5:58–61.
38 Sanada S, Murakami N, Ohtahara S: Changes in blood flow of the middle cerebral artery during absence seizures. Pediatr Neurol 1988;4:158–161.
39 Nehlig A, Vergnes M, Waydelich R, Hirsch E, Charbonne R, Marescaux C, Seylaz J: Absence seizures induce a decrease in cerebral blood flow: Human and animal data. J Cereb Blood Flow Metab 1996;16:147–155.

40 Diehl B, Diehl RR, Stodieck SR, Ringelstein EB: Spontaneous oscillations in cerebral blood flow velocities in middle cerebral arteries in control subjects and patients with epilepsy. Stroke 1997;28:2457–2459.
41 De Simone R, Silvestrini M, Marciani MG, Curatolo P: Changes in cerebral blood flow velocities during childhood absence seizures. Pediatr Neurol 1998;18:132–135.
42 Diehl B, Knecht S, Deppe M, Young C, Stodieck SR: Cerebral hemodynamic response to generalized spike-wave discharges. Epilepsia 1998;39:1284–1289.
43 Grubb ABP, Gerard G, Wolfe DA, Samoil D, Davenport CW, Homan RW, Temesy-Armos P: Syncope and seizures of psychogenic origin: Identification with head-upright tilt table testing. Clin Cardiol 1992;15:839–842.
44 Sturzenegger M, Donati F, Weiss M, Hess CW: Syncope of unclear origin – Role of 2 diagnostic tests with high specificity. Schweiz Med Wochenschr 1996;126:674–681.

Dr. med. Arto C. Nirkko
Department of Neurology, University Hospital, Inselspital
CH–3010 Bern (Switzerland)
Tel. +41 31 632 3332, Fax +41 31 632 9679, E-Mail arto.nirkko@insel.ch

Baumgartner RW (ed): Handbook on Neurovascular Ultrasound.
Front Neurol Neurosci. Basel, Karger, 2006, vol 21, pp 251–260

Functional Transcranial Doppler Sonography

Hubertus Lohmann, E. Bernd Ringelstein, Stefan Knecht

Department of Neurology, University of Münster, Münster, Germany

Abstract

Functional transcranial Doppler sonography (fTCD) constitutes a complementary neuroimaging tool measuring cerebral perfusion changes due to neural activation. Functional TCD utilizes pulse-wave Doppler technology to record blood flow velocities in the anterior, middle, and posterior cerebral arteries. Comparable to other perfusion-sensitive neuroimaging techniques like functional magnetic resonance imaging or positron emission tomography, fTCD is based on a close coupling between regional cerebral blood flow changes and neural activation. Due to a continuous registration of blood flow, TCD offers an excellent temporal resolution in comparison to other neuroimaging techniques. The technique is noninvasive and easy to apply. Blood flow measurements are robust against movement artifacts. Thus, fTCD is predestinated for follow-up investigations, especially in individuals with diminished ability to cooperate, like patients or children. Since its introduction the technique has contributed substantially to the elucidation of the hemispheric organization of cognitive, motor, and sensory functions in adults and children. This chapter delineates the physical and physiological principles of the technique. A prototypical experimental setup and analysis techniques are described. Scientific and clinical applications of fTCD are presented.

Since the first demonstration of noninvasive Doppler ultrasound pericranial recordings of the cerebral blood flow velocities (CBFV) in the basal cerebral arteries by Aaslid et al. [1], functional transcranial Doppler sonography (fTCD) has been established as a complementary perfusion-sensitive neuroimaging tool. Like functional magnetic resonance imaging (fMRI) and positron emission tomography, fTCD is based on the close linkage between local neural activity and regional cerebral blood flow (rCBF) changes (neurovascular coupling) [2]. rCBF changes result in CBFV alterations in the supplying basal cerebral arteries, which can be continuously monitored by fTCD. In contrast to fMRI and positron emission tomography, fTCD provides high temporal resolution, which allows the assessment of fast changes in flow parameters resulting from changes in neural activity. Additional advantages of the technique are its noninvasiveness, low costs, and mobility, which makes it ideal for follow-up investigations in adult and pediatric patients or healthy subjects. One major disadvantage is the limited spatial resolution of the technique. fTCD usually compares relative perfusion differences between homolog areas in the hemispheres by measuring CBFV in the supplying arteries (bilateral fTCD monitoring). This means that spatial resolution is restricted to the vascular territories of the insonated vessels. Additionally, about 5% of the healthy population exhibits an insufficient temporal ultrasound window. This means that the ultrasound beam cannot penetrate the skull due to an increased bone thickness.

Recent advances in the technique have produced a large number of fTCD studies on the organization of sensory, motor, and cognitive functions in the brain [for a review, see 3]. Especially, the hemispheric lateralization of language function has been a major field of investigation.

Physical and Technical Principles

fTCD measures blood flow velocities in the basal cerebral arteries as a perfusion correlate of changes in local neural activity. Blood flow recordings are based on the so-called *Doppler shift* (or *Doppler effect*). Aaslid et al. [1] introduced the principle of noninvasive pericranial recording of the CBFV in basal brain arteries. In fTCD, commercially available ultrasound devices with (bilateral) pulse-wave 2-MHz-ultrasonic probes (pw-ultrasonography) are used for blood flow recordings. In contrast to continuous-wave ultrasonography, pw-ultrasonography allows an adjustment of the insonation depth and sample volume (pulse length). This way, a selective segment within a given vessel can be insonated. Signal artifacts resulting from reflections by the skull can thus be eliminated effectively.

In fTCD studies, mainly the temporal window is used for blood flow recordings. This window allows the insonation of basal cerebral arteries, the M1- and M2-segment of the middle cerebral artery (MCA), and the proximal segments of the anterior and posterior cerebral arteries. Three important aspects of fTCD blood flow velocity recording warrant the validity and reliability of the subsequent outcome, for example, the lateralization of function being monitored.

First, in fTCD measurements a physiological flow pattern in the insonated vessel segment is a prerequisite for a reliable estimation of rCBF. This prerequisite is most likely violated when fTCD measurements are performed in or in proximity of stenotic vessels. Therefore, sound knowledge about vessel anatomy, insonation techniques, and flow characteristics of the basal cerebral arteries in healthy and pathological conditions are requested [4].

Second, fTCD measurements require a continuous blood flow recording over a longer period of time. Due to the small stimulus-evoked CBFV changes and in dependency of the given experimental task, a single measurement thus may last 20–90 min. Therefore, the ultrasonic probes are attached on a flexible fixation system, which allows the stable positioning of the probes on the bone window. This way, fTCD is fairly robust against signal artifacts resulting from moderate mechanical impact on the probes provoked by ordinary head movements. However, frequent coughing, sneezing, or yawning may considerably add nonsystematic signal artifacts, which can result in a reduced signal-to-noise ratio. Speaking aloud may also constitute a source of artifacts. In many experimental tasks subjects are requested to speak in order to demonstrate task compliance. This, however, may produce systematic signal artifacts, which can affect the reliability and validity of fTCD measurements. Therefore, the use of covert ('silent') task performance in combination with a subsequent task to control for compliance is recommended [5]. Alternatively, verbalizing in a low voice can reduce the risk of signal artifacts.

Third, the assessment of the absolute value of blood flow by fTCD is not possible: Due to the interindividual variability in vessel course and morphology the angle varies by which the ultrasound is directed onto the insonated segment (insonation angle). Under physiological conditions, insonation angles between 0–30° have been observed. This leads a negative deviation of the assessed velocity of up to 15% (given an insonation angle of 30°) since the Doppler shift depends on the cosine function of the insonation angle (see also figure 1 for an example). The insonation angle cannot be estimated by outer anatomical landmarks or corrected technically. As a consequence, when CBFV values are used in fTCD studies normalized, i.e., relative velocity changes are analyzed.

CBFV Data Recording

As mentioned above, the calculation of flow velocity by the Doppler shift presumes that a single moving blood particle passes the ultrasound beam. However, blood flow is characterized by a parabolic flow profile, i.e., blood particles display a spectrum of different velocities. In TCD this leads to a composite frequency (shift) in which the blood particles differentially contribute to the signal. In TCD devices the composite frequency is submitted to a so-called fast Fourier transformation. This way the contributions of different velocities can be calculated. The *Doppler spectrum* (sonogram) visualizes the spectrum of all different flow velocities at a given time point. The intensity of each velocity

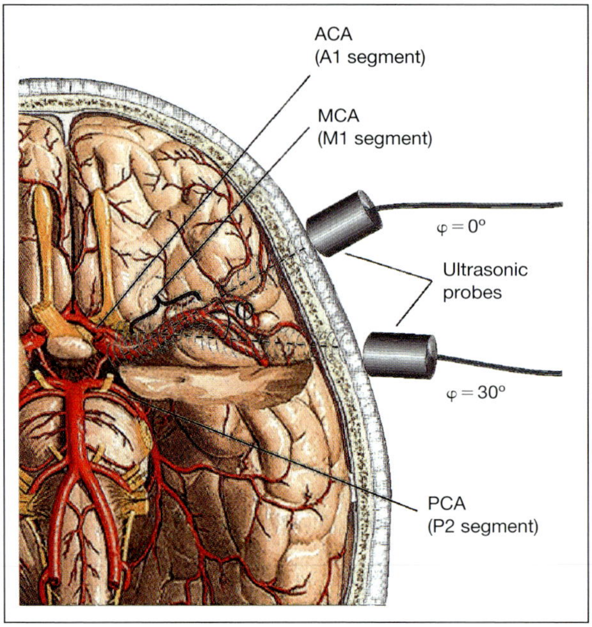

Fig. 1. Measurement of the CBFV in the basal arteries through the transtemporal cranial window: in most fTCD studies the M1-segment of the MCA is insonated at a depth of 40–60 mm. The two probe positions illustrate the dependency of the recorded flow velocity as a cosine function of the insonation angle. In case of the lower probe position, this results in a negative deviation of 15% of the absolute velocity in the insonated vessel segment. ACA, MCA, and PCA = Anterior, middle, and posterior cerebral arteries.

is color-coded. Figure 2 depicts a sonogram by a screen shot of an ultrasonic device (DWL Multidop T2; www.compumedics.com). The envelope curve represents the maximal flow velocity, which is usually at the center of the vessel and is calculated in centimeters per second. Depending on the ultrasonic device this envelope curve or a different perfusion parameter (e.g., intensity-weighted mean velocities) is exported for further data analysis.

Measuring Neural Activity by fTCD: Physiological Basics

Like other perfusion-sensitive neuroimaging techniques, fTCD is based on a close linkage between changes of neural activity and rCBF. Local neural activity, in response to a cognitive task, results in an augmentation of glucose and oxygen consumption, which is compensated by an increase of rCBF (neurovascular coupling). The rCBF increase is regulated by alteration of the

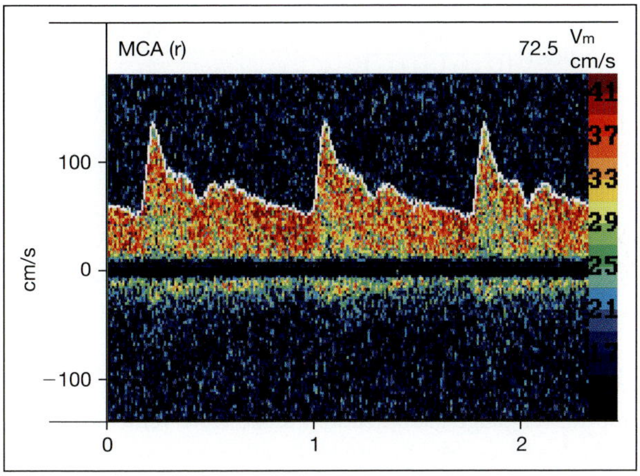

Fig. 2. Doppler spectrum and envelope curve extracted by insonation of the middle cerebral artery as a function of time (here in seconds): The y-axis indicates the different velocities at the insonated segment of the vessel. Signal intensity (amplitude) of each recorded velocity is color-coded. The envelope curve refers to the maximum blood flow velocities following the cardiac cycle. For data analysis, most studies use the maximal CBFV.

cerebrovascular resistance. This is accomplished by a dilatation of the arterioles in the precapillary bed mediated by several vasoactive substances. Functional MRI or fTCD measure a distinct correlate of rCBF changes. Whereas fMRI uses a local shift in the ratio of deoxygenated and oxygenated blood as an intrinsic magnetic resonance signal, fTCD relies on CBFV changes in the supplying basal cerebral arteries, which correspond to alterations in rCBF. The proportionality between CBFV and rCBF in the supplying arteries can be deduced mathematically, under the assumption that several flow and vessel characteristics, such as constancy of blood viscosity, laminar flow, stable vessel diameter, and circular configuration of the vessel, are present [6]. Although these prerequisites cannot be assumed under physiological conditions entirely, a close relationship between rCBF changes due to local neural activity and corresponding CBFV alterations has been demonstrated [7]. In contrast, pathological conditions in the vessel configuration can lead to altered flow characteristics. For example, it is known that in and in the vicinity of stenotic vessels there is a risk of a non-laminary (turbulent) flow pattern depending on the degree of the stenosis and the perfusion pressure. If fTCD is applied in vessel segments with a risk of a non-laminary flow, proportionality of CBFV and rCBF is not assured.

CBFV modulations due to a defined stimulus (i.e., an experimental task) are small in contrast to spontaneous fluctuations of the blood flow velocity resulting from autonomic processes like arousal, respiration, ventricular

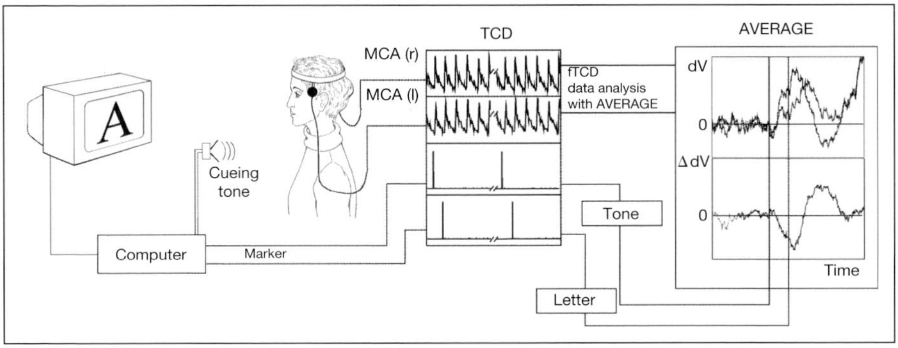

Fig. 3. Prototype fTCD setup for language lateralization: blood flow velocities in the basal arteries (here the middle cerebral arteries; MCAs) are bilaterally monitored by a commercially available TCD device. Stimulus presentation is accomplished by computer display. CBFV envelope curve are stored with the simultaneously recorded marker signal for segmentation of event-related signal intervals. Offline analysis is performed by AVERAGE, a program for automated blood flow data analysis (figure from [4]).

contractions, and other slow periodical oscillations. Together, these nonspecific modulations can exceed the stimulus-related response in CBFV up to ten times [8]. As a consequence, data analysis in fTCD studies investigating cognitive functions is dependent on averaging stimulus-related CBFV modulations across subjects or across multiple trials within a subject.

Prototype Examination Setup and Analysis

In the following we describe a prototypic examination setup for the investigation of language lateralization and quantitative offline data analysis the way it is used in our laboratory. Hardware requirements comprise a commercially available two-channel pw-ultrasonic device with a monitoring operation mode for continuous CBFV registration and a conventional personal computer for stimulus sequencing and presentation (fig. 3). CBFV in the insonated basal cerebral arteries are recorded bilaterally at a sample rate of at least 20 Hz.

For language lateralization subjects perform a covert word generation task: 5 s after a cueing tone a letter is presented for 2.5 s on the personal computer display. The subjects are then requested to silently find as many words as possible with a given letter for 15 s. To control for compliance, the subjects are subsequently asked to report the words found before for 5 s. The word generation task is followed by a resting period of 32.5 s, resulting in total

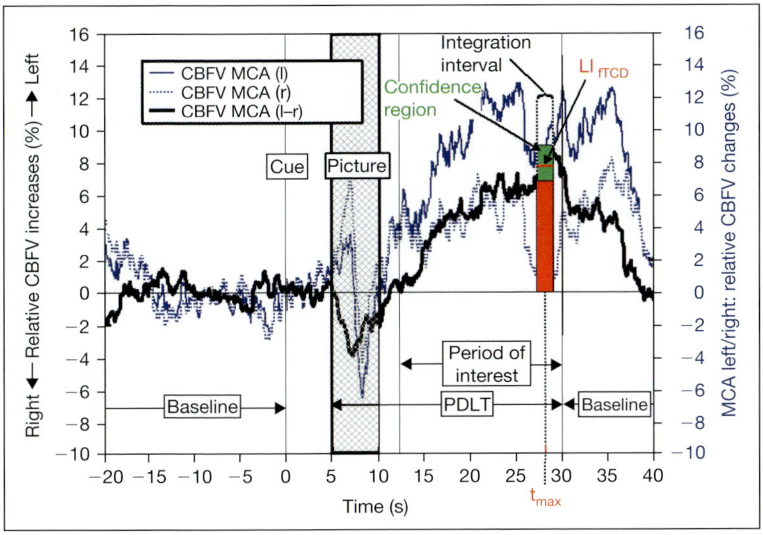

Fig. 4. Averaged event-related CBFV modulations resulting from 30 repetitions of a language lateralization paradigm (PDLT; picture description language task) in an 8-year-old child. The left y-axis indicates the relative perfusion increases between the left and right middle cerebral arteries (MCAs) during resting period (baseline) and task performance (PDLT) as the difference between the averaged relative perfusion changes in the left and right MCA (right y-axis in blue). Positive values by calculation indicate left hemispheric dominance and vice versa. An fTCD language lateralization index (LI; red column; +7.8%) with confidence bands (indicated in green) is calculated by the maximum increase during a defined period of interest (figure from [16]).

duration of one minute of each trial. fTCD investigations in language lateralization usually consist of 20–30 trials in succession (box-car design).

A trigger signal generated by the presentation personal computer that is stored together with the CBFV data indicates the beginning of each trial. For offline blood flow data analysis, bilateral CBFV data and the trigger signal are stored in numerical file format (e.g., ASCII), which can be imported by the blood flow analysis software.

Data analysis is performed by the computer program AVERAGE, which allows the automated analysis of event-related blood flow compatible with various TCD devices [9]. The program provides several steps of data preprocessing, i.e., data normalization, artifact management, noise reduction, and heart beat analysis. For quantification of relative perfusion increases between the insonated arteries in a given period of interest, a lateralization index can be calculated (fig. 4). The program offers parametric and nonparametric statistical procedures by which task-related differences in perfusion between the hemispheres can be analyzed.

Scientific and Clinical Applications of fTCD

Since the 1980s a large number of fTCD studies have investigated the dynamics and lateralization effects of CBFV changes in response to sensory, motor, and cognitive tasks. The majority of fTCD studies have focused on the lateralization of functions mediated by distinct brain regions within the vascular territories of the MCA. Among these, different language-related functions have been most intensively investigated (for a review, see [3] or [10]).

Language is a prototypical lateralized brain function. Lateralization of functions in the brain is conceived as an essential principle of neural organization based on phylogenetic roots and formed by the interaction of genetics and environmental influences during ontogeny. Therefore, the development of a fTCD technique investigating language function in children and adults seems to be most relevant for the investigation of a genetic component of cerebral lateralization [11], neural plasticity during ontogeny (i.e., potential shifts in lateralization) [12], and reorganization processes after brain damage (i.e., recruitment of the nondominant hemisphere).

However, validity and reliability of the procedure must be warranted. Therefore, a number of fTCD studies on language functions in adults and children were cross-validated with the gold standard, the Wada test and fMRI [13–15]. Reproducibility of the technique for language lateralization was assessed in adults and children [12, 16]. The studies show the potential of fTCD in assessing language function accurately and reproducibly. From a technical point of view, fTCD avoids a number of problems that fMRI encounters. In fMRI, different calculation methods exist to describe lateralization. So far the 'optimal' method to establish lateralization measures remains controversial. Many of the current approaches do not fulfill the criteria of robustness and reproducibility. Many measures depend on external parameters, e.g., the statistical threshold applied in the data analysis [17].

Due to its noninvasiveness and availability, a clinical application of fTCD is the implementation of the technique in preoperative assessment of patients who will undergo neurosurgery. In contrast, conducting the Wada test, currently standard procedure for mapping language function, bears the risk of physical distress and increased morbidity in up to 5% [18, 19]. Functional TCD is capable of assessing higher language functions in patients with intractable temporal lobe epilepsy [20]. Thus, fTCD provides a less risky method for lateralization procedures in patients undergoing neurosurgery.

Outlook

Recent developments in fTCD have shown that the technique can assess language function reliably in adults and children. Functional TCD thus has the potential to assess hemispheric differences in activation for a wide range of brain functions in normal subjects and patients. Experienced clinicians now possess an easy applicable and fast method to investigate lateralization of functions. This way, for example, large cohorts of specific clinical and normal populations can be monitored to elucidate different influences of brain lateralization.

References

1 Aaslid R, Markwalder TM, Nornes H: Noninvasive transcranial Doppler ultrasound recording of flow velocity in basal cerebral arteries. J Neurosurg 1982;57:769–774.

2 Kuschinsky W: Regulation of cerebral blood flow; in Moonen CTW, Bandettini PA (eds). Functional MRI. Berlin, Heidelberg, New York, Springer-Verlag, 2000, pp 15–24.

3 Duschek S, Schandry R: Functional transcranial Doppler sonography as a tool in psychophysiological research. Psychophysiology 2003;40:436–454.

4 Ringelstein EB, Otis SM, Niggemeyer E, Kahlscheuer B: Transcranial Doppler sonography: Anatomical landmarks and normal velocity values. Ultrasound Med Biol 1990;16:745–761.

5 Knecht S, Henningsen H, Deppe M, Huber T, Ebner A, Ringelstein EB: Successive activation of both cerebral hemispheres during cued word generation. Neuroreport 1996;7:820–824.

6 Deppe M, Ringelstein EB, Knecht S: The investigation of functional brain lateralization by transcranial Doppler sonography. NeuroImage 2004;21:1124–1146.

7 Clark JM, Skolnick BE, Gelfand R, Farber RE, Stierheim M, Stevens WC, Beck G Jr, Lambertsen CJ: Relationship of 133Xe cerebral blood flow to middle cerebral arterial flow velocity in men at rest. J Cereb Blood Flow Metab 1996;16:1255–1262.

8 Diehl RR, Diehl B, Sitzer M, Hennerici M: Spontaneous oscillations in cerebral blood flow velocity in normal humans and in patients with carotid artery disease. Neurosci Lett 1991;127: 5–8.

9 Deppe M, Knecht S, Henningsen H, Ringelstein EB: AVERAGE: A Windows program for automated analysis of event related cerebral blood flow. J Neurosci Methods 1997;75:147–154.

10 Stroobant N, Vingerhoets G: Transcranial Doppler ultrasonography monitoring of cerebral hemodynamics during performance of cognitive tasks: A review. Neuropsychol Rev 2000;10:213–231.

11 Anneken K, Konrad C, Drager B, Breitenstein C, Kennerknecht I, Ringelstein EB, Knecht S: Familial aggregation of strong hemispheric language lateralization. Neurology 2004;63: 2433–2435.

12 Lohmann H, Dräger B, Müller-Ehrenberg S, Deppe M, Knecht S: Language lateralization in young children assessed by functional transcranial Doppler sonography (fTCD). NeuroImage 2005;24:780–790.

13 Rihs F, Sturzenegger M, Gutbrod K, Schroth G, Mattle HP: Determination of language dominance: Wada test confirms functional transcranial Doppler sonography. Neurology 1999;52:1591–1596.

14 Knecht S, Deppe M, Ebner A, Henningsen H, Huber T, Jokeit H, Ringelstein EB: Non-invasive determination of hemispheric language dominance using functional transcranial Doppler sonography: A comparison with the Wada test. Stroke 1998;29:82–86.

15 Deppe M, Knecht S, Papke K, Lohmann H, Fleischer H, Heindel W, Ringelstein EB, Henningsen H: Assessment of hemispheric language lateralization: A comparison between fMRI and fTCD. J Cereb Blood Flow Metab 2000;20:263–268.

16 Knecht S, Deppe M, Ringelstein EB, Wirtz M, Lohmann H, Dräger B, Huber T, Henningsen H: Reproducibility of functional transcranial Doppler sonography in determining hemispheric language lateralization. Stroke 1998;29:1155–1159.
17 Jansen A, Menke R, Förster AF, Bruchmann S, Sommer J, Weber B, Knecht S: Reproducibility, information content and robustness of quantitative fMRI measures for the lateralization of cognitive brain funtions (in preparation).
18 Lee GP, Loring DW, Meador KJ, Flanigin HF, Brooks BS: Severe behavioral complications following intracarotid sodium amobarbital injection: Implications for hemispheric asymmetry of emotion. Neurology 1988;38:1233–1236.
19 Loring DW, Meador KJ, Lee GP, King DW: Amobarbital effects and lateralized brain function: The Wada test. New York, Springer Verlag, 1992.
20 Knake S, Haag A, Hamer HM, Dittmer C, Bien S, Oertel WH, Rosenow F: Language lateralization in patients with temporal lobe epilepsy: A comparison of functional transcranial Doppler sonography and the Wada test. NeuroImage 2003;19:1228–1232.

Hubertus Lohmann
Department of Neurology, University of Münster
Albert-Schweitzer-Strasse 33
DE–48145 Münster (Germany)
Tel. +49 251 8345306, Fax +49 251 8345313, E-Mail H.Lohmann@uni-muenster.de

Baumgartner RW (ed): Handbook on Neurovascular Ultrasound.
Front Neurol Neurosci. Basel, Karger, 2006, vol 21, pp 261–268

Future Developments in Neurovascular Ultrasound

Stephen Meairs, Michael Hennerici

Department of Neurology, University of Heidelberg, Universitätsklinikum Mannheim, Mannheim, Germany

Abstract

Significant new developments in neurovascular ultrasound include molecular approaches to diagnostics and therapy. Addition of targeted ligands to microbubbles, has opened new avenues for the identification of vascular injury. This is because the molecular signatures of overexpressed adhesion molecules such as the integrin $\alpha_v\beta_3$, ICAM-1, and fibrinogen receptor GPIIb/II can be used to localize contrast agents through the use of complementary receptor ligands. Recent experiments have demonstrated the feasibility of microbubble-ultrasound-enhanced gene therapy to the brain. This new technology holds the promise of delivering genes more selectively than other methods and less invasively than direct injection. Microbubbles may also be employed as carriers of gene agents. The ability to focus ultrasound and cause local cavitation with these carriers may provide a new tool for gene therapy. Fortuitously, the intact blood-brain barrier (BBB), a major limitation in using genes for therapy of brain disease, can be opened with ultrasound. This localized, transient, and reversible opening of the BBB with ultrasound can provide an anatomically selective and targeted gene delivery. Future developments in neurovascular ultrasound will include improvements in technologies for ligand attachment to microbubbles, better methods for imaging targeted ultrasound agents in the brain, and optimization of ultrasound-mediated gene delivery.

New developments have significantly expanded the horizon of neurovascular ultrasound. These include diverse applications using contrast agents to provide avenues for increasing diagnostic confidence and for characterizing brain perfusion deficits. Further advances have expanded the field of neurovascular ultrasound beyond the diagnostic realm. Emergent treatment of acute ischemic stroke now includes the possibility of using ultrasound to enhance rt-PA thrombolysis, although specific conditions and recommendations have not yet been established [1, 2]. Moreover, recent studies show that intravenous microbubbles combined with transcranial ultrasound can rapidly open acute intracranial thrombotic occlusions [3]. These advances may have important implications for future treatment of stroke patients. Significant new developments in neurovascular ultrasound involve molecular approaches to diagnostics and therapy. This chapter will discuss the role of ultrasound in neurovascular molecular imaging, in opening the blood-brain barrier (BBB) for selective drug therapy, and in targeting gene therapy to the brain.

Neurovascular Molecular Imaging with Ultrasound

Molecular imaging can be defined as the characterization and measurement of biological processes at the cellular and molecular level using remote imaging detectors. Key goals of molecular imaging include noninvasive detection of pathology using disease-associated molecular signatures, in vivo delineation of complex molecular mechanisms of disease, and detection of gene expression [4]. Targeted ultrasound techniques combine ultrasound imaging technology with specific contrast agents for the assessment of molecular or genetic signatures for disease. Because of the high echogenicity of ultrasound contrast agents as compared to tissue or plasma, the echo from a single microbubble can be detected with ultrasonographic imaging techniques. This means that ultrasound can interrogate a volume in the order of 0.004 pL, thus offering a high level of resolution for detection of molecular signatures [5].

There are several strategies for targeting microbubble contrast agents to specific regions of disease. A first approach takes advantage of inherent chemical or electrostatic properties of the microbubble shell, resulting in arrest of microbubbles within the microcirculation. This method ('passive targeting') relies on the disease-related upregulation of receptors that bind nonspecifically to either albumin or lipid components of the microbubble shell. The second approach is referred to as 'active targeting' or 'specific targeting'. This involves deliberate attachment of specific antibodies or other ligands to the microbubble surface, leading to the accumulation of targeted contrast agents at a specific site. This is due to the use of adhesion ligands, which recognize disease antigens. A number of different adhesive ligands have been explored that specifically bind to cellular receptors indicative of disease. These include antibodies, peptides, and polysaccharides. Most targeted ultrasound contrast agents are microbubbles, but other vehicles can be used, including acoustically active liposomes and perfluorocarbon emulsions.

Addition of targeted ligands to microbubbles opens new avenues for the identification of vascular occlusion or areas of vascular injury. Adhesion molecules such as the integrin $\alpha_v\beta_3$, intercellular adhesion molecule-1, and fibrinogen receptor GPIIb/IIIa are overexpressed in regions of angiogenesis, inflammation, or thrombus, respectively. These molecular signatures can be used to localize ultrasound contrast agents through the use of complementary receptor ligands. This approach has recently been demonstrated for imaging of angiogenesis using microbubbles targeted to α_v-integrins [6]. Likewise, lipid-based perfluorobutane-filled microbubbles have been synthesized with various densities of anti-intercellular adhesion molecule-1 monoclonal antibodies conjugated to the bubble shell to investigate early stages of atherosclerosis [7]. Targeted microbubbles directed to the GPIIb/IIIa receptor of activated platelets have also been developed for visualization of thrombus [8, 9] and leukocyte-targeted microbubbles can be used to characterize inflammation [10] and to identify inflamed plaques [11]. Although application of targeted contrast-enhanced ultrasound for molecular imaging is at the early stages of development, it is potentially easily translatable to routine clinical practice because the technique is relatively inexpensive, portable, and uses technology that is widely used to evaluate vascular disease.

Ultrasound-Mediated Gene Therapy

A number of preclinical studies have begun to address the feasibility of gene therapy for stroke. This is because the molecular pathophysiology of stroke can be altered by the expression of key genes in a time interval, cell population, and quantities that are sufficient to alter the response to ischemic injury in the brain. One possibility for gene therapy in stroke lies in the potential to increase the brain's resistance to ischemic damage by upregulating genes known to improve cell survival. This may be accomplished by incorporating genes into neurons already suffering from an ischemic insult or into those in which such an event is anticipated.

A central question is whether direct gene delivery of proteins offers an advantage over other molecular pharmaceutics, including small-molecule protein activators and inhibitors or systemic protein delivery itself. Gene therapy necessarily incurs a delay between gene delivery and expression. This delay in expression makes genetic therapies less attractive as an acute-phase therapy for neuroprotection. Nonetheless, early delivery of gene products may mitigate the ongoing molecular cascade leading to cell death that occurs over a period of several days in the ischemic penumbra.

Although most therapeutic drugs are relatively low-molecular-weight compounds, gene-based therapeutic agents are much larger molecules. Therapeutic genes are macromolecules with several thousand base pairs and molecular weights over 1 million daltons (Da). Although most conventional therapeutic agents are relatively stable in the blood, genetic materials are rapidly metabolized by serum esterases, and are therefore not stable to intravenous administration unless the genetic material is stabilized in some fashion. Moreover, genes are usually too large to pass across the capillary fenestrations of blood vessels unless they are assisted by some mechanism. After genes reach the brain tissue, they must pass across cell membranes and enter the cell nucleus. This is not easy, since cells have designed efficient mechanisms for processing exogenous molecules. Once cells take up macromolecules, these are generally digested by lysosomes within the cells. Therefore, successful clinical gene therapy requires effective gene delivery. Recent work suggests that ultrasound may play a key role in the development of new approaches for gene delivery in stroke patients.

There is now considerable evidence that ultrasound can enhance transgene expression. Simple exposure to ultrasound has been shown to increase transgene expression in vascular cells by up to 10-fold after naked DNA transfection. Likewise, transfection studies performed using marker genes that do not exert a therapeutic effect, i.e., *p*-chloramphenicol acetyltransferase, β-galactosidase, and green fluorescent protein, demonstrated that ultrasound consistently increased gene expression in cell lines such as HeLa, NIH t-3, and COS-1 cells [12]. The enhancement of transfection occurred at levels of ultrasound of about 0.5 W/cm^2, and duration of exposure of only about 15 s, and did not appreciably heat the cells nor adversely affect their survival. The mechanism by which ultrasound enhances transfection is mostly likely through cavitation, which in turn increases microvascular permeability. This effect can be dramatically increased in the presence of ultrasound contrast agents [13]. As microbubbles are cavitated by ultrasound, local shock waves increase capillary permeability. This process increases transcapillary passage of macromolecules or nanospheres codelivered with the microbubbles [14]. Cavitation probably opens micropores in small blood vessel walls, making the vessels more passable to molecules and nanoparticles. Therefore, microvascular permeability caused by cavitation of microbubbles may be exploited therapeutically to increase local delivery of therapeutic materials such as genes.

Not only can microbubbles be used to enhance the effects of ultrasound on gene expression. They may also be employed as carriers of gene therapeutic agents [12, 15]. There are a number of ways to entrap drugs with microbubbles. One technique is to incorporate them into the membrane that stabilize microbubbles. Charged drugs can be stabilized in or onto the surfaces of microbubbles by virtue of electrostatic interactions. In this way, cationic lipid-coated microbubbles can bind DNA. This is because DNA is a polyanion and binds avidly to cationic (positively charged) microbubbles. Drugs can also be incorporated into the interior of microbubbles. Another way to entrap drugs in microbubbles is to create a layer of oil to stabilize the outer surface of the bubble. Hydrophobic drugs can then be incorporated into the oil layer. Regardless of the technique used to incorporate the drugs, they are released when ultrasound energy cavitates the microbubble. These methods for making drug-carrying microbubbles are most applicable to drugs that are highly active. This is the case for gene-based drugs, in which the amount of gene injected is usually on the order of micrograms or milligrams. Therefore, large volumes of bubbles are not required to deliver highly active drugs such as genes.

Recent in vitro and in vivo animal experiments have demonstrated the feasibility of microbubble-ultrasound-enhanced gene therapy to the brain. After intracisternal injection of microbubbles and plasmid DNA, the reporter gene was detected in meningeal cells exposed to ultrasound (1 MHz continuous wave, duty cycle 26%, pulse repetition frequency 2 Hz, 5 W/cm^2, acoustic pressure 0.55 MPa) [16]. Likewise, following intrastriatal injection of microbubbles and naked plasmid DNA, significantly increased gene transfer was demonstrated in glial cells [16]. In another recent study 210 kHz ultrasound and 5.0 W /cm^2 of insonation for 5 s effectively transfected plasmid DNA into culture slices of mouse brain (nearly 150-fold increase). The effect was reinforced by 5-fold using a combination with the echo contrast agent, Levovist. When DNA was intracranially injected, Levovist also enhanced gene transfection in newborn mice [17].

In summary, ultrasound may be used to enhance gene expression. In the presence of microbubbles, a synergistic effect is attained, and cavitation is a likely mechanism. Acoustically active materials that bind or entrap genetic materials have a potential role for gene delivery. These materials can be injected intravenously, and targeted gene delivery is attained within the tissue exposed to ultrasound. This new technology holds the promise of delivering genes more selectively than other methods and less invasively than direct injection. The ability to focus ultrasound and cause local cavitation with these gene carriers may provide a new tool for gene therapy of a variety of brain diseases. However, as opposed to other organs, gene therapy to the brain using high-molecular-weight complexes of plasmid DNA and microbubbles must overcome the blood-brain barrier (BBB). Fortuitously, recent studies indicate that ultrasound can also be used to facilitate drug delivery across the BBB.

Permeating the Blood-Brain Barrier with Ultrasound

In addition to the physiological barrier at the level of basal lamina, the BBB is formed by the endothelial cells of the cerebral microvessels that connect to each other by means of intracellular attachments known as tight junctions. The factors that determine penetration of substances from the blood to the central nervous system are lipid solubility, molecular size, and charge. The BBB prevents penetration of ionized water-soluble materials with a molecular weight greater than 18Da. Chemical modification of drugs to make them lipophilic or the use of other carriers, such as amino acid and peptide carriers, are ways to support propagation through the barrier. Another possibility is to diffusely alter the function of the BBB by temporarily opening the tight junctions, which is now possible with an increasing number of chemicals.

The BBB can be opened with intra-arterial injection of hyperosmotic solutions such as mannitol. This causes the endothelial cells to shrink, which results in an opening of the tight junctions that lasts for a few hours. Both osmotic and chemical methods require invasive intra-arterial catheterization and produce diffuse, transient BBB opening within the entire tissue volume supplied by the arterial branch that is injected. A more localized drug delivery method can be accomplished only by injecting directly into the targeted brain area through a needle or catheter. Such direct injections are invasive and require opening the skull, cause penetration of nontargeted brain tissue, and carry the risk of brain damage, bleeding, and infection.

There is now good evidence that ultrasound can be used to permeate blood-tissue barriers. Large molecules and genes can cross the plasma membrane of cultured cells after application of acoustic energy [18]. Indeed, electron microscopy has revealed ultrasound-induced membrane porosity in both in vitro and in vivo experiments [19]. High-intensity focused ultrasound allows selective and nondestructive disruption of the BBB in rats [20]. If preformed gas bubbles are introduced to the blood stream prior to focused ultrasound exposure, the BBB can be transiently opened at the ultrasound focus without acute neuronal damage [21]. The introduction of cavitation sites into the blood stream confines the ultrasound effects to the vasculature and reduces the power needed to produce BBB opening by a factor of two orders of magnitude. This diminishes the risk of tissue damage and makes this technique more easily applied through the intact skull.

Several avenues of transcapillary passage after ultrasound sonication have been identified. These included transcytosis, passage through endothelial cell cytoplasmic openings, opening of tight junctions, and free passage through injured endothelium [22]. However, the exact mechanism of how ultrasound affects the BBB is unclear. Previous experiments suggest that BBB opening is mainly the result of an interaction between ultrasound waves and microbubbles. There appear to be several ways in which this interaction could produce disruption of the BBB. An ultrasound wave causes bubbles to expand and contract in the capillaries. The expansion of larger bubbles can fill the entire capillary lumen, resulting in a mechanical stretching of the vessel wall. This in turn may result in the opening of the tight junctions. This interaction can also create a change in the pressure in the capillary to evoke biochemical reactions that trigger the opening of the BBB. Bubble oscillation may also reduce the local blood flow and induce transient ischemia, which could trigger BBB opening. Finally, the bubbles can collapse during sonication, causing localized shock waves and fluid jets. Such mechanical effects are likely responsible for the opening of the BBB, and may play an important role in tissue damage induced at high-pressure amplitudes.

In summary, the intact BBB, a major limitation in using genes for therapy of brain disease, can be opened with ultrasound. This allows a localized, transient, and reversible opening to provide anatomically selective targeted drug delivery. This approach will likely be used in conjunction with ultrasound-mediated gene delivery to the brain. Future developments in neurovascular imaging will likely include improvements in technologies for ligand attachment to microbubbles, better methods for imaging targeted ultrasound agents in the brain, and optimization of ultrasound-mediated gene delivery.

References

1 Alexandrov AV, Molina CA, Grotta JC, Garami Z, Ford SR, Alvarez-Sabin J, Montaner J, Saqqur M, Demchuk AM, Moye LA, Hill MD, Wojner AW: Ultrasound-enhanced systemic thrombolysis for acute ischemic stroke. N Engl J Med 2004;351:2170–2178.

2 Daffertshofer M, Gass A, Ringleb P, Sitzer M, Sliwka U, Els T, Sedlaczek O, Koroshetz WJ, Hennerici MG: Transcranial low-frequency ultrasound-mediated thrombolysis in brain ischemia: Increased risk of hemorrhage with combined ultrasound and tissue plasminogen activator: Results of a phase II clinical trial. Stroke 2005;36:1441–1446.

3 Culp WC, Porter TR, Lowery J, Xie F, Roberson PK, Marky L: Intracranial clot lysis with intravenous microbubbles and transcranial ultrasound in swine. Stroke 2004;35:2407–2411.

4 Weissleder R, Mahmood U: Molecular imaging. Radiology 2001;219:316–333.

5 Dayton PA, Ferrara KW: Targeted imaging using ultrasound. J Magn Reson Imaging 2002;16: 362–377.

6 Leong-Poi H, Christiansen JP, Klibanov AL, Kaul S, Lindner JR: Noninvasive assessment of angiogenesis by ultrasound and microbubbles targeted to alpha(v)-integrins. Circulation 2003;107:455–460.

7 Weller GE, Villanueva FS, Klibanov AL, Wagner WR: Modulating targeted adhesion of an ultrasound contrast agent to dysfunctional endothelium. Ann Biomed Eng 2002;30:1012–1019.

8 Schumann PA, Christiansen JP, Quigley RM, McCreery TP, Sweitzer RH, Unger EC, Lindner JR, Matsunaga TO: Targeted-microbubble binding selectively to GPIIb IIIa receptors of platelet thrombi. Invest Radiol 2002;37:587–593.

9 Tardy I, Pochon S, Theraulaz M, Nanjappan P, Schneider M: In vivo ultrasound imaging of thrombi using a target-specific contrast agent. Acad Radiol 2002;9(suppl 2):S294–S296.

10 Christiansen JP, Leong-Poi H, Klibanov AL, Kaul S, Lindner JR: Noninvasive imaging of myocardial reperfusion injury using leukocyte-targeted contrast echocardiography. Circulation 2002;105: 1764–1767.

11 Lindner JR: Detection of inflamed plaques with contrast ultrasound. Am J Cardiol 2002;90: 32L–35L.

12 Unger EC, Hersh E, Vannan M, Matsunaga TO, McCreery T: Local drug and gene delivery through microbubbles. Prog Cardiovasc Dis 2001;44:45–54.

13 Lawrie A, Brisken AF, Francis SE, Cumberland DC, Crossman DC, Newman CM: Microbubble-enhanced ultrasound for vascular gene delivery. Gene Ther 2000;7:2023–2027.

14 Skyba DM, Price RJ, Linka AZ, Skalak TC, Kaul S: Direct in vivo visualization of intravascular destruction of microbubbles by ultrasound and its local effects on tissue. Circulation 1998;98: 290–293.
15 Shohet RV, Chen S, Zhou YT, Wang Z, Meidell RS, Unger RH, Grayburn PA: Echocardiographic destruction of albumin microbubbles directs gene delivery to the myocardium. Circulation 2000;101:2554–2556.
16 Shimamura M, Sato N, Taniyama Y, Yamamoto S, Endoh M, Kurinami H, Aoki M, Ogihara T, Kaneda Y, Morishita R: Development of efficient plasmid DNA transfer into adult rat central nervous system using microbubble-enhanced ultrasound. Gene Ther 2004;11:1532–1539.
17 Manome Y, Nakayama N, Nakayama K, Furuhata H: Insonation facilitates plasmid DNA transfection into the central nervous system and microbubbles enhance the effect. Ultrasound Med Biol 2005;31:693–702.
18 Taniyama Y, Tachibana K, Hiraoka K, Namba T, Yamasaki K, Hashiya N, Aoki M, Ogihara T, Yasufumi K, Morishita R: Local delivery of plasmid DNA into rat carotid artery using ultrasound. Circulation 2002;105:1233–1239.
19 Ogawa K, Tachibana K, Uchida T, Tai T, Yamashita N, Tsujita N, Miyauchi R: High-resolution scanning electron microscopic evaluation of cell-membrane porosity by ultrasound. Med Electron Microsc 2001;34:249–253.
20 Mesiwala AH, Farrell L, Wenzel HJ, Silbergeld DL, Crum LA, Winn HR, Mourad PD: High-intensity focused ultrasound selectively disrupts the blood-brain barrier in vivo. Ultrasound Med Biol 2002;28:389–400.
21 Hynynen K, McDannold N, Vykhodtseva N, Jolesz FA: Noninvasive MR imaging-guided focal opening of the blood-brain barrier in rabbits. Radiology 2001;220:640–646.
22 Sheikov N, McDannold N, Vykhodtseva N, Jolesz F, Hynynen K: Cellular mechanisms of the blood-brain barrier opening induced by ultrasound in presence of microbubbles. Ultrasound Med Biol 2004;30:979–989.

Prof. Dr. Stephen Meairs
Neurologische Klinik, Ruprecht-Karls-Universität Heidelberg
Universitätsklinikum Mannheim
DE–68167 Mannheim (Germany)
Tel. +49 621 383 3550, Fax +49 621 383 3807, E-Mail meairs@neuro.ma.uni-heidelberg.de

Author Index

Subject Index